Recovery, Analysis, and Identification of Commingled Human Remains

Recovery, Analysis, and Identification of Commingled Human Remains

Bradley J. Adams, PhD
Editor
Office of Chief Medical Examiner
New York, NY

John E. Byrd, PhD
Editor
Joint POW/MIA Accounting Command
Central Identification Laboratory
Hickam AFB, HI

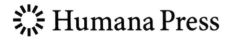 Humana Press

Editors

Bradley J. Adams
Office of Chief Medical Examiner
New York, NY
BAdams@ocme.nyc.gov

John E. Byrd
Joint POW/MIA Accounting Command
Central Identification Laboratory
Hickam AFB, HI
john.byrd@jpac.pacom.mil

ISBN: 978-1-58829-769-3   e-ISBN: 978-1-59745-316-5

Library of Congress Control Number: 2007939412

Cover illustration: Courtesy of John E. Byrd, PhD, editor

Printed on acid-free paper

9 8 7 6 5 4 3 2 1

springer.com

Preface

Public fascination with the rapid developments of forensic science in recent years has led to greater expectations of success in the field of human identification. This relates to field recovery, laboratory analysis, and analytical findings. Mass fatality events can result in the intermixing, or commingling, of human remains from numerous individuals. As the number of individuals increases, so does the complexity of the forensic investigation and the skills needed for case resolution. Body fragmentation adds an even further level of difficulty since each separate fragment initially has to be treated independently until it can be proven to link to another. With forensic investigations, commingling must be resolved to the greatest extent possible since it impairs personal identification of the decedents and prevents the return of remains to next of kin. Even in the archaeological context when personal identification is not an issue, accurate sorting and reliable estimates of the number of individuals are critical to an understanding of the population demographics and cultural practices.

The treatment of these complex scenarios and the science of identification have benefited tremendously from advancements in basic research, improvements in crime scene procedures, development of reference databases, improvements in computer technology, the addition of molecular biology, and more. *Recovery, Analysis, and Identification of Commingled Human Remains* is a collection of chapters dedicated to the description of many of these tools, as well as more general discussions of ethics, policy, logistics, documentation, and other more administrative issues that relate to the challenges associated with the recovery, analysis, and identification of commingled human remains.

In Chapter 1, Ubelaker provides an historical overview of the anthropological attention given to commingled human remains. As he points out, the issue of commingling has only been glossed over in forensic anthropology textbooks until recently. Greater attention to this topic has been recognized as the discipline experiences an increasing emphasis on mass fatality events such as aircraft crashes, terrorist attacks, natural disasters, human rights violations, and other contexts where human remains are apt to be commingled. This chapter also sets the stage for the diverse topics covered throughout the rest of this volume.

The next chapters (2 and 3) discuss field recovery techniques and present case examples involving commingled remains. Although field context has always played an informal role in the process of sorting remains, Tuller et al. (Chapter 2) and

Reineke and Hochrein (Chapter 3) provide convincing arguments that field context is a significant line of evidence that must be captured by appropriate field recovery procedures. Proper training and experience with archaeological techniques are essential for personnel tasked with the recovery of commingled human remains. Field data and spatial relationships can potentially indicate associations of fragmentary remains with each other, as well as other evidence critical to case resolution. Failure to adequately document field context can jeopardize all phases of the investigation. In Chapter 2, Tuller et al. present an example from a human rights investigation of a mass grave in Serbia, while in Chapter 3, Reineke and Hochrein use case examples to outline the protocols employed by the Federal Bureau of Investigation's Evidence Response Teams.

Chapters 4 through 6 present diverse case examples involving commingled human remains. The state of the art for resolving commingling incorporates a mix of traditional methods (e.g., gross techniques) and cutting-edge technology (e.g., DNA testing). In Chapter 4, Egaña and colleagues present several challenging cases associated with international human rights investigations in El Salvador, Zimbabwe, and Argentina. These examples by the Equipo Argentino de Antropología Forense (EAAF) describe not only difficulties in the field, but also obstacles with identification. It is through research, controlled field recovery, and laboratory analysis that many of these cases can be resolved. In Chapter 5, Steadman et al. present a look into one of the most bizarre forensic situations to occur in the United States, the Tri-State Crematorium in Noble, Georgia. In this case, hundreds of bodies intended for commercial cremation were discarded by an unethical crematorium owner on his wooded grounds. As a result, bodies and body parts in varying states of decomposition were dispersed across many acres. Members of the Disaster Mortuary Operational Response Team (DMORT) worked with the Georgia Bureau of Investigation to deal with the unique recovery and identification challenges. Not surprisingly, questions were also raised by families that had received cremated remains processed at the Tri-State Crematorium, and a subsequent analysis of numerous urn contents was undertaken. Chapter 6 by Ubelaker and Rife presents an archaeological perspective of the recovery and analysis of commingled human remains from Greek tombs. While decedent identification is not an issue, these findings are important for paleodemographic reconstructions and an understanding of mortuary behavior. As the authors demonstrate, many of the challenges related to recovery and analysis faced in this context are the same as those encountered in modern forensic contexts.

Chapters 7 though 13 deal mainly with laboratory and morgue analysis of commingled remains. Chapter 7 by Mundorff highlights the role of anthropologists in mass fatality events, specifically the triage of remains at the morgue. It is during the initial triage that commingling problems are likely to be recognized, and the skills of an anthropologist are well suited for this task. Three distinct incidents that occurred in New York City are discussed (the 9/11 attacks on the World Trade Center, the crash of Flight 587, and the crash of the Staten Island Ferry). The similarities and differences between them are highlighted, and the role of the anthropologist in morgue triage is discussed for each of these very different disasters. In Chapter 8, Viner provides an overview of the role of radiology in mass fatality events and the various technological options currently available. Radiology plays an important role from triage through the final stages of identification. Radiology is one of the best means of recognizing the presence of commingling, especially in cases of extreme fragmentation, when body parts of different people may become embedded within each other. It is also a critical component in the identification process. Case examples, including the London bombings of July 7, 2005, and human rights investigations by the International Criminal Tribunal for the Former Yugoslavia (ICTY), show the role of radiology in the analysis of mass fatalities.

Chapter 9 by Warren outlines laboratory procedures for assessing commercially cremated remains for the presence of commingling. Due to the extreme fragmentation associated with commercial cremation, this can be very challenging. Often times these types of cases involve litigation when families suspect the mishandling of bodies by funeral homes. Due to the nature of commercial cremation, some degree of commingling is inevitable in every case. A jury will make a determination as to whether or not there was negligence in the cremation practice largely based on the anthropological findings. Chapter 10 by Byrd explores laboratory methods for sorting remains; in essence, "rebuilding" individuals. This chapter extends the method of osteometric sorting to paired elements and adjoining bones that articulate. New statistical models are provided for application to forensic cases. In Chapter 11, Schaefer provides yet another technique for recognizing commingling and for sorting remains. In this case, stages of epiphyseal fusion are used to identify relationships that are incongruous and indicative of commingling. Typical fusion patterns are identified and methods are presented to statistically evaluate fusion stages between various elements.

Chapter 12 by Adams and Konigsberg describes the best methods for estimation of the number of individuals (i.e., the death population) represented by skeletal remains. This issue can be of great importance when there are a large number of individuals represented and an accurate estimate of the dead is needed. An archaeological example is presented, but these techniques are amenable to both modern and prehistoric contexts. While the techniques for quantification outlined in Chapter 12 are mainly for well-preserved bones, a quantification technique suitable for fragmentary remains is presented by Herrmann and Devlin in Chapter 13. This innovative method uses geographic information systems and treats individual bone specimens as though they were geographic regions. Application of the method permits one to systematically evaluate which bone portions are duplicated in a large assemblage and derive a count of the minimum number of individuals represented.

The introduction of DNA technology into forensic science has revolutionized the process of identification. It has also proven essential to the process of sorting commingled remains, especially those that are too fragmentary to be suitable for gross techniques. However, excitement over the boost we have enjoyed as a result of the introduction of DNA testing can promote naïveté on the part of administrators and the general public as to the reality of these capabilities. It is easy to presume that use of DNA testing renders other methods superfluous. Chapters 14 through 16 reveal that DNA testing is most powerful when utilized in the context of all the evidence and in conjunction with other methods. In Chapter 14, Yazedjian and Kešetović describe the successful DNA-led program of identification at the International Commission on Missing Persons (ICMP) in Bosnia-Herzegovina. It is estimated that as many as 40,000 people went missing as a result of conflicts in the former Yugoslavia. Many of the missing individuals highlighted in this chapter are young men, and there is a lack of reliable antemortem data. The similarity of the biological profile and the lack of antemortem records severely limit the role of anthropology in the identification effort, but its overall importance is not diminished. This chapter details the importance of DNA in the identification effort and the collaborative role played by anthropology in ensuring quality control measures and validation of the DNA results. In Chapter 15, Mundorff et al. discuss identification efforts at the New York City Medical Examiner's Office with more than 20,000 human remains from the World Trade Center attacks of September 11, 2001. Similar to the previous chapter, the WTC examples show the complementary relationship between anthropology and DNA analysis in the quality control of the identification effort. This chapter highlights the advantages and caveats of the heavy reliance on DNA testing for the resolution of commingling. Case examples are presented that show how mistakes were made and how these problems were subsequently recognized and resolved. The lessons learned in the efforts of the New York City Medical Examiner's Office are certain to benefit other forensic organizations for years to come. In Chapter 16, Damann and Edson showcase the benefits of collaboration among various specialists, including anthropologists, odontologists, pathologists, and molecular biologists. They describe the process employed by the most successful sustained program of identification utilizing DNA testing, that of the U.S. Department of Defense. The experiences of the Joint POW/MIA Accounting Command's Central Identification Laboratory and the Armed Forces DNA Identification Laboratory have led to the development of a model program of DNA sampling and processing.

The final two chapters cover more general issues, including the nexus between policy and method and between condition of remains and administrative procedures. In Chapter 17, Kontanis and Sledzik discuss the special problems encountered when mass fatality incidents result in commingled remains. Of particular interest are the severity of body fragmentation and the overall effect on incident resolution (e.g., time involved in decedent identification). They present data from several disasters ("open" and "closed" populations) and discuss the numerous challenges associated with each one. In any of these scenarios, it is critical that goals and guidelines must be established at the onset. These protocols relate to the identification of bodies and body parts, as well as policies regarding "common tissue." To help in these assessments, Kontanis and Sledzik propose a "probative index" that is applied to individual bodies or body portions to prioritize analytical work for each specimen. In Chapter 18, Hennessey treats a topic seldom discussed in the literature: commingling of data. The forensic identification process is data-intensive, particularly when confronted with mass fatalities. Information from a plethora of analyses crossing disciplinary boundaries must be collated and stored in searchable databases. Antemortem information for the missing is often collected in an *ad hoc* manner, including inputs from doctors, dentists, family members, and friends. This information comes in a variety of formats, ranging from antemortem radiographs and dental charts to descriptions of tattoos. Analysts can be easily overwhelmed by the volume, variety, and inconsistencies of data. Standardization and quality control of the data are critical. Hennessey shares his considerable experience in coping with the inevitable errors and provides guidance as to how they can be minimized in future operations.

The chapters in *Recovery, Analysis, and Identification of Commingled Human Remains* reveal that the public's heightened expectations for quality in forensic recovery and identification of the dead have a legitimate basis. Novel methods and increased rigor in analysis and data management have led to significant gains in our ability to deal with commingled remains. We are confident that the reader will find many new tools to add to his or her analytical toolkit in the pages that follow.

Bradley J. Adams and John E. Byrd

Contents

Contributors

Bradley J. Adams
Office of Chief Medical Examiner, New York, NY

Patricia Bernardi
Equipo Argentino de Antropología Forense, Buenos Aires, Argentina

Erik Bieschke
Office of Chief Medical Examiner, New York, NY

John E. Byrd
Joint POW/MIA Accounting Command, Central Identification Laboratory, Hickam AFB, HI

Emily Craig
Kentucky Medical Examiner's Office, Frankfort, KY

Sharna Daley
International Commission on Missing Persons, Sarajevo, Bosnia and Herzegovina

Franklin E. Damann
National Museum of Health and Medicine, Armed Forces Institute of Pathology, Washington, DC

Joanne Bennett Devlin
Department of Anthropology, University of Tennessee, Knoxville, TN

Mercedes Doretti
Equipo Argentino de Antropología Forense, Buenos Aires, Argentina, and New York, NY

Suni M. Edson
Armed Forces DNA Identification Laboratory, Rockville, MD

Sofía Egaña
Equipo Argentino de Antropología Forense, Buenos Aires, Argentina

Laura Fulginiti
Maricopa County Forensic Science Center, Phoenix, AZ

Anahí Ginarte
Equipo Argentino de Antropología Forense, Buenos Aires, Argentina

Michael Hennessey
Gene Codes Forensics, Ann Arbor, MI

Nicholas P. Herrmann
Department of Anthropology, University of Tennessee, Knoxville, TN

Michael J. Hochrein
Laurel Highlands Resident Agency, Federal Bureau of Investigation, Pittsburgh, PA

Ute Hofmeister
International Committee of the Red Cross, Geneva, Switzerland

Rifat Kešetović
International Commission on Missing Persons, Sarajevo, Bosnia and Herzegovina

Lyle W. Konigsberg
Department of Anthropology, University of Illinois, Urbana-Champaign, IL

Elias J. Kontanis
Joint POW/MIA Accounting Command, Central Identification Laboratory, Hickam
AFB, HI

Elaine Mar-Cash
Office of Chief Medical Examiner (1998–2006), New York, NY

Amy Z. Mundorff
Department of Archaeology, Simon Fraser University, Burnaby, British Columbia,
Canada

Gary W. Reinecke
Laboratory Division, Evidence Response Team Unit, Federal Bureau
of Investigation, Quantico, VA

Joseph L. Rife
Classics Department, Macalester College, St. Paul, MN

Maureen Schaefer
Anatomy and Forensic Anthropology, Faculty of Life Sciences, University
of Dundee, Dundee, Scotland, United Kingdom

Robert Shaler
Forensic Science Program, The Pennsylvania State University, University Park, PA

Paul S. Sledzik
Office of Transportation Disaster Assistance, National Transportation Safety Board,
Washington, DC

Frederick Snow
Georgia Bureau of Investigation, Decatur, GA

Kris Sperry
Georgia Bureau of Investigation, Decatur, GA

Dawnie Wolfe Steadman
Department of Anthropology, Binghamton University, State University
of New York, Binghamton, NY

Hugh Tuller
Joint POW/MIA Accounting Command, Central Identification Laboratory, Hickam
AFB, HI

Silvana Turner
Equipo Argentino de Antropología Forense, Buenos Aires, Argentina

Douglas H. Ubelaker
Department of Anthropology, Smithsonian Institution, MNNH, Washington, DC

Mark D. Viner
INFORCE Foundation, Bournemouth, UK, and St. Bartholomew's and The Royal
London Hospitals, London, United Kingdom

Michael Warren
Department of Anthropology, University of Florida, Gainesville, FL

Laura Yazedjian
International Commission on Missing Persons, Sarajevo, Bosnia and Herzegovina

Chapter 1
Methodology in Commingling Analysis: An Historical Overview

Douglas H. Ubelaker

In 1962, Wilton Krogman published the first major text focusing specifically on forensic anthropology. Although his *The Human Skeleton in Forensic Medicine* is widely recognized as a classic historical text, it presents little discussion of issues of commingling in the analysis of human remains. The more focused 1979 follow-up text by T. Dale Stewart devoted only 2 of its 300 pages to commingling topics despite existing publications that focused on bone weight analysis (Baker and Newman 1957), ultraviolet fluorescence (Eyman 1965; McKern 1958), forensic neutron activation (Guinn 1970), statistical approaches to commingling issues (Snow and Folk 1965), and other considerations (Kerley 1972). Stewart noted (1979: 38) that most remains studied by forensic anthropologists at that time had been found as primary skeletons. For such cases, context and field documentation indicated that commingling likely was not a major issue.

In 2005, many skeletons studied by forensic anthropologists also were found as primary interments. Increasingly, however, cases are presented involving commingling issues. Mass disasters (Stewart 1970), cremation litigation (Murray and Rose 1993), human rights investigations, separation of recent from ancient remains, and many other types of modern cases raise questions such as, "How many individuals are represented in a group of remains?" and "How can remains of single individuals be identified within collections of remains from multiple individuals?" Cases and questions involving commingling issues are highly variable and problem-specific in modern forensic anthropology (Ubelaker 2002).

The methodology employed in answering these questions also can be highly variable (Rösing and Pischtschan 1995). As with most analysis in forensic anthropology, there is no "cookbook" approach to commingling issues. Practitioners must be aware of the myriad of techniques available and craft a case-specific protocol to address the specific problems at hand.

The chapters assembled in this volume represent a testimony to the growing need for commingling analysis within forensic anthropology and to the vast array of approaches available now to meet that need. Although basic inventory and documentation techniques are desirable in all cases, specific problems call for the selection of particular methods. This volume provides the reader with an overview of both the problems and the solutions.

From: *Recovery, Analysis, and Identification of Commingled Human Remains*
Edited by: B. Adams and J. Byrd © Humana Press, Totowa, NJ

Separation of Bone and Tooth from Other Materials

Some problem applications call for identification of bone and tooth materials and their separation from other, similarly appearing items. These issues emerge particularly in small particle analysis of fragmentary and/or burned materials. Since DNA analysis can be employed even with small, fragmentary evidence to contribute to identification, many submitted cases involve such evidence. Particles of drywall, plastic, geological materials, and many other items can resemble bone and tooth, especially after exposure to intense heat or other taphonomic factors. Likewise, bone and tooth can be difficult to recognize as such after taphonomic alteration.

When gross morphology is inadequate to distinguish materials in such cases, microscopy can be useful. A high-quality dissecting microscope may allow detection of structure unique to bone and tooth (Ubelaker 1998). However, lack of such detail may be problematic since some bone and tooth fragments can be altered to the extent that surface diagnostic features may be lacking. Thin sections may be useful in such cases, but preparation techniques are destructive and may preclude molecular analysis with very small fragments.

Scanning electron microscopy/energy dispersive spectroscopy (SEM/EDS) provides a useful new tool in separating nonbone and tooth material (Ubelaker et al. 2002). Analysis presents not only a highly magnified surface image, which may in itself be useful, but compositional spectra that can be identified as elements. The presence and relative proportions of the constituent elements can be useful to distinguish bone and tooth from other materials. A comparative database of analyses of many known materials, including bones and teeth representing a variety of conditions, is now available to provide the probabilities of association. This system is especially useful to exclude materials from being bone or tooth but also can be helpful in the diagnosis of their presence (Ubelaker et al. 2002).

Recognition of Nonhuman Animal

In some commingling cases it may be necessary to document the presence of non-human animals or even determine species. Again, morphological assessment is the initial method of choice if the materials present diagnostic information. If bone and tooth fragments lack the necessary morphological features due to fragmentation or taphonomic alteration (Haglund and Sorg 1997), then microscopy may prove helpful. If sufficient material is present to support preparation of ground thin sections, the occurrence of plexiform bone or a characteristic osteon banding pattern may rule out a human origin (Mulhern and Ubelaker 2001). However, the presence of a typical human microscopic pattern is not necessarily diagnostic for human origin since that general pattern can be shared with some other animals (Mulhern and Ubelaker 2003).

In such cases, the technique of choice likely would be protein radio-immunoassay (pRIA). Very small samples (200 mg or less) can be utilized not only to conclusively and quantitatively separate human from nonhuman but also to identify nonhuman species (usually at the family level) if necessary (Ubelaker et al. 2004). The technique involves protein extraction followed by a solid-phase double-antibody radio-immunossay utilizing controls of antisera (raised in rabbits) and radioactive (iodine-125) marked antibody of rabbit gamma globulin developed in donkeys.

Separation of Ancient and Modern Remains

Case analysis may call for the separation of remains of recently deceased individuals from those who died long ago. Scenarios calling for such analysis might include a collection of remains found in the possession of an individual suspected of both grave-robbing and homicide, remains of a potential homicide victim found in an old cemetery with evidence of looting, or a mass disaster with modern victims at the site of a cemetery, or another such collection of older remains.

Presented with such problems, authorities might consider radiocarbon dating, focusing particularly on artificial radiocarbon. Atmospheric testing of thermonuclear devices beginning in the early 1950s produced abnormally high levels of artificial radiocarbon that, through the food chain, were incorporated into the tissues of all living things, including humans (Taylor 1987).

Levels increased steadily until about 1963 when international test ban agreements ceased the practice. Atmospheric levels of artificial radiocarbon have subsequently declined but still remain above pre-1950 levels. If analysis detects elevated levels of radiocarbon, the investigator knows that the individual was alive after 1950. Analysis of different tissues and consideration of the age at death of the individual may help pinpoint the birth dates and the death dates of the individual within the bomb-curve period (Ubelaker 2001; Ubelaker and Houck 2002).

Sorting Procedures

Once nonhuman materials have been separated out, analysis of the human remains usually begins with careful inventory (Buikstra and Ubelaker 1994). The extent and nature of the inventory typically are problem-driven but should document in appropriate detail what bones or parts of bone are present, approximate ages at death, and bone side (left or right). Other observations that may prove relevant include bone morphology, bone size, and articulation patterns (Buikstra and Gordon 1980; Buikstra et al. 1984; Kerley 1972; London and Curran 1986; London and Hunt 1998). Inventory and morphological assessment may be supplemented with such techniques as ultraviolet fluorescence (Eyman 1965; McKern 1958), radiography, serological testing, neutron activation, trace element analysis (Finnegan 1988; Finnegan and Chaudhuri 1990; Fulton et al. 1986; Guinn 1970), and bone weight (Baker and Newman 1957) and density studies (Galloway et al. 1997; Lyman 1993; Willey et al. 1997).

Modern DNA techniques increasingly are employed in commingling cases, especially to identify fragmentary evidence and assemble separated remains of single individuals following mass disasters. As noted in this volume, DNA technology and other complex approaches are best used in consideration of context and the prudent use of resources. Selection of remains to be analyzed for DNA should be driven by context, morphological analysis, and available resources. It would not be logical to obtain DNA profiles from more than one bone in an assemblage if they all were found in articulation. Similarly, it would not be necessary to have DNA data from more than one bone fragment of several found in separate locations if morphological study found that they fit together and originated from a single bone.

Approaches to documenting the minimum number of individuals present (MNI) have evolved beyond simple counts of elements present and their duplication (Allen and Guy 1984; Casteel 1972, 1977; Chase and Hagaman 1987; Steele and Parama 1981; Wild and Nichol 1983). Methodological and statistical approaches available include computer procedures for matching bones by size (Gilbert et al. 1981), a modified mark-capture procedure (LeCren 1965), the Lincoln Index based on matching pairs of bones (Winder 1992), and the more complex Lincoln/Peterson Index (Adams 1996; Adams and Konigsberg 2004). These approaches not only refine the estimation of the MNI but also seek to establish the MLNI (most likely number of individuals present).

The chapters in this volume explore the issues discussed above in great depth. They present the range of problems encountered in modern forensic anthropology that call for commingling analysis. They also present the growing methodology to address these problems. Anthropologists continue to study remains in their laboratories brought to them by law enforcement officials, similar to the way it was done when Wilton Krogman and T. Dale Stewart were publishing their volumes over two decades ago. However, today anthropologists deal with commingling issues at crash sites, makeshift morgues, and medical examiner's offices, frequently working alongside other professionals as part of analysis teams. The nature of the cases and the format and methodology for their analysis continue to evolve. This volume documents important aspects of that evolution and provides the reader with the information needed for successful resolution of commingling issues.

References Cited

Adams, B. J. 1996 The Use of the Lincoln/Peterson Index for Quantification and Interpretation of Commingled Human Remains. Department of Anthropology, University of Tennessee, Knoxville.

Adams, B. J. and L. W. Konigsberg 2004 Estimation of the most likely number of individuals from commingled human skeletal remains. *Am. J. Phys. Anthropol.* 125(2):138–151.

Allen, J. and J. B. M. Guy 1984 Optimal estimations of individuals in archaeological faunal assemblages: How minimal is the MNI? *Archaeol. Oceania* 19:41–47.

Baker, P. T. and R. W. Newman 1957 The use of bone weight for human identification. *Am. J. Phys. Anthropol.* 15(4):601–618.

Buikstra, J. E. and C. C. Gordon 1980 Individuation in forensic science study: Decapitation. *J. Forensic Sci.* 25(1):246–259.

Buikstra, J. E., C. C. Gordon, and L. St. Hoyme 1984 The case of the severed skull: Individuation in forensic anthropology. In *Human Identification: Case Studies in Forensic Anthropology*, T. A. Rathbun and J. E. Buikstra, eds. Charles C. Thomas, Springfield, IL.

Buikstra, J. E. and D. H. Ubelaker (editors) 1994 *Standards for Data Collection from Human Skeletal Remains, Proceedings of a Seminar at The Field Museum of Natural History (Arkansas Archeological Survey Research Series No. 44)*. Spiral ed. Arkansas Archeological Survey, Fayetteville.

Casteel, R. W. 1972 Some biases in the recovery of archaeological faunal remains. *Proc. Prehistoric Soc.* (38):382–388.

Casteel, R. W. 1977 Characterization of faunal assemblages and the minimum number of individuals determined from paired elements: Continuing problems in archaeology. *J. Archaeol. Sci.* (4):125–134.

Chase, P. G. and R. M. Hagaman 1987 Minimum number of individuals and its alternatives: A probability theory perspective. *OSSA* 13:75–86.

Eyman, C. E. 1965 Ultraviolet fluorescence as a means of skeletal identification. *Am. Antiquity* 31(1):109–112.

Finnegan, M. 1988 Variation of Trace Elements Within and Between Skeletons Using Multiple Sample Sites. Paper presented at the 15th Annual Meeting of the Paleopathology Association, Kansas City, MO.

Finnegan, M. and S. Chaudhuri 1990 Identification of Commingled Skeletal Remains Using Isotopic Strontium. Paper presented at the 42nd Annual Meeting of the American Academy of Forensic Science, Cincinnati, OH.

Fulton, B. A., C. E. Meloan, and M. Finnegan 1986 Reassembling scattered and mixed human bones by trace element ratios. *J. Forensic Sci.* 31(4):1455–1462.

Galloway, A. P., P. Willey, and L. Snyder 1997 Human bone mineral densities and survival of bone elements: A contemporary sample. In *Forensic Taphonomy: The Postmortem Fate of Human Remains*, W. D. Haglund and M. H. Sorg, eds., pp. 295–317. CRC Press, Boca Raton, FL.

Gilbert, A. S., B. H. Singer, and D. J. Perkins 1981 Quantification experiments on computer-simulated faunal collections. *OSSA* 8:79–94.

Guinn, V. P. 1970 Forensic neutron activation analysis. In *Personal Identification in Mass Disasters*, T. D. Stewart, ed., pp. 25–35. Smithsonian Institution, Washington, DC.

Haglund, W. D. and M. H. Sorg (editors) 1997 *Forensic Taphonomy: The Postmortem Fate of Human Remains*. CRC Press, Boca Raton, FL.

Kerley, E. R. 1972 Special observations in skeletal identification. *J. Forensic Sci.* 17(3):349–357.

Krogman, W. M. 1962 *The Human Skeleton in Forensic Medicine*. Charles C. Thomas, Springfield, IL.

LeCren, E. D. 1965 A note on the history of mark-recapture population estimates. *J. Anim. Ecol.* 34:453–454.

London, M. R. and B. K. Curran 1986 The use of the hip joint in the separation of commingled remains (abstract). *Am. J. Phys. Anthropol.* 69:231.

London, M. R. and D. R. Hunt 1998 Morphometric segregation of commingled remains using the femoral head and acetabulum (abstract). *Am. J. Phys. Anthropol.* 26(Suppl):152.

Lyman, R. L. 1993 Density-mediated attrition of bone assemblages: New insights. In *From Bones to Behavior*, J. Hudson, ed., pp. 324–341. Center for Archaeological Investigations, Carbondale, IL.

McKern, T. W. 1958 *The Use of Shortwave Ultraviolet Rays for the Segregation of Commingled Skeletal Remains*. Environmental Protection Research and Developments Command, Quartermaster Research and Development Center Environmental Protection Research Division, Natick, MA.

Mulhern, D. M. and D. H. Ubelaker 2001 Differences in osteon banding between human and nonhuman bone. *J. Forensic Sci.* 46(2):220–222.

Mulhern, D. M. and D. H. Ubelaker 2003 Histologic examination of bone development in juvenile chimpanzees. *Am. J. Phys. Anthropol.* 122(2):127–133.

Murray, K. A. and J. C. Rose 1993 The analysis of cremains: A case study involving the inappropriate disposal of mortuary remains. *J. Forensic Sci.* 38(1):98–103.

Rösing, F. W. and E. Pischtschan 1995 Re-individualisation of commingled skeletal remains. In *Advances in Forensic Sciences*, B. Jacob and W. Bonte, eds. Verlag, Berlin.

Snow, C. and E. D. Folk 1965 Statistical assessment of commingled skeletal remains. *Am. J. Phys. Anthropol.* 32:423–427.

Steele, D. G. and W. D. Parama 1981 Frequencies of dental anomalies and their potential effect on determining MNI counts. *Plains Anthropologist* 26(91):51–54.

Stewart, T. D. (editor) 1970 *Personal Identification in Mass Disasters*. Smithsonian Institution, Washington, DC.

Stewart, T. D. 1979 *Essentials of Forensic Anthropology*. Charles C. Thomas, Springfield. IL.

Taylor, R. E. 1987 *Radiocarbon Dating: An Archaeological Perspective*. Academic Press, Orlando, FL.

Ubelaker, D. H. 1998 The evolving role of the microscope in forensic anthropology. In *Forensic Osteology, Advances in the Identification of Human Remains*, K. J. Reichs, ed., pp. 514–532. Charles C. Thomas, Springfield, IL.

Ubelaker, D. H. 2001 Artificial radiocarbon as an indicator of recent origin of organic remains in forensic cases. *J. Forensic Sci.* 46(6):1285–1287.

Ubelaker, D. H. 2002 Approaches to the study of commingling in human skeletal biology. In *Advances in Forensic Taphonomy: Method, Theory, and Archaeological Perspectives*, W. D. Haglund and M. H. Sorg, eds. CRC Press, Boca Raton, FL.

Ubelaker, D. H. and M. M. Houck 2002 Using radiocarbon dating and paleontological extraction techniques in the analysis of a human skull in an unusual context. *Forensic Sci. Comm.* (4):4.

Ubelaker, D. H., J. M. Lowenstein, and D. G. Hood 2004 Use of solid-phase double-antibody radioimmunoassay to identify species from small skeletal fragments. *J. Forensic Sci.* 49(5):924–929.

Ubelaker, D. H., D. C. Ward, V. S. Braz, and J. Stewart 2002 The use of SEM/EDS analysis to distinguish dental and osseos tissue from other materials. *J. Forensic Sci.* 47(5):940–943.

Wild, L. and R. Nichol 1983 Estimation of the original number of individuals using estimators of the Krantz type. *J. Field Archeol.* (10):337–344.

Willey, P., A. Galloway, and L. Snyder 1997 Bone mineral density and survival of elements and element portions in the bones of the Crow Creek Massacre victims. *Am. J. Phys. Anthropol.* 104:513–528.

Winder, N. P. 1992 The removal estimator: A "probable numbers" statistic that requires no matching. *Int. J. Osteoarchaeol.* (2):15–18.

Chapter 2
Spatial Analysis of Mass Grave Mapping Data to Assist in the Reassociation of Disarticulated and Commingled Human Remains

Hugh Tuller, Ute Hofmeister, and Sharna Daley

Introduction

When considering possible solutions to the problem of sorting commingled human remains from a mass grave context, one is inclined to think of methods conducted within a laboratory setting (Dirkmaat et al. 2005), such as physical pair-matching of skeletal elements, evaluating articulation of elements, statistical analysis of measurements taken from the elements, or other such techniques that use data generated during mortuary analysis (Buikstra et al. 1984; Byrd and Adams 2003); in short, techniques that focus on the remains well after they have been recovered from the grave. Data generated during the excavation of a mass grave unfortunately are not often consulted when attempting to tackle problems of commingling. Nevertheless, observations and recordings taken during proper excavation can directly assist in the reassociation of disarticulated and commingled remains. In particular, mapping data and grave depositional event recording can be valuable information for use in the reassociation of disarticulated body parts to their corresponding bodies.

The potential of disarticulation and commingling of bodies and body parts is an issue in every mass grave. Not only are bodies initially commingled as they are deposited in the grave, but the condition of the bodies prior to burial, decomposition processes, taphonomic conditions within the grave, and the intentional destruction and/or tampering with the bodies by those who buried them contribute to the eventual disarticulation and mixing of elements, more so when an initial (primary) mass grave is disturbed and bodies are moved to a secondary mass grave(s). Care in exposing and removal of remains from a grave by an observant excavator, knowledgeable in human skeletal anatomy, is the single most important step limiting (and hopefully eliminating) further disarticulation during the recovery. Without a controlled excavation, disarticulation will be compounded, further adding to the already confused mix within the grave. Yet careful exposure and removal of remains does not have to be the only contribution a proper excavation makes. A well-documented, archaeologically led excavation generates data that may be used not only for prevention of further commingling, but also for resolving commingled remains.

Recognition of archaeological techniques and observations as potential key elements in assisting forensic case work has been acknowledged in the past (Dirkmaat

From: *Recovery, Analysis, and Identification of Commingled Human Remains*
Edited by: B. Adams and J. Byrd © Humana Press, Totowa, NJ

and Adovasio 1997; Morse et al. 1976; Owsley 2001; Skinner 1987). Nevertheless, no suggestion has been proposed as to how archaeological observations can be logically and consistently utilized within mortuaries, especially those processing hundreds of remains from mass graves. Unfortunately, mass grave investigation is often sharply divided between two activities, recovery operations (grave excavation) and mortuary examination (autopsy), with neither activity having much contact with the other. While the forensic anthropologist or pathologist in charge of the mortuary may fully respect the contributions archaeology makes during the recovery operations, he may be unaware of the potential role archaeology can play in sorting commingled remains *after* the excavation. Archaeology, for the most part, is still very much viewed by mission planners as an outdoor (or at least out-of-mortuary) activity with no further connection to the mortuary other than delivering remains and associated evidence as intact as possible. Only under unusual circumstances does archaeology seem to be consulted during mortuary examination.

For example, Haglund (2001) describes a circumstance where excavation maps displaying the position of remains within a mass grave were used to help sort out fragmented crania superimposed upon each other. While Haglund uses this example as one of several positive contributions archaeology can bring to the investigation of mass graves, he unfortunately does not detail how the maps were used. It is assumed that the physical maps, not the recorded spatial data used to create the maps, were consulted to help rectify the commingling issue. Furthermore, it seems that this use of excavation maps may have been an isolated example; that the maps were consulted only after the commingling issue with this particular case was recognized in the mortuary, and the use of maps was not a standard aspect of their mortuary operation. No further reference to map use within their mortuary was mentioned.

In our study, a computer program is used to analyze spatial relationships between disarticulated and commingled remains within a mass grave. Similar to Haglund's example using maps to assist in sorting commingled crania to adjacent bodies, the computer program examines the spatial data generated during the electronic survey of body and body parts within a grave and comparing the locations of disarticulated elements to all possible matching points. The hypothesis is that a disarticulated body part closest to the point on the body missing that part is the most likely correct match out of all other possible matching body parts within the grave. Such a program can be run prior to or during mortuary examination, providing mortuary personnel with immediate suggestions as to which disarticulated body part(s) may belong to a particular body. When confronted with hundreds of bodies and body parts from a mass grave to sort through, prior knowledge of potential matching elements can be an effective starting point for rectifying commingling issues. Although not a definitive method or technique for reassociation, spatial analysis provides an objective and systematic approach based on the nature of the grave that may aid in reassociations.

In addition to generating data that can be analyzed spatially, an archaeological approach to mass grave excavation can identify events in the creation of the grave, which, in turn, has the potential to assist in resolving commingling issues. Specifically, the identification of depositional events of human remains within a grave, when combined with spatial analysis, can narrow the search parameters of possible matching disarticulated body parts within a group of recovered remains.

Materials and Methods

The focus of this study is on the largest of a series of mass graves excavated during 2002 on the Special Police Training Grounds in Batajnica, a suburb of Belgrade, in Serbia. Victims in the grave have thus far proved to be Kosovar Albanians killed in the spring of 1999 and transported to Belgrade for disposal. As of this writing, the majority of the remains have been identified. While overall control of the site and the associated evidence belonged to the Belgrade District Court, the actual excavation of the grave was conducted by forensic archaeologists from the International Commission for Missing Persons (ICMP) assisted by a crew of archaeologists from the University of Belgrade. All authors were employed by ICMP at the time of this excavation.

The grave in discussion, designated BA05 (Batajnica 05), was approximately 25 meters long, 3 meters wide, and 2 meters deep. We can deduce from the archaeological findings that a front-end loader-type construction machine dug the grave, creating a ramp down into the earth at one end as it removed soil (Fig. 2.1). BA05 was a complex mass grave in that it consisted of elements of both primary and secondary depositions as well as having areas within the grave where attempts were made at cremating the grave contents. Furthermore, we can infer that while many of the bodies transported to Belgrade from areas in Kosovo were gathered off the surface of the ground and loaded onto trucks; some were even wrapped in blankets or plastic sheeting, others were dug up from graves where they were originally buried. A situation occurred where, on one extreme, a number of trucks likely carried neatly packaged bodies, while others contained jumbled mixes of soil, bodies, and even some pieces of coffin. Before the trucks deposited their loads into the grave, the base of the grave was lined with old vehicle tires and pieces of lumber. The first trucks appear to have backed into the grave, where they dumped their loads. Later trucks dumped their contents on the surface of the ground next to the grave, where the remains either were directly pushed into the grave from the side or were first set afire and allowed to burn for a time before being pushed in. As remains and backfill were deposited into the grave, gasoline and additional tires were added to the mix in an apparent attempt to keep the fires going.

The perpetrators, however, were not as methodological in the destruction of the bodies as they had planned. Perhaps because of fear of ongoing NATO bombing strikes in the area at the time, or simply because those carrying out the orders to make the graves were not enthusiastic about their assigned task, the bodies appear to have been buried shortly after they were deposited in the grave, putting many of the fires out almost as quickly as they were started. As bodies mounded up over the edge of the grave, a construction machine repeatedly drove over the top of remains, crushing them down into the grave as it deposited more soil. The combined activities

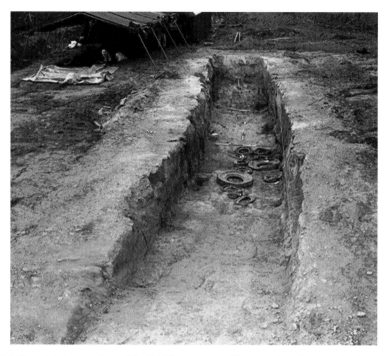

Fig. 2.1 Completed excavation of the BA05 mass grave. The ramp into the grave begins near the bottom of the photograph. Note vehicle tires on the base of the grave

of different body collection strategies in Kosovo, the act of transporting them to Belgrade by truck, attempts at destroying them by fire, and machine activities made the excavation, recording, and recovery of the human remains within this grave extremely challenging.

In order to accurately map spatial relations within and around the grave, the ICMP archaeologists employed an electronic Sokkia set 600 total station equipped with a Sokkia SDR 31 data logger. Total stations, which are being used increasingly at archaeological sites and outdoor crime scenes, are becoming familiar equipment at mass grave excavation sites. Capable of recording position points in three dimensions in a fraction of the time traditional tape measure and transits take, a total station's data can be downloaded by computer programs and rendered into three-dimensional maps illustrating the exposed human remains, artifacts, and grave features, in any imaginable combination (Wright et al. 2005). What would have taken days to map by hand can now be accomplished in a few hours.

While a single point recorded from a complete body or disarticulated body part in a grave can be used to represent those remains on a map, excavators of mass graves using total stations typically record a series of points to represent a set of remains. This series of points can then be connected in stick-figure manner in a geographic information systems (GIS) program, to represent a body for map purposes. Points recorded on a complete body are typically the head of the body and all major limb joints. During the excavation of mass grave BA05, a total of 15 points for a complete body was recorded. In addition to the head and joint points mentioned, a central pelvis, central body mass, and, when found in isolation, the mandible had points taken on them. While the amount of points recorded may seem excessive, we have found that it takes only 3–4 minutes to survey a complete body and does not interfere with the flow of work. Indeed, by recording the series of points, it forces the person recovering the body to check that all the major elements are present, helps to eliminate possible commingling mistakes during the recovery, and ensures an accurate field inventory of the remains.

Many current total stations and/or related data loggers have limited capacity for recording text to describe the points recorded. The Sokkia data loggers used by ICMP could only accommodate up to 16 characters and spaces in their description field. Although this limits the amount of text that may be attached to a particular record, one would not necessarily want to be slowed down inputting long, descriptive text during the excavation. It may be possible to preprogram an alternative data logger such as a tablet PC or laptop with these codes to operate in a quicker usable format, but standard data loggers are currently incapable of doing this alone.

To bypass the lack of available space and ensure speedy input of text, short descriptive codes, adopted from the International Criminal Tribunal for the former Yugoslavia's mass grave survey procedures (Hanson et al. 2000), were used to identify the points taken. Points recorded on a body received a four-letter code beginning with the side from where the point is being taken, followed by the first three letters of the body element. A left shoulder would be recorded as LSHO. Elements such as the cranium (CRAN) that does not have a side used the first four letters of the name of element. Table 2.1 lists the codes and elements they represent used during the excavation of BA05.

Table 2.1 Body Points Recorded and Their Associated Total Station Codes

Code Entry	Description
CRAN	Cranium
RSHO	Right shoulder
RELB	Right elbow
RWRI	Right wrist
LSHO	Left shoulder
LELB	Left elbow
LWRI	Left wrist
CPEL	Central pelvis point
RPEL	Right pelvis point
LPEL	Left pelvis point
RKNE	Right knee
RANK	Right ankle
LKNE	Left knee
LANK	Left ankle
CPOI	Central point—body
MAND	Mandible (if disarticulated)

A total station records the location of a given point in X, Y, and Z (e.g., north, east, and elevation) coordinate format. Each body or body part uncovered in the grave received a unique evidence number. This evidence number was added to the mass grave identifier (BA05) along with the four-letter body location code. A string of recorded total station code for a single point taken on a body may read BA05 123B RELB followed by the X, Y, and Z numerical coordinates. In this example, BA05 represents the grave number at Batajnica, 123B is the individual body evidence number (B = body), and RELB indicates the point recorded was the right elbow. A complete body would be represented by 15 sets of these codes, while an individual body part (BP = body part), for example, an unassociated disarticulated left arm, would have only three points recorded: the shoulder (LSHO), elbow (LELB), and wrist (LWRI). Figure 2.2 is an example of what a complete body may look like after exposure in a grave and then rendered in a map as a stick figure, each position point taken labeled with the appropriate code. It should be noted here that while 15 points were taken on a complete body, the central point (CPOI) taken on a body was not used in our spatial analysis for reasons explained in the Discussion section.

A word regarding body (B) vs. body parts (BP) classifications. There is currently no standard used in the international community of mass grave investigators regarding the definition of what constitutes a body or body part. Indeed, this is a constant source of debate among practitioners—debates that unfortunately often take place at the graveside as the first disarticulated remains are about to be removed. While it may seem obvious that a complete articulated body can be defined as a body (B), it becomes less clear how to classify a body in progressively disarticulated condition. At what point does a body become categorized as a body part? It is easy to imagine that an unassociated disarticulated limb or skull will be categorized as a body part (BP), but should remains consisting of a torso missing its head and a leg be considered a body part or a body? What if it is also missing the other leg

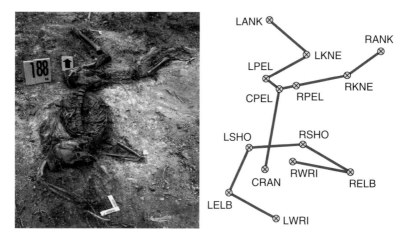

Fig. 2.2 Body 188B *in situ* and represented in map form

and an arm? Or if, as regularly happens, the remains become disarticulated at the lumbar vertebrae and the upper half is missing a limb or two? Proposals such as "If 75% of the remains are present it can be categorized as a B and less than 75% a BP" promote disagreements in the grave between recovery team members over how much of the body is present. Currently, the categorization of remains is usually left up to the lead recovery leader or individual team member removing the remains from the grave. This is often without thought regarding how the categorization may affect mortuary operations. There is a need to standardize these categorizations in a comprehensive manner that assists mortuary analysis.

In mass grave BA05, as with most excavated graves, the categorization occurred in an ad hoc fashion. While most of the remains were intact enough to be classified as Bs, on occasion it was unclear and the lead archaeologist made the call. In general, if 50% or more of a body was present, then it was classified as a B. Fortunately, most BPs tended to be disarticulated limbs consisting of at least two articulating bones. Single disarticulated bones without association were categorized as "general bones" (GB) and were not recorded by the total station (as a result of this study, we now advocate the recording of all long bones as well as a carefully planned classification system for potential spatial analysis). Only complete hands and feet were recorded as body parts; two or more of these "minor" bones recovered in articulation were categorized as GBs. It should be recognized that while it is desirable to reassociate as many disarticulated elements back to their bodies, a number of elements such as unassociated ribs and the bones of the hands and feet are often beyond the capacity of anthropology to reassociate given the number of remains within large mass graves. Until DNA technology becomes easier and less expensive, the possibility of reassociating such elements with limited funding and time constraints is economically out of reach. Numerous GBs as well as hands, feet, and sections of torso will not be reassociated because of these reasons, and so mission planners, with relevant governmental bodies and family associations, will have to decide what to do with these "extra" elements.

In addition to recording points on a body/body part for spatial analysis, surveying the remains also renders a basic skeletal inventory of that case. At the completion of an excavation, the total station data can act as a backup to any evidence/photographic log or other documentation source. In addition, all the individual body or body part points can be downloaded to provide an instant inventory for mortuary use. A quick glance at a case's code will indicate not only if it is a body (B) or body part (BP), but what elements that case consists of. Elements absent from the inventory represent disarticulated elements—an important heads-up for an anthropologist or pathologist getting ready to begin an autopsy.

Within the BA05 mass grave, according to records, 378 cases comprising 289 Bs and 89 BPs, and 594 single disarticulated bones and bone fragments (GBs), were recovered from 12 separate deposits of human remains. Each deposit, identified through archaeological techniques, represents a truck load dumped into the grave, or a collection of bodies dumped on the surface beside the grave and then pushed into the grave by a construction machine. The excavation team recorded location points on all body and body parts, as described. In addition, the individual deposit within the grave from which the remains were recovered was noted. As mentioned, the single disarticulated bone and bone fragments (GBs) were not recorded by the total station, but instead were gathered in separate bags according to the deposit from which they were recovered. As no points were recorded from these elements, they are not included in this study. Again, as a result of this analysis we would suggest that single disarticulated long bones receive the same attention as Bs and BPs if spatial analysis is to be conducted.

All Bs, BPs, and artifacts were assigned an individual, sequentially assigned evidence number. The remains and artifacts were placed in separate body bags or plastic bags depending upon their size. The evidence number was recorded in an evidence log book and written on the outside of the body/evidence bag. A separate slip of paper with the evidence number was sealed in a Ziploc-type bag and placed inside the body bag with the remains. The remains were then transferred to a storage area to await autopsy. The mortuary/evidence personnel were provided a copy of the evidence log.

Autopsies were conducted on site while the excavation of the Batajnica mass graves was ongoing. This manner of operation precluded most reassociation efforts. Reassociation can only be attempted after a grave is completely excavated and a remains inventory established, or you risk the chance of missing a matching element still buried within the grave. Due to both legal and political considerations between the Belgrade authorities and ICMP, DNA took the lead in identification and reassociation of recovered remains. During autopsy, hard-tissue samples were taken from all bodies and body parts and later processed through ICMP DNA laboratories. It was through DNA results that reassociations were eventually established. Not only did positive results assist in identification, but identical sequences between disarticulated body parts and bodies allowed for reassociation of 41 disarticulated elements from the BA05 mass grave.

As there was little opportunity for reassociation methodologies to be applied at Batajnica, analysis of the spatial relationship of remains within BA05 presented here was done at a much later time and was not part of the original mortuary effort. The spatial analysis was performed without prior knowledge of ICMP DNA reassociation results, which serve as a control.

A spatial analysis program, derived from Microsoft Access, was used on the BA05 survey data to calculate the distance between bodies missing elements and potential matching body parts in the mass grave. The formula used for this analysis calculates the distance between two points in three-dimensional space and then produces a list of potential matches in order from nearest to furthest. It is important to use three-dimensional distances and not, as is sometimes done, two-dimensional maps, which distort the real relationships between elements. The idea of using mass grave mapping data to search for nearest probable matches has most likely occurred to many people in the past. However, few seem to have actually gone as far as to develop the idea. One person who has attempted to use mass grave mapping data in this manner is Richard Wright.

Wright kindly provided ICMP with a program for spatial analysis (Wright 2003), which he adapted from his earlier cranial morphometric research (Wright 1992). However, Wright's spatial analysis program lacked the option to narrow the search to only those elements that could potentially match the remains being examined. Instead it computes the distance from the point you wish to search from, say a RELB for a missing lower right arm, to *all* other points recorded within the grave regardless of whether or not those points are lower right arm points. What you want is a list of potential disarticulated right lower arms. However, you end up with a list, organized by distance, of crania, shoulders, knees, wrists, and all the other points recorded within the grave, as well as the potential matching lower right arms. Although Wright's program allows the number of points displayed to be limited, this does not diminish the fact that numerous points with no relationship to the remains being examined must be filtered through to reveal those that do represent potential matches.

The spatial analysis program designed for this study is based on a number of SQL Queries in Microsoft Access and allows data gathered from the total station or GIS software to be imported in various formats. Unlike Wright's program, only potential matches are listed in the results of a query. All other points are ignored, and thus filtering is automatic.

We currently do not offer our spatial program for public use. However, it must be emphasized that a number of commercially available database programs are able to perform spatial analysis. As mentioned, we used Microsoft Access, already available on most PCs. Anyone experienced in creating SQL Queries in Microsoft Access or a similar program should be able to make a program capable of spatially analyzing total station data given the parameters described below. This study's aim is to inform the reader of the potential of spatial analysis of mapping data, not to provide step-by-step guidance on how to create their own Microsoft Access (or other program) database. Such guidance could not keep up with computer program technology, and it is certain that anyone wishing to use such a program would want to tailor it to his specific needs. If no current member on your team is experienced in database management, we suggest an Information Technology (IT) specialist be employed to create your queries and train your staff on the program's operation. Database managing is one of many aspects of mass grave investigation that must be planned for in advance. A spatial analysis program to be used in the mortuary can be created at the same time and incorporated into your overall operating procedures.

For this study, the steps for running searches in our spatial analysis program are as follows:

From a given case, the code of the specific point where disarticulation occurs is entered. For a body (e.g., case 030B) missing a right lower leg, this would be "030B RKNE." Next, possible codes of matching elements are entered. In this case of mass grave BA05, it would have been another "RKNE." As a result of this study, the point codes have been modified to perform more detailed queries as later detailed in the Discussion section. In addition to searching for elements with matching code, a wildcard can be used in the search, e.g., to find both left and right lower legs, in case they have been sided wrongly during excavation. If desired, the search may further be limited to a certain deposit of human remains within the grave, thus narrowing the possibilities even more. Tables 2.2 and 2.3 display results of a spatial analysis query for the example case.

The result of this query is a list of potential matching elements, ranked by three-dimensional distance from nearest to furthest (Table 2.2). Displayed in the table is the target point (the right knee of case 030B, in this example), the deposit from which the remains were recovered (if applicable), the case number of the possible matching body part, the distance in meters between the targeted point, the element of the body part queried for (right knee in this example), and the ranking of the possible matching body part. The ranks are according to distance; rank 1 being the closest, rank 2 the second closest, and so on.

It is also possible to include the inventory on all the points surveyed on each body or body part, so as to give an idea of which elements are present in each case. In this manner, when the potential matching part inventory shows the body part to have repeated elements with the case body, the potential matching part may be removed from initial consideration. This could eliminate the need to physically retrieve the possible matching body part from the collective remains in storage (no small task when you have hundreds of remains to sort through) while those body parts that better match with the body are examined.

For example, in Table 2.3 the first (and thus closest) body part to the targeted 030B RKNE is case number 058BP at just under 0.25 meter's distance. Examination of all the points recorded on 058BP reveals that it consists of both left and right lower legs. Both knee and ankle points are present (RKNE, LKNE, RANK, and LANK) but no pelvic points, which would indicate if the presence of a femur was recorded. If case 030B has a left lower leg, 058BP can be excluded as a potential match. On the other hand, if the body is missing both lower legs, 058BP should be considered as the best possible match according to distance.

For the 378 cases (289 Bs and 89BPs) recovered from BA05 mass grave at the time of the study, 46 reassociations had been completed on the basis of matching DNA. Out of these, five were excluded from this study because the matching DNA samples had been taken from the same cases and thus only corroborated original association. Nine more matches were excluded because of lack of sufficient data for the queries. The lacking data were in part information on what body elements

Table 2.2 Example Results of Spatial Query Showing Possible Matches, Listed in Order of Distance from the Targeted Point (030B RKNE), When Searching for a Right Lower Leg

Body Survey Code	Deposit Number	Case Number	Distance in Meters	Element	Rank
030B RKNE	1	058BP	0.24866	RKNE	1
	1	067BP	0.89834	RKNE	2
	8	225BP	3.62864	RKNE	3
	9	300BP	5.525004	RKNE	4
	9	425BP	5.646783	RKNE	5
	11	347BP	10.35154	RKNE	6

Table 2.3 Detailed Query Result Showing Four Possible Lower Leg Matches, by Distance, to case 030B with All Recorded Points Displayed

Case Number	Distance in Meters	Deposit Number	Recorded Code Present
058BP	0.24866	1	058BP RKNE
			058BP LKNE
			058BP RANK
			058BP LANK
067BP	0.89834	1	067BP RKNE
			067BP LKNE
			067BP RANK
			067BP LANK
225BP	3.62864	8	225BP RKNE
			225BP RANK
300BP	5.525004	9	300BP RKNE
			300BP LKNE
			300BP RANK
			300BP LANK

the matching parts consist of (due to unclarity in the field and the inaccessibility of certain anthropological data at the time of this study) and in part missing spatial data (coordinates). For each of the remaining 32 cases, a query was run, producing a list of possible matches. As stated before, these lists display the possible matching cases in an order from closest to furthest, thus ranking them according to distance. From this list of possible matches, the true matches, as corroborated by the DNA analysis, were marked. On each list, the ranks were numbered and the match that was actually corroborated by DNA was marked.

Again, the hypothesis is that the nearest-ordered disarticulated body part is more likely to be the matching element than all other possible matching body parts within the grave. This hypothesis should certainly be expected to be valid in a simple primary mass grave. On the other hand, it is likely that the stronger the commingling, as we find in complex secondary mass graves or cases of intentional commingling of remains, the less likely the hypothesis is to be true. However, running the analysis against disarticulated remains from the *same deposit* should help alleviate this problem, even in a secondary mass grave, especially if it consists of clearly defined deposits from different primary sites.

As explained, spatial analysis will produce a list, ordered by distance, of every possible match within grave. Yet, as noted, many mass graves are made of separate deposits of bodies, often gathered from different geographic locations. Remains recovered from BA05, for example, came primarily from three different municipalities in Kosovo. Analysis of the spatial relationships between all remains within BA05 would produce a list that contains possible matches of body parts originating from different municipalities. By narrowing the search to the separate deposits within the grave, particularly complex graves such as secondary burials, the accuracy of the list produced by the spatial analysis program should increase.

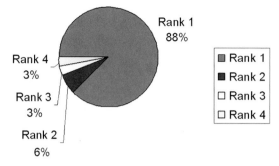

Fig. 2.3 Distribution of confirmed matching elements by their rank in the list of possible matching elements

Results

From the 32 DNA reassociated body parts, 88% (28 reassociations) of the total were first in rank. That is, the actual matching body part was closer to the body it belonged to than all other potential matching parts. Six percent (2 reassociations) were second in rank, the third and fourth ranked cases were each represented by one reassociation (3 percent each) (Fig. 2.3).

The resulting lists of potential matches produced by the spatial analysis averaged 10 or more candidates long and often the number of candidates reached 20 or more. These large lists of possible matches indicate that the demonstrated results are not simply due to a lack of alternative matches in the grave.

As to be expected in a predominately primary grave, the distance between most matching body parts was considerably less than 1 meter: The median distance between the matching elements, from one mapped articulation point to the other,

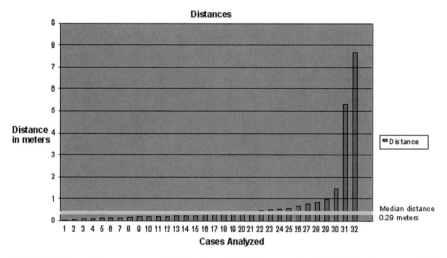

Fig. 2.4 Distances between reassociated body parts, listed by case (median 0.29 meters, mean 0.75 meters)

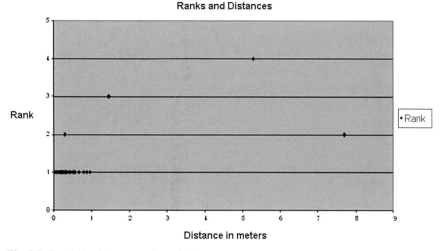

Fig. 2.5 Correlation between ranks and distances

was 0.29 meters (Fig. 2.4). In two cases, the matching elements were over 5 and 7 meters away. These outliers may be explained by machine action within the grave, which probably moved these body parts when going back and forth, or by the described cremation activities that took place beside the grave before remains were pushed in. The correlation between rank on the spatial analysis results list and distance is shown in Fig. 2.5. Again, it shows most DNA reassociated elements high in rank on the list and in close distance to the matching body. A higher rank, on the other hand, it seems—at least in these very few cases—does not necessarily indicate a proportionate increase in distance, and vice versa.

Discussion

The results indicate that spatial analysis of the distribution of disarticulated remains within a mass grave may help solve commingling problems by suggesting probable reassociation matches in ranked order. Minimally, it will provide an objective testing strategy to implement during laboratory analysis. Spatial analysis of excavation survey data from mass grave BA05 found that 88% of the DNA reassociated matches were the closest in physical distance to each other, and the median between the disarticulated parts was only 0.29 meters. It may be assumed that most matching disarticulated remains that have so far failed to produce a DNA sequence in BA05 likewise are ranked high on the generated lists and were recovered near their matching element. When considering the numerous possible matches for each body part within BA05, narrowing down the possibilities to a few most likely matching candidates could dramatically assist reassociation efforts. The same would hold true for all mass graves, especially primary ones, excavated and recorded in a similar manner.

Without knowledge of the spatial relationships of the body parts, mortuary personnel will be unaware of which disarticulated remains were near each other in the grave. In the authors' experiences, either mortuary personnel examine remains recovered from mass graves in a more or less random fashion as the cases are removed from storage—often starting with complete bodies then moving to body parts where little or no reassociation is attempted—or the entire collection of hundreds (or thousands) of elements is laid out so the examiner can walk around between cases trying to piece disarticulated parts together. In this manner, reassociation possibilities rely primarily on the examiner's memory and is limited by how much space is available. These methods are not a prudent use of time and energy, and under such circumstance managers are forced to consider the benefits of reassociation efforts.

While spatial analysis cannot identify matching body parts on its own, it does provide a list of the most likely candidates in ranked order. A focused effort can then be made where the nearest disarticulated body part is examined first, the next-closest second, and so on. Or, depending upon what additional reassociation methods (e.g., pair-matching, conjoining fracture, articular surface comparison, metric analysis, etc.) the examiner wishes to employ, the first several most likely candidates could be removed from storage and examined together. In addition, the recovery data itself provide an electronic remains inventory that, at bare minimum, will give mortuary personnel an idea of the number and type of remains that may be related to the case they are working on.

Logically, spatial analysis would have more success with remains recovered from primary graves than those recovered from secondary deposits where remains were removed from their original context and further disarticulated. Further research into spatial distribution in secondary graves will give a better estimate of the probabilities encountered in such cases. The more intentional commingling a group of bodies is subjected to, the more difficult it will be to reassociate disarticulated body parts. In addition, greater numbers of commingled remains will require greater effort to resolve the problem. While a large number of bodies may have been disposed of in a mass grave, the number of remains that need to be queried during spatial analysis may be reduced through careful recording of body depositional events. A query run on remains from within a single deposit, instead of the whole grave, may prove to be very helpful in narrowing down the number of probable matching remains. Indeed, with the exception of testing all recovered remains for DNA matches, focusing attention on remains from a single deposit at a time would assist all methods of reassociation.

Survey Codes

The use of excavation survey data (originally intended for the production of maps and a basic grave inventory) for spatial analysis requires coding that is specifically adapted to this purpose. ICTY total station survey codes were used to record body and body part positions during the excavation of mass grave BA05. Afterwards, a spatial analysis of the remains distribution within the grave was conducted in which certain limitations of the adopted ICTY codes were made apparent.

While the ICTY codes are proficient enough for mapping purposes, they were found at times to be misleading when presenting an inventory of incomplete remains. For example, using the ICTY codes, a leg disarticulated due to a mid-shaft fracture of the femur would only have two points taken on it—the ankle and knee—while the fracture point of the distal femur would not be recorded (the ICTY codes only provide codes for joints and not the end points of disarticulated limbs). A later review of the codes for this body part would mislead one to assume only the lower leg is present, although half the femur is actually present.

Not only did the ICTY codes create inaccurate inventories, they also caused some confusion during spatial analysis requiring additional research in the excavation logs, sketches, and photos. As a result, the ICTY codes have since been augmented with additional codes (Table 2.4) that are now used in ICMP's standard operating procedures for surveying of mass graves. Limitations of the ICTY codes and the additions made for accurate inventory and smooth running of the spatial analysis are detailed below. The standard ICTY codes are still used, with the exception of the central body point (CPOI)—omitted as it really does not assist in mapping or spatial analysis. This set of 14 codes makes up the standard points taken. The additional codes in Table 2.4 are used to clarify the inventory and assist spatial analysis in the case of incomplete remains.

Table 2.4 Additional Suggested Total Station Survey Codes

Code Entry	Element
CFRG	Cranial fragments
MAND	Mandible
RHUM	Right humerus
RULN	Right ulna
RRAD	Right radius
LHUM	Left humerus
LULN	Left ulna
LRAD	Left radius
RFEM	Right femur
RTIB	Right tibia
RFIB	Right fibula
LFEM	Left femur
LTIB	Left tibia
LFIB	Left fibula
- - - - P	Proximal end
- - - - D	Distal end
- - - - F	Fracture point
- - - - V	Virtual point*
SPINT	Spine top
SPINB	Spine bottom
SPINI	Spine inflection point
- - - - FI	Fracture inflection

*Used only for shoulder and pelvic points (e.g., LSHOV, RPELV).

To better represent a cranium that is fragmented, the code CFRG (**Cranial Fragm**ents) is used. Coding in this manner will notify both a surveyor who is later making a map, and mortuary personnel that what is present is a fractured and possibly incomplete skull. The code MAND is used for a disarticulated, unassociated **Mand**ible. If only a portion of the mandible is recovered, a left/right designation can be added.

As noted, one problem with the ICTY codes found during the spatial analysis of BA05 is that incomplete or disarticulated limb ends are not clearly defined. With the ICTY codes, the humeral head of a complete disarticulated left arm would be recorded as a left shoulder (LSHO). A body missing the lower portion of its right leg would have a point recorded on the distal end of the right femur as a right knee (RKNE). Neither of these points is technically the joint it is recorded to represent. The other bones that make up the joint are absent. While the codes are adequate for mapping purposes, they force extra steps to be taken during analysis of the spatial relationships between disarticulated remains.

For example, when using the ICTY code system to generate a list of bodies that a disarticulated left arm may belong to, a query between that arm's humeral head data point (LSHO) would be run against the other LSHO data points in the grave. Results would include not only the potential bodies missing a left arm, but all the other disarticulated left arms in the grave (added to the results because of their recorded LSHO codes). These other arms would then have to be filtered out of the results.

To get around this additional step and make the spatial analysis program more user-friendly, additions to the coding system for incomplete or disarticulated limbs must be made. Similar to the ICTY code system, when the end of a long bone needs to be recorded, a four-letter code is generated starting with the side that element is from followed by the first three letters of the name of that bone. This is followed by either the suffix of "P" for "proximal" or "D" for "distal" to indicate which end of the bone the point is being recorded. The proximal end of the left humerus in the above example, instead of being recorded as LSHO, would have the code of LHUMP (**L**eft **Hum**erus **P**roximal). The elbow and wrist of a left disarticulated arm would be recorded in the standard method (LELB and LWRI). The distal end of the right femur in the above example would be RFEMD (**R**ight **Fem**ur **D**istal), instead of RKNE. To locate possible matches for the disarticulated arm example, the LHUMP data would be run against all LSHOV data points from the grave (only body trunks would have this code virtual points are discussed below). For the body missing the lower right leg, its RFEMD data point would be run against RTIBP (**R**ight **Tib**ia **P**roximal) data points of disarticulated lower legs within the grave.

The additional codes listed in Table 2.4 better define disarticulated and fractured elements, allowing for a more accurate field inventory, and narrow the search parameters of potential reassociations by excluding misleading data points from the search. These codes should only be used to record disarticulated limb ends, while the standard 14 ICTY codes should be used for articulating joints. In this manner it will be readily apparent which point on the limb needs to be used in the spatial analysis program and creates a more accurate inventory. Lower arms and legs consist of two long bones. If you need to record a point on a disarticulated lower limb where both bones are present, it is suggested that the ulna and tibia are used, as these bones best articulate to their upper limb counterparts. The fibula and radius should be used if the other bone is absent.

Disarticulation may also occur at fracture points. The ICTY codes are incapable of demonstrating such trauma, forcing the surveyor to stop the recording points at the last joint prior to reaching the fracture. This gives an inaccurate representation of the remains present and will muddy all spatial analysis results. To overcome this, fracture data points should be recorded from long bones that are missing one end. These codes are to be understood as the end point of a long bone where the remainder of the bone is missing, and thus no joint, proximal, or distal long bone point could be taken. The fracture point will again be coded by using the side from where the arm came from, the first three letters of the fractured long bone, then the letter "F" to indicate it is a fracture point, and followed by a "P" of "D" suffix denoting the point as the proximal or distal end of that bone segment (Table 2.4). As spatial analysis is aimed at assisting in the reassociation of disarticulated remains, perimortem and postmortem fractures are coded the same way. Trauma analysis, as well as all final remains analysis, should be conducted during mortuary analysis.

Figure 2.6 illustrates a hypothetical example of how these fracture codes are used. An otherwise complete body is missing a right arm from mid-shaft humerus down. The regular shoulder point is taken on the body (RSHO) but the elbow is missing— only half the humerus is present. In such a case, a point will be taken on the distal end of the existing proximal section of humerus where the fracture/disarticulation took place. Thus, that point on the body would be recorded as RHUMFD (**R**ight

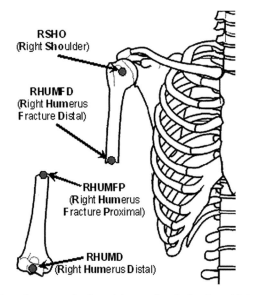

Fig. 2.6 Demonstration of survey codes for a right arm disarticulated at mid-shaft humerus due to a fracture. A spatial query search for the missing distal humerus would involve the codes RHUMFD and RHUMFP

Hum**erus F**racture **D**istal end of bone). It is important to understand that a distal designation is given to this fracture point as it represents the most distal end of that section of right humerus. The proximal end of this proximal section of humerus has already been recorded as the right shoulder (RSHO) because it articulates with the body and so does not receive a "proximal" designated point. In an effort to try to locate the missing lower portion of arm, a spatial analysis query would be run from the body's RHUMFD point to all RHUMFP (**R**ight **Hum**erus **F**racture **P**roximal end of bone) points recorded in the grave. This point represents the fracture (and most proximal point) on the disarticulated distal section of a humerus. Only distal sections of humeri disarticulated due to a fracture of the shaft can have this proximal code. In this example, the lower arm is missing so the distal section of the right humerus would receive the code RHUMD (**R**ight **Hum**erus **D**istal end of bone).

The query that is run to try to match the disarticulated bone is therefore between the fracture points on the humerus shaft—the point of separation (Fig. 2.6). If the fracture was clean on both bone ends, the fracture pattern can be articulated and all other possible disarticulated fractured distal humeri can be excluded from consideration. As the articulating distal humerus is absent the lower arm, a second query can be run, this time searching from the distal end of the right humerus (RHUMD) to all possible right proximal ulnae (RULNP) and perhaps radii (RRADP).

In the BA05 inventory data, it was noted that sometimes shoulder and pelvic points on bodies were absent. These survey points were not recorded sometimes because the surveyor felt that not enough of the joint remained present on the body to justify its recording. For example, a surveyor may have omitted taking a shoulder point from a body missing its left arm and scapula. As the body physically did not have a complete shoulder (only the clavicle remained), no point was taken. This scenario does not present too difficult a problem for mapping purposes, but without a left shoulder data point recorded from the body, reassociation analysis cannot be attempted. While disarticulated left arms have data points recorded from their proximal ends, there is no corresponding shoulder point on the body available for the spatial analysis program to be queried against. The same would hold true for a body missing one side of its pelvis.

To overcome the lack of a shoulder or pelvic joint to query during spatial analysis, it will be necessary to record a "virtual point" on the body where the joint would have been. Minor location inaccuracies should present little if any difference in the generated list of possible matches from a spatial analysis of the data. To denote the presence of a virtual point, the regular code is followed by the suffix "V" (e.g., LSHOV, RPELV) (Table 2.2).

An additional concern was how to accurately record the bodies that separated at the spine. From the authors' experience working in mass graves, disarticulation of the spinal column often occurs at the cervical and lumbar regions. Disarticulation occurs regularly enough at the lumbar or lower thoracic region that bodies will often be categorized in evidence logs as "upper" or "lower" bodies (to further confuse the body vs. body part classification debate). Likewise, heads often disarticulate with a couple of cervical vertebrae attached. Vertebral shape and checking the articulation between vertebrae offer a good platform for reassociating upper and lower bodies and cranium. To assist mortuary workers in these efforts of reassociation, it is suggested that the additional total station codes, listed in Table 2.4, be used to identify the points of disarticulation on a spine: SPINT (**Spin**e **T**op) and SPINB (**Spin**e **B**ottom).

Determination of "top" or "bottom" depends on the anatomical orientation of the body part in question. A lower body consisting of legs, a complete pelvis, and several vertebrae would have an SPINT point recorded on the uppermost vertebra. A thorax consisting of only thoracic vertebrae and ribs would have an SPINT point recorded on its T1 and an SPINB on T12. A cranium with a couple of cervical vertebrae attached would have the following points recorded on it: CRAN (**Cran**ium) and SPINB (indicating the last attached vertebra). The presence of SPIN points would indicate to mortuary personnel that reassociation via vertebrae may be possible.

A final suggestion to augment the ICTY codes is the inclusion of an "inflection point." At times spinal columns and fractured long bones are bent in such a manner that a surveyor making a map may question the accuracy of a recorded point. If a body is bent double over itself in the grave, the mapped connection line made between the cranial point and the central pelvis point representing the spinal column would look absurdly short, perhaps only several centimeters long. The same would hold true for a fractured long bone in a limb radically bent at an impossible angle.

The inclusion of a point where the spinal column or radically bent long bone doubles back on itself would create a more understandable map. While inflection codes are not used for spatial analysis (radical inflection may be present, but disarticulation is not), the inclusion of an inflection point will denote the presence of the extreme bend, possibly assisting mortuary personnel in their postmortem analysis. For indicating a spinal column inflection point, as indicated in Table 2.2, an "I" is added to the end of the regular SPIN code (SPINI). In an effort to keep survey time short, fracture inflection points should only be recorded when the bend is so great that the surveyor knows it may cause confusion during mapping. A fracture inflection point is recorded by adding an "I" instead of a distal or proximal suffix after the regular fracture code (e.g., RFEMFI).

Figure 2.7 illustrates the approximate location of most of the additional survey codes described above. As explained, some of the codes can be combined when confronted with fractures and inflection points. While not all of the combinations are reflected in the figure, the illustration serves as a reference to help visualize survey possibilities. Although the list of combined ICTY and suggested augmented survey codes appears lengthy, ICMP personnel using the new code system during excavation of several mass graves have found them to be very manageable. Most recorded points on a body will consist of the original 14 ICTY codes. The additional codes we suggest here are only used when remains are disarticulated or when the standard codes cannot accurately represent the elements present. It is suggested that a list of the codes and an illustration like Fig. 2.7 be used as a reference by the surveyor in the field. We have found it convenient to hang the codes directly on the total station tripod for quick reference.

All codes suggested here are just those: suggestions. We have found these codes to work satisfactorily in *realistic* international situations involving complex mass

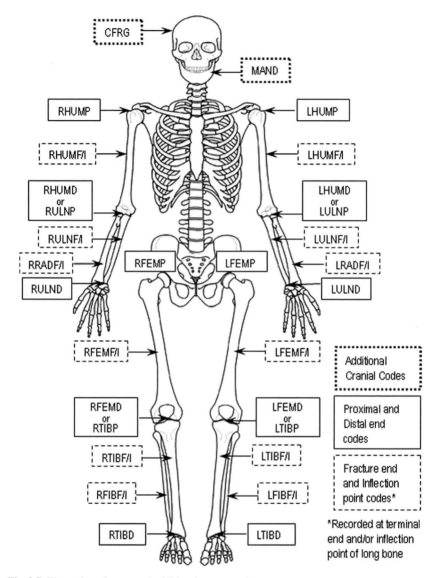

Fig. 2.7 Illustration of suggested additional survey codes

graves, and we feel they reach a level of accuracy that serves both the investigation and identification goals of the various organizations we have worked for without exceeding timelines and budgets. However, if investigation organizers decide that smaller elements, not represented within our suggested coding system, are to receive the same attention as larger, more complete elements, additional codes could be created by using the same system proposed here. For example, a disarticulated **left hand** may be coded LHAN.

Whatever the codes decided upon, the important thing to keep in mind is that all codes must be *consistently* applied to all remains recovered in order for your spatial analysis program to be *consistently* helpful. The same coding system should be consistently applied to all the graves scheduled for excavation. If all graves created during a conflict are to be excavated, then the work will most likely take several years and be done by different personnel making up the excavation teams. Thus, standard survey codes must be decided upon prior to excavation of the first grave and consistently applied over the entire course of work or there will be a buildup of conflicting codes. Changes in survey codes will only complicate the identification process, inhibit accurate spatial analysis, and create inconsistencies in the evidence log.

Inconsistent recording of survey points are akin to inconstancies of recording evidence at a crime scene; the more inconsistency introduced, the weaker the evidence. The old adage of "garbage in, garbage out" applies.

It should be noted that spatial analysis can be run using data containing only ICTY-type codes. However, as shown, these codes are limited. The analyst will have to spend extra time filtering the data, which would most likely involve searching through secondary sources such as field exhumation notes/body exhumation forms and photographs. Ideally, the analyst would be someone working in the mortuary who could run a spatial query on a particular case immediately after it is found to be missing an element. It is postulated that the use of only ICTY coded data would slow such a process down to the point where running a query in the mortuary would not be beneficial. While this does not exclude the possibility of running queries outside the mortuary prior to autopsy, the suggested additional codes proposed here, if properly implemented during excavation, would allow for direct field data transfer into the mortuary.

Conclusion

The combination of numerous bodies, taphonomic conditions, time afforded to decomposition, and intentional disturbance or destruction of remains within a mass grave context can all contribute to disarticulation and commingling. While there is wide agreement that careful excavation is necessary and can contribute to mortuary analysis of remains, few examples exist of excavation data being applied within the laboratory. The spatial analysis of remains distribution within a grave is one method of bridging the gap between field and mortuary activities. By providing a list that ranks the most likely reassociations by distance from each other, spatial analysis can assist mortuary personnel with the reassociation of disarticulated body parts.

During the excavation of mass grave BA05, ICTY survey codes were used to record body and body part positions. A spatial analysis of the remains distribution within the grave was conducted using DNA matching results as a control. Results for the relatively complex grave show that the spatial analysis provides good evidence that certain bodies and body parts belong together. In secondary mass graves or other complex situations, the probability would be expected to be less. In such complex cases, analysis by separate deposits of human remains within the grave, as opposed to spatial searches involving all elements within the whole grave, will most likely prove to be a useful strategy. To create a more accurate inventory and easier spatial analysis queries, a number of additional survey codes to augment the standard ICTY codes have been suggested.

It is essential to implement a good documentation process in the field as well as good data flow from field to the mortuary. This will result in a detailed field inventory of recovered remains—useful as evidence, for planning of mortuary processes, and to develop rough estimates of remains represented in a grave. It will also assist in the reassociation of disarticulated remains.

The concept of using spatial data to help assist problems of commingled remains is not mind-boggling, nor should its implementation be complex. The only necessary elements are consistent code recording during survey of remains with an eye toward spatial analysis and a plan to use the analysis during autopsy.

Acknowledgments All authors were employed by the International Commission on Missing Persons (ICMP) during the initial development of this study. Although two of the authors have since moved on, we would all like to thank ICMP for the continued cooperation and interest that led to completion of this work. The principal author would also like to acknowledge the support received from the Oak Ridge Institute of Science and Education during the writing of this chapter.

References Cited

Buikstra, J. E., C. C. Gordon, and L. St. Hoyme 1984 The case of the severed skull: Individuation in forensic anthropology. In *Human Identification: Case Studies in Forensic Anthropology*, T. A. Rathbun and J. E. Buikstra, eds., pp. 121–135. Charles C. Thomas, Springfield, IL.

Byrd, J. E. and B. J. Adams 2003 Osteometric sorting of commingled human remains. *J. Forensic Sci.* 48(4):717–24.

Dirkmaat, D. C. and J. M. Adovasio 1997 The role of archaeology in the recovery and interpretation of human remains from an outdoor forensic setting. In *Forensic Taphonomy*, W. H. Haglund and M. H. Sorg, eds., pp. 39–64. CRC Press, Boca Raton, FL.

Dirkmaat, D. C., J. M. Adovasio, L. Cabo, and V. Rozas 2005 Mass Graves, Human Rights and Commingled Remains: Considering the Benefits of Forensic Archaeology. Paper presented at the 57th Annual Meeting of the American Academy of Forensic Science, New Orleans.

Haglund, W. D. 2001 Archaeology and forensic death investigations. *Historical Archaeol.* (35): 35–38.

Hanson, I., J. Sterenberg, and R. Wessling 2000 *Survey Procedures: ICTY Forensic Field Team Bosnia: 2000 Field Season*. Manuscript on file, Exhumation and Examination Division, International Commission on Missing Persons, Sarajevo, Bosnia and Herzegovina.

Morse, D., D. Crusoe, and H. G. Smith 1976 Forensic archaeology. *J. Forensic Sci.* 21(2):323–332.

Owsley, D. W. 2001 Why the forensic anthropologist needs the archaeologist. *Historical Archaeol.* 35(1):35–38.

Skinner, M. 1987 Planning the archaeological recovery of evidence from recent mass graves. *Forensic Sci. Int.* 34(4):267–287.

Wright, R. 2003 Program NN_ICMP.EXE: A Computer Program for Nearest Neighbours Spatial Analysis of Forensic Exhumations. Manuscript on file, Exhumation and Examination Division: International Commission on Missing Persons, Sarajevo, Bosnia and Herzegovina.

Wright, R., I. Hanson, and J. Sterenberg 2005 The archaeology of mass graves. In *Forensic Archaeology: Advances in Theory and Practice*, J. Hunter and M. Cox, eds., pp. 137–158. Routledge, New York.

Wright, R. V. S. 1992 Correlation between cranial form and geography in Homo sapiens. *Archaeol. Oceania* (27):128–134.

Chapter 3
Pieces of the Puzzle: FBI Evidence Response Team Approaches to Scenes with Commingled Evidence

Gary W. Reinecke and Michael J. Hochrein

Introduction

Since the establishment of the Federal Bureau of Investigation's (FBI's) Evidence Response Team (ERT) Unit in 1993, ERTs across the United States have been involved in the collection of evidence from scenes large and small. One hundred forty-one teams, composed of more than 1,100 members, have been formed within the 56 FBI Field Offices, or Divisions. Single or combined teams, in either Federal cases or as requested assistance in State or local investigations, have participated in over 2,000 crime or search scenes. FBI ERTs have been deployed internationally to sites in Africa, the Middle East, the Balkans, Central Asia, and Southeast Asia. Those domestic and international deployments have included bombings, terrestrial crashes, and mass graves in which the remains of the victims are intrinsically commingled. Regardless of the size of the scenes, similar fundamental approaches toward scene management and evidence collection have proven imperative in making sense of sometimes confusing situations.

Perhaps there is no other crime scene setting where the documentation of the three-dimensional position of fragmented and commingled evidence is more critical than that involving multiple or mass deaths. Such scenes may consist of the burial of two or more homicide victims in a common grave; or they could entail extremely fragmented remains over several acres of a crash scene. In both types of scenes, the identification of individual pieces in their environmental contexts preserves the patterns and relationships between evidence. These relationships, and patterns formed, are defined during the final stages of actions, which were physically or behaviorally controlled. The act, or reason for the final position of the evidence or remains, is initially controlled by human behavior and/or natural laws. Both controls have been the subject of a myriad of research. For example, the positioning of victims' bodies is many times the result of conscious or subconscious efforts of the killer(s). Brooks (1985), Burgess and Ressler (1985), Douglas et al. (1986), Douglas and Munn (1992a, b), Keppel (2005), Lundrigan and Canter (2001), Rajs et al. (1998), Ressler et al. (1985), and Rossi (1982) are just a representative few of the studies addressing the psychology behind victim selection, crime scene selection, and victim treatment that are ultimately reflected in the positioning of a body and other evidence. In cases involving clandestine burials, suspects

From: *Recovery, Analysis, and Identification of Commingled Human Remains*
Edited by: B. Adams and J. Byrd © Humana Press, Totowa, NJ

go beyond affecting site selection and victim body position to also create and affect the space in which the body(ies) is(are) concealed. Hochrein (1997, 2002) discusses spatial evidence, or geotaphonomic characteristics, which are created and influenced by conscious and subconscious subject behavior. The physics behind the patterned distribution of evidence in explosive or collision events has been discussed by several authors, including Anker and Taylor (1989), Barrie and Hodson-Walker (1970), Bergen-Henengouwan (1973), Gable (1968), Hellerich and Pollak (1995), Hill (1989), Kreft (1970), Matteson (1974), Min and Jia (1992), Steele (1983), and Swegennis (1987), to, again, name a few. In postblast, or postcrash, settings, the controlling factor is, at some point, the physical dynamics of explosion, which involve known forces on known volumes and materials resulting in predictable patterns in which exploded materials are distributed. In the absence of explosion, forces of momentum will still affect evidence distributions. By precisely recording the final position of crash debris and human remains, as well as environmental features that could have affected their flight on the way to those positions, research and predictive models represented by the aforementioned references are possible or confirmed. In the same vein, the precise mapping of body position and associated evidence in a multiple-victim interment may reveal the human behavior that affected when, why, and how each individual was placed in the common burial. Often, however, crime scene investigators are faced with pressure from superiors or co-workers who believe the piece-plotting of evidence is pointless because they believe fragmentation occurs randomly, or all evidence in a clandestine grave was deposited contemporaneously. In order to overcome outside pressures to compromise during collection efforts, FBI ERT members receive training throughout their Bureau careers that emphasizes the efficient yet complete recovery of evidence. Regardless of the magnitude of the scene, the same efforts toward quality and quantity of information gathering are attempted.

In this chapter, the authors will present the FBI ERT concept and basic protocols. Two cases are then presented to illustrate how those protocols were followed and how the extra effort toward three-dimensional mapping of human remains and associated evidence can aid in the interpretation, reconstruction, and presentation of a crime or disaster scene. Both cases involve multiple victims and represent a middle ground between cases of a single victim and those constituting large-scale mass disasters.

FBI Evidence Response Team Protocols and Responsibilities

The quality and quantity of evidence collected at any crime scene are directly impacted by the amount of preparation by crime scene investigators toward potential responses. As mentioned above, FBI ERT members are required to apply fundamental techniques of crime scene management, evidence collection, and documentation to each and every site they process. In large and small scenes, personnel duties and responsibilities are clearly defined and basic stages involving the organization of the search for potential evidence are well known to all ERT members. The size and magnitude of the crime scene may affect the number of personnel deployed to the scene, and the type of crime being investigated may require different forensic tools, but the basis for duties and assignments and organization of the search remain the same. The processing of a vehicle used in a crime may take only a handful of personnel to process. A major postblast, or -crash, scene could involve multiple teams from numerous field offices. For example, 137 ERT members were utilized toward the collection of evidence from the Pentagon crime scene in the aftermath of the September 11, 2001, terrorist attacks. In response to the events of that same day, 480 FBI ERT members worked over 10 months with other Federal, State, and local investigators in processing debris from the World Trade Center in New York City. At the same time 96 ERT team members were utilized at the crash of Flight 93 near Shanksville, Pennsylvania.

Certain personnel duties and responsibilities are necessary in almost any major search operation. The following duties and responsibilities are typically crucial to ensure that search efforts are conducted in an organized and methodical fashion. It is important to note it may not be feasible to have one person assigned to each duty. It is relatively common for one person to accomplish two or more. For all positions, the interest and attitude of personnel are paramount concerns. Training and experience will only be used to best potential when team members possess a positive attitude. This human side of evidence response teams is significant due to the long hours and attention to detail often required of personnel. The following lists the major assignments as well as corresponding general duties and responsibilities:

1. Team leader
2. Photographer and photographic log recorder
3. Sketch preparer
4. Evidence recorder/custodian
5. Evidence recovery personnel
6. Specialists (as required)

Team Leader

The team leader has the overall responsibility at the scene to ensure that communication, assessments, and responsibilities are conducted thoroughly and completely. The team leader assumes control upon arrival at the scene and is cognizant of safety issues that may affect team members. This may be as simple as having extra police officers or agents at the scene or may be as complex as prearranging military assets and personnel in a war-torn region. Once the scene is secured and any safety issues are addressed, the team leader, usually assisted by the photographer, will conduct a preliminary walkthrough of the scene with the purpose of evaluating potential evidence and preparing a written narrative. Once the scene has been evaluated, the team leader will brief other members of the team, will establish a search pattern, and will make appropriate assignments to team members. A command post should be created outside the crime scene. The command post could be located in a building, under a pop-up tent, or inside a motor vehicle or could even be located under a shady tree. The purpose of the command post is to maintain a designated area where the exchange of information can take place between the team leader and investigative personnel. The command post is also the point where coordination between all law enforcement agencies occurs. The team leader maintains these responsibilities throughout the entire process and should continually reevaluate the efficiency of the search during the entire course of the operation. Once the search has been completed and a final survey and inventory review has been completed, it is the team leader's responsibility to release the scene.

Photographer and Photographic Log Recorder

The photographer should make every effort to document the scene before it is entered by other team members. This should include the photography of any victims, crowds, or motor vehicles that may be considered part of the scene. The photographer is required to photograph the entire scene with overall, medium, and close-up coverage, using measurement scales when appropriate. All items of evidence must be photographed before they are moved. This will require communication and cooperation between other team components to include the sketch preparer, evidence recorder/custodian, and evidence recovery personnel. Cooperation among these team components remains important when numbering and identifying items of evidence. Each item of evidence collected will have one number assigned to the item and should be identified using the same nomenclature on all logs created at the scene. Using a different description on logs can become confusing when testifying in court. A room described on a log as the family room and later described as a den on another log can lead one to wonder if there were actually two rooms. In the case of multiple skeletal remains, the confusion could be even greater. All latent fingerprints and other impression evidence are photographed with and without scale before any lifts and/or casts are removed. Every photograph must be documented by the photographic log recorder on a photo log, which should also include a photo sketch. The photo sketch depicts the item photographed and its relationship within the scene along with the angle and direction of the camera at the time of the photograph.

Sketch Preparer

The sketch preparer is responsible for determining the scope of the scene and the selection of equipment used for mapping. The sketch preparer determines if two-dimensional measurements are sufficient or if three-dimensional documentation is required. The sketch preparer determines if hand tools, total station, or three-dimensional scanning equipment is utilized. The availability of the equipment, the environment being mapped, and the type of presentation required in court will assist the sketch preparer in determining the suitable method. Regardless of the type of sketch or equipment used, any prepared sketch must follow certain protocols and contain specific information. The sketch preparer must diagram the immediate scene and orient the sketch with north. Evidence item numbers and nomenclature must be coordinated with the other team components. Adjacent buildings, rooms, furniture, etc. need to be indicated as appropriate. The sketch preparer should obtain appropriate assistance for operating equipment such as total stations and three-dimensional scanners. It is very difficult for one person to operate this equipment, and training is necessary for all operators. Even simple measuring with hand tools is more efficient with assistance. The sketch preparer will determine the scale to be utilized. Whether the scene is depicted in feet and inches or it is determined that metric measurements will be used, measurements must be consistent and the sketch preparer must ensure consistency throughout the mapping process.

Evidence Recorder/Custodian

The evidence recorder/custodian is responsible for the overall coordination of the documentation, packaging, and preservation of all evidence obtained at the scene. The evidence recorder/custodian is responsible for maintaining an evidence recovery log, which reflects the description, date, times, location, and individual collecting of each item of evidence. The evidence recorder/custodian receives and records all evidence from the evidence recovery personnel and is responsible for coordinating numbering and nomenclature of items with all other components of the team. The evidence recorder/custodian maintains the chain of custody by maintaining control of the evidence from the scene to the transmittal of the evidence to the case investigator, property room, or crime lab, per agency guidelines.

Evidence Recovery Personnel

The evidence recovery personnel are responsible for locating and collecting items of evidence at the scene. They are also responsible for ensuring that each item collected has been photographed and placed in the sketch before it is moved from the scene and that the numbering and nomenclature of evidence are consistent with the other components. The evidence recovery personnel mark each item of evidence with their initials and date when collecting items. This is normally witnessed by a second individual who also initials and dates the item. This process ensures the availability of at least one evidence recovery member if testimony is later required at a court hearing or trial. The evidence recovery personnel are required to keep the team leader apprised of any significant evidence located throughout the search. The evidence recovery personnel ensure they are appropriately dressed (gloves, Tyvek, mask, etc.) to avoid any contamination issues while operating within the crime scene.

Specialists

It is sometimes necessary and prudent to bring in expertise from outside services. The field of forensic science is so broad today that no agency will have every form of specialty service available from among its ranks. Typically, specialists are brought in from industry, the academic community, private scientific laboratories, and similar concerns. The Evidence Response Team program has over 1,100 members nationwide, and several members have formal education in more than one listed specialty, but these individuals are not always available or in a specific geographic area where they can respond to every case. When dealing with outside specialists, some pertinent aspects to consider are

- The competency and reliability of the specialist
- The ability of the specialist to work within law enforcement guidelines at a scene
- The role of the specialist in presenting expert testimony in court

Specialists should be identified before they are needed in an actual case. A current contact list should be maintained if possible. The agency should meet with these individuals to determine the best manner to jointly conduct search planning, operations, and follow-up activity. Some examples of specialty assistance to be considered are described next.

Medical Examiner/Pathologist/Coroner

The medical examiner/pathologist/coroner role at a crime scene will vary by jurisdiction. Some states and counties are part of the coroner system. The coroner may or may not have a medical background and may have a staff to include pathologists or may contract out the work. It is important to be familiar with the system responsible for your crime scene. In some jurisdictions a pathologist will respond to the scene, in some jurisdictions the Medical Examiner's office will send one of its investigators, and in some jurisdictions there is no response to the scene. The important point to remember in all these scenarios is that the deceased is the responsibility of those medical examiner/pathologist/coroner jurisdictions and that the remains should not be touched without their approval. Regardless of which system is in place, the medical examiner/pathologist/coroner is responsible for the postmortem examination.

Odontologist

The odontologist can be very useful in the identification of the victim. The odontologist is capable of comparing ante- and postmortem dental records and rendering identification. The odontologist is extremely useful when dealing with skeletal and decomposed remains. The odontologist normally conducts these comparisons at the morgue or a dental office. The odontologist should be utilized at the scene of arson where burned teeth can be preserved before transport of the remains. The teeth of victims in post-arson scenes can be easily destroyed and lost during movement of the remains. The odontologist can preserve the teeth for transport and is able to more easily identify burned teeth within the scene. Odontologists responded to the Tsunami disaster in Phuket, Thailand, and assisted in many of the identifications made there. Three acceptable methods of identification were accepted in Thailand for the Tsunami victims: dental, DNA, and fingerprint comparisons.

Anthropologist

The anthropologist can identify skeletal portions of human remains and, using the skeletal remains, can determine factors such as age, race, stature, and gender, which are very useful in the identification of the remains. The anthropologist can also assist in determining if skeletal remains are human or animal. In the case of mass or commingled graves, the anthropologist can sort the skeletal remains and group the remains by victim. Anthropologists can assist in identifying tool marks on bone and in determining whether they are caused by animals or weapons. They can assist in determining whether damage to the skeletal remains occurred ante-, peri- or post-mortem.

Entomologist

The entomologist is useful in the collection, preservation, and identification of various insects located within the general area of the human remains. The entomologist is able to assist in determining the time of death by studying the development of the collected specimens and determining the environmental conditions over a specified period of time.

Botanist

The botanist, like the entomologist, is able to assist in determining the time of death after collecting and identifying plant life found within the general area of human remains. The botanist also requires local environmental conditions to assist in the determination of time of death. The botanist can further assist in determining plant material associated with the remains that is not consistent with the area where the remains were recovered.

Blood Pattern Analyst

Using acceptable scientific methods, the blood pattern analyst is able to enter a bloody crime scene and analyze various groups and shapes of bloodstains. Through this analysis, identification of various types of stains, the velocity required to create the stain, and the direction of travel can be determined. The blood pattern analyst can assist the investigation by offering a recreation of the events and identifying types of instruments used to create the pattern.

Geologist

The geologist can assist the investigation with issues relating to rock and soil. During the recovery of human remains, the geologist can advise on the consistency of soil as the grave is excavated and identify any soil and/or rock that is not consistent with the local region. A geologist can be useful in determining data obtained through the use of ground-penetrating radar or other geophysical prospecting methods.

Surveyor

A surveyor or surveying crew is useful in mapping utilizing the total station. A surveyor can also assist in locating local maps and topographic maps.

Engineer

Engineers can be of assistance in cases such as postblast scenes where large structures have collapsed or partially collapsed. They have expertise in shoring, bracing, evaluating, and lifting structural components.

Bomb Technician

The bomb technician can be called to assist in cases where an explosive device is present or intelligence reports the possibility of such devices. The bomb technician can sweep the scene for primary and secondary devices. The bomb technician has render-safe capability and can conduct the render-safe technique at the site or transport the device to another location for detonation.

Crime Laboratory Examiner

The crime laboratory examiner is generally trained in several or one specific discipline such as DNA, trace evidence, firearms and toolmarks, chemistry, etc. Depending on the circumstances of the case and local policy, it may be advantageous to request a crime laboratory examiner to respond to the scene or to consult with the examiner over the telephone. The crime laboratory examiner can assist in providing information on the proper collecting, packaging, and transmittal of specific types of evidence.

Safety Officer

The safety officer is trained in the use of various detection devices to measure hazardous gases such as carbon monoxide and methane. The safety officer is also OSHA trained and can advise team members regarding the mandate to wear steel-toed shoes, helmets, protective eyewear, levels of Tyvek, etc. The safety officer receives training in confined space and, like the engineer, can assist in partial or full building collapses.

Hazmat Specialist

The Hazmat specialist is trained in the detection and mitigation of all hazardous materials, including chemical, biological, and nuclear materials. No suspected scene should be entered by personnel before it has been cleared by a Hazmat specialist. The Hazmat specialist is also trained in the collecting and shipping of evidence in a hazardous environment.

Organization of the crime scene search process is paramount to any successful search. The FBI Evidence Response Teams are trained in a basic 12-step process as described below:

1. Preparation: Preparation requires training and maintaining adequate supplies and equipment to conduct the crime scene search. Teams are required to accumulate packaging and collection materials necessary for typical search circumstances. A list of required supplies and equipment is maintained, and teams put together response kits for various type scenes such as Latents, recovery of human remains, DNA collection, etc. Each team member receives training in completing computerized and preformatted logs and administrative work sheets. Prior to the search, legal documents and ramifications are discussed among the team. This may involve reviewing the search warrant for familiarization of the items and types of items to be seized. The team leader is preselected, and assignments to other positions are generally predetermined. Specialized vehicles are stocked with supplies and equipment to handle a variety of circumstances to include communications, shelter, lighting, etc. Each team member is issued a variety of clothing to cover a wide range of weather conditions. Safety equipment such as steel-toed boots, gloves, helmets, eye protection, and respirators is issued to each team member. In the event of extended searches, a rotation of teams is developed. On several remote and overseas deployments, food and water were made part of the load-out package. Several teams maintain their own medically trained personnel or draw medical personnel from other entities within the FBI. Local medical resources and adequate hospitals are identified prior to all deployments. Prior to arrival at the scene, communication is usually established with services of an ancillary nature (e.g., medical examiner, prosecuting attorney, and other specialists as required) so that questions that surface during the investigation may be resolved.

2. Approach scene: Upon initial arrival at the scene, be alert for evidence and be cautious concerning transient evidence, foot/tire impressions, and trace evidence. Make certain to protect evidence if necessary from contamination or loss. Extensive notes should be taken immediately; the notes can be written or dictated. Consideration of the safety of all personnel is paramount.

3. Secure and protect: Take control of the scene immediately, and determine the extent to which the scene has been protected. Obtain information from personnel who have knowledge of the original condition of the scene, including first responders, medical personnel, any witnesses, and/or surviving victims. Designate one person in charge for final decision making and problem resolution. Take

extensive notes, and do not rely on memory. Keep out unauthorized personnel and record times and names of all personnel entering or leaving the scene.

4. Preliminary survey: Cautiously walk through the scene, and maintain administrative and emotional control. Select a narrative technique (written, audio, or video). Have preliminary photographs taken by the designated photographer. Delineate the extent of the search area, and initially expand the perimeter. Organize methods and procedures to be utilized, and recognize special problem areas. Identify, protect, and document transient physical evidence. Determine personnel and equipment needs, and make specific assignments. Develop a general theory of the crime based on current information. Take extensive notes to document the scene, and describe the physical and environmental conditions as well as personnel movements.

5. Evaluate physical evidence possibilities: This evaluation begins upon the arrival at the scene and becomes detailed in the preliminary survey stage. Ensure that the collection and packaging materials and equipment are sufficient. Focus first on evidence that could be lost and leave the least transient last. Ensure all personnel consider the variety of possible evidence, not only evidence within their specialties. Search the easily accessible areas and progress out to view locations, always being aware of hidden items. Evaluate whether evidence appears to have been moved inadvertently or whether the scene appears to be contrived.

6. Narrative: The narrative is a running, general-terms description of the condition of the crime scene. The narrative describes the scene in a "general to specific" reference scheme. Use a systematic approach in narrative. Nothing is insignificant to record if it catches one's attention. Under most circumstances, do not collect evidence during the narrative. Use photographs and sketches to supplement, not substitute, for the narrative. The narrative should include case identifier; date, time, and location; weather and lighting conditions; condition and position of evidence.

7. Photography: Photograph the crime scene as soon as possible and prepare a photographic log that records all photographs and a description and location of evidence. Establish a progression of overall, medium, and close-up views of the crime scene. Photograph from eye level to represent the normal view. Photograph the most fragile areas of the crime scene first. Photograph all stages of the crime scene investigation including discoveries before the evidenced is moved. Photograph the evidence in detail, and include a scale with the photographer's name and the date. When a scale is used, first take the photograph without the scale. Photograph the interior crime scene in an overlapping series using a normal lens, if possible. Overall photographs may be taken using a wide-angle lens. Photograph the exterior crime scene, establishing the location of the scene by a series of overall photographs including a landmark. Photographs should have 360 degrees of coverage. Consider aerial photography when possible. Photograph entrances and exits from the inside and the outside. Photograph important evidence twice, taking a medium-distance photograph that shows the evidence and its position to other evidence. The second photograph is a close-up photograph

that includes a scale and fills the frame. Prior to entering the scene, attempt to acquire prior photographs, blueprints, or maps of the scene.

8. Sketch: The sketch establishes a permanent record of items, conditions, and distance and size relationships. Sketches supplement the scene photographs and the narrative description. Sketch number designations should coordinate with the evidence log number designations. Sketches are normally not drawn to scale; however, the sketch should have measurements and details to complete a drawn-to-scale diagram if necessary. The sketch should include case identifier; date, time, and location; identity and assignments of personnel involved in the sketch; dimensions of the rooms, furniture, doors, and windows; distances between objects, persons, bodies, entrances, and exits; measurements showing the location of evidence; key, legend, compass orientation, scale, scale disclaimer, or a combination of these features.

9. Conduct crime scene search: Use a search pattern (grid, strip, or spiral) and search from the general to the specific for evidence. Be alert for all evidence, and carefully search entrances and exits. Wear latex or cotton gloves to avoid leaving fingerprints. To avoid contamination, do not excessively handle the evidence after recovery. Label and seal all evidence packages at the crime scene. Obtain known standards (e.g., fiber samples from a known carpet). Make a complete evaluation of the crime scene.

10. Record and collect physical evidence: Photograph all items before collection, and document on the photographic log. Mark evidence locations on the sketch, and complete the evidence log with notations for each item of evidence. As previously set forth, have one person serve as evidence custodian. Two persons should observe the evidence in place during recovery and mark evidence for identification. Mark directly on the evidence when feasible; otherwise, place identifying marks on packaging. Constantly check paperwork, packaging, and other information for errors.

11. Final survey: The final survey is a review of all aspects of the search. Discuss the search with all personnel and ensure that all documentation is correct and complete. Photograph the scene showing the final condition. Ensure that all evidence is secured and that all equipment is retrieved. Ensure that hiding places or difficult access areas have not been overlooked.

12. Release: Release the crime scene after the final survey. Documentation for the release of the crime scene should include the time and date of release, to whom released, and by whom released. Ensure that the evidence is collected according to legal requirements, documented and marked for identification. If a search warrant was used, leave a copy of the warrant and receipt. Consider the need for specialists (e.g., a blood pattern analyst or medical examiner) to observe the scene before it is released. Once the scene is released, reentry may require a warrant, so the scene should be released only when all personnel are satisfied that the scene was searched correctly and completely. Only the person in charge should release the scene.

The following case histories are typical of situations to which FBI ERTs as well as other law enforcement agencies respond on a daily basis across the world. They serve here to present the applications of the above protocols and responsibilities toward efficiently and accurately putting together the often mixed and confusing pieces of crime scene puzzles.

Recovery of a Multiple Victim Burial

Recent American history mercifully lacks a chapter involving mass genocide or the clandestine, mass internment of homicide victims. Obviously, the histories of Western Europe (Abarinov 1993), the Balkans (Bax 1997; Calabrese 1994; Cigar 1995; Djuric 2004; Komar 2003; Primorac et al. 1996; Skinner et al. 2003), Southeast Asia (Dodd 2000), Central and South America (Binford 1996; Danner 1993; Doretti and Snow 2002; La Fundación de Antropologia Forense de Guatemala 2000; Manuel and Stover 1991; McCleskey 1983), as well as Africa (Connor 1996a, b; Haglund 1997; PHR 1996; Snow 1994) and the Middle East (Briscoe and Snow 1993; PHR 1992; Scott and Connor 1997; Stover et al. 2003) do not share this attribute. The above-mentioned works have documented the recovery and forensic examination of victims from the mass graves of the Holocaust to the horrors of 1994 Rwanda, and more recent atrocities uncovered in Iraq.

The closest we come in the contemporary United States to mass graves are investigations of homicides in which two or more victims were killed and interred contemporaneously. In ongoing research first presented in 1999, one of the authors has reviewed 920 homicide cases in which victims' remains have been reported as buried (Hochrein et al. 1999). Of those 920 cases dating from 1951 to 1997, 143 (15%) were reported as involving the burial of two or more persons. Of those 143 cases, 55 (6% of the total cases reviewed and 38% of those involving multiple homicides) described the burial of multiple victims in common graves. Examples include the triple homicide committed by Christopher Hightower in 1991. The common grave of two of his victims was found near Barrington, Rhode Island, two months after their murders. Tony Carruthers used a recently dug grave shaft in a Memphis, Tennessee cemetery to conceal the bodies of three of his victims beneath a legitimate burial in 1994. In 1990, cult leader Jeffrey Lundgren directed the murders and mass burial of five of his followers on a Kirkland, Ohio, farm. And serial killers Dean Corll and Elmar Henley buried 17 of their 26 victims beneath a Galveston, Texas, boat shed during the early 1970s.

Among the multiple victim interments excavated by one of the authors was that of four victims associated with the subject of an illegal drug investigation. The forensic recovery of remains in that case demonstrates how proper forensic archaeological techniques, applied in the scheme of the overall ERT protocols outlined above, can lessen complications during their forensic physical anthropological analyses and create a more meaningful product for courtroom presentation. In that case a drug dealer learned that one of his partners had provided information to law enforcement investigators and would testify against him in an upcoming trial. With the assistance of a girlfriend, the drug dealer drove the partner, his girlfriend, and her two children to a rural wooded setting and shot them. The girlfriend and her 6- and

10-year-old daughters were innocent victims. The dealer's partner came to live with them a week before their murders. All of the bodies were then buried in a common grave. Seven years later the events of that night were described for investigators by a jailhouse informant who had heard them from the dealer's girlfriend. Using hand-drawn sketches and the verbal description given to the informant, investigators were able to locate two graves containing a total of five victims. One was a single grave located near the edge of a Midwest cornfield containing the body of a second partner. The other, holding the remains of the four victims described above, was found in a wooded flood plain along a country road. The searches of both scenes were coordinated with local, State, and Federal case investigators while following the ERT protocols.

Evidence Response Teams from the FBI's Omaha and St. Louis Divisions were requested to assist in the location and excavation of the graves. Initially unable to find that of the second partner, buried alone, the team concentrated its efforts on the grave, which would eventually be found to contain the remains of two adults and two children identified as the first partner, his girlfriend, and her 6- and 10-year-old daughters. The FBI ERT protocol used in this and other forensic archaeological excavations entailed the use of minimally intrusive techniques to first confirm the presence of buried evidence. This was followed by the systematic excavation, documentation, and removal of biological, cultural, and geotaphonomic evidence from the grave. Throughout that process team members trained in specific techniques were assigned duties of photography, excavation, mapping, inventory/packaging, etc. Overseeing the safety and needs of the team members and assisting personnel was the team leader. Among the team leader's responsibilities were ensuring site security and arranging work shifts, water, meals, and accommodations in order that the crime scene could be processed over two days without interruption. The team that addressed this site consisted of members from two different FBI Divisions and a supervisor for the Evidence Response Team Unit. The ERT Unit also provided geophysical prospecting equipment and operators. The excavation was directed by a team member who had postgraduate training and professional experience as an archaeologist before joining the FBI. Two assistant excavators and two photographers documented the scene in diagrams and photographs. Three additional team members and three non-ERT investigators shared responsibilities of screening, evidence packaging and logging, supply requests, etc.

Following the confirmation of a buried anomaly using ground-penetrating radar and soil core sampling, a small pit or "window" was excavated in the approximate center of the grave to determine the depth and nature of the buried evidence. This preliminary, or exploratory, excavation also demonstrated one problem commonly encountered with commingled skeletal elements whether buried or deposited on the surface: mixed nonhuman and human bones (Outram et al. 2005). The excavation window not only confirmed the presence of human remains but also those lying in direct association that were clearly of nonhuman origin. They would later be identified as those of a short-tailed shrew (*Blarina brevicauda*) and opossum (*Didelphis virginiana*) (Fig. 3.1).

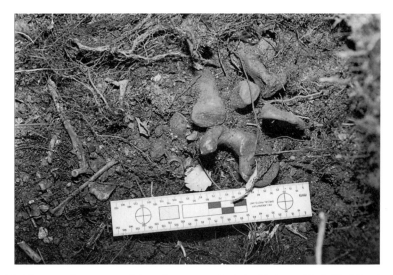

Fig. 3.1 Close-up of opossum and shrew bones commingled with those of Individual 1 at the base of the test excavation window (photo by Lavone Tienken)

A nonforensic, nonarchaeological, less systematic excavation of the grave may have resulted in the collection of both the human and nonhuman bones, which could be separated later. What would have been lost, however, would have been the contextual explanation for how the opossum and shrew came to be buried with the human victims. In this case, the excavation and three-dimensional mapping revealed, and allowed documentation of, an in-filled burrow, or krotovina, which extended from above the torso of Individual number 1 (later identified as the first partner mentioned above), toward and through the northeast corner of the grave. It was above Individual 1's chest that the opossum and shrew bones were excavated in what was identified as a chamber in the in-filled krotovina (Fig. 3.2). With the geotaphonomic and archaeological information preserved, it was possible to reconstruct how an abandoned burrow was used by a wintering opossum, which then died. Without the use of strict archaeological protocols, the commingled bones could have easily been misinterpreted as an intentional placement of road kill over the bodies to further conceal them from humans or animals curious about the disturbed ground.

Once a clandestine human burial was confirmed through the excavation window, a grid system for three-dimensional mapping and photographic purposes was established over the grave. Using the grid units, initially, as arbitrary boundaries, the excavation window was expanded across the grave at 5- to 10-centimeter (1.97- to 3.94-inch) arbitrary levels until the outline of the feature was visible. This was the point at which a system of krotovinas, which explained the commingled nonhuman and human remains, was first realized and recorded.

The second hazard of commingled remains in this case involved the excavation and collection of the victims' remains. Although each of the victims was clothed at the time of burial, the years that had lapsed until their recovery allowed time for

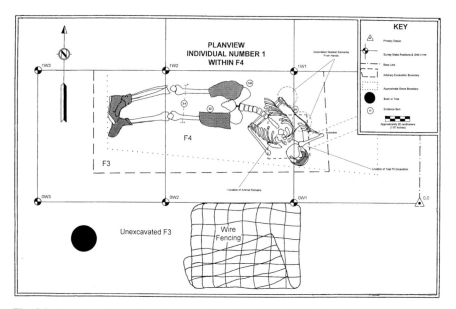

Fig. 3.2 Planview of Individual No. 1 showing the position of the krotovina in relationship to human remains and the excavation test window

the natural fibers of shirts and pants to disintegrate. With the exception of Individual 4 (later identified as the 6-year-old daughter), buried at the bottom of the pit with her head covered by a shirt, there was very little soft tissue present. Without any soil thrown into the pit between each victim, the skeletal elements from one were in direct contact with those beneath or above. An unfortunate fact of forensic archaeology, unlike the archaeology of funded academic research projects, is that they more often than not fall under relatively severe time and budgetary constraints. In spite of their relationship to cases of life and death, pressures are placed on the crime scene investigators to collect evidence as quickly as possible. Combined with limited manpower and supplies, this often calls for developing "shortcuts" to increase efficiency during the excavation. The author made the decision in this case to collect the small skeletal elements comprising victims' hands and feet en masse rather than the detailed and time-consuming excavation and mapping of individual carpal and phalangeal bones. Once uncovered, the area of each hand or foot was minimally revealed, and then the matrix or block of soil containing exposed bones and fingernails was removed, screened separately through ¹/₄-inch hardware cloth and, at times, the smaller-gauge mesh of geology sieves. The items recovered from the screen were then packaged separately as coming from respective victims. Using this technique, some of the elements from different individuals' hands became mixed because of their close proximity to another's. That tradeoff of lessened time in the field versus extra time spent by the forensic physical anthropologist in the morgue or laboratory is often associated with situations of commingled remains.

For the crime scene reconstructionist and criminal investigator, the exact position of each victim's hands and fingers may be a critical piece of the investigative puzzle they are tasked with putting together. The position and orientation of such elements to weapons or terminal ballistic evidence obviously impact scene interpretations and therefore legal strategies. The intentional positioning, or staging, of bodies has been documented as a signature used by killers and could include the victim's hands. The position of the hands in relation to other areas of the body such as the head or face could be interpreted as defensive posture. In hindsight, the position of the victims' hands in the presented case could have impacted what the jury imagined may have taken place at the time of death and burial. Valid or not, the image of a mother's hand touching or holding those of her child in the same grave could have tremendous impact among some jury members. The mapping of each phalange or carpal bone may not be necessary in the documentation of every clandestine burial but should not be ruled out as nonprobative. That determination can only be made when the case detectives or agents consider all of the physical, testimonial, and circumstantial evidence they have available. The forensic archaeologist or crime scene technician is not in a position to make that decision and should always try to collect the maximum amount of information without assumptions.

In the instant case, the practice of using outside specialists was demonstrated through consultations with a forensic mammalogist from the Department of the Interior, Fish and Wildlife Service and botanists from the Missouri Botanical Gardens and the University of Missouri. It continued with the medical examiner's employ of a qualified and experienced forensic physical anthropologist and odontologist. As assistance to those specialists, and especially the forensic anthropologist, the human remains were transferred from the grave, following photography and mapping, to steriles white fabric sheets in the same position they were revealed through excavation. All clothing, ligatures, gags, etc. were maintained as found over or among the skeletal elements of respective individuals. If possible, arm, leg, and other anatomical positioning was preserved as the remains were placed on the sterile sheet. Associated remains such as the bones of the hands or feet, which were excavated and screened en bloc, were packaged separately and then wrapped with the individual with whom they were associated. Once wrapped in the fabric sheet, an additional plastic sheet was used to package and label each victim's remains. (Note: Packaging of biological evidence in plastic is generally not recommended unless, as in this situation, the evidence was immediately transported to a laboratory setting and examined soon after.)

The expert examinations of the remains were accomplished by a forensic anthropologist, forensic odontologist, and DNA specialist as coordinated by the direction of the Medical Examiner's Office. Their analyses confirmed the identities of the victims as the drug dealer's partners, his girlfriend, and her two daughters. The demographic differences between the victims assisted not only in their identifications but also in the separation of skeletal elements commingled during burial and excavation. In spite of commingling of some of the smaller skeletal elements, the careful, systematic excavation and packaging preserved trace evidence and ballistic evidence

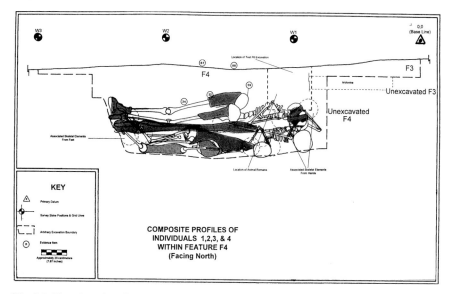

Fig. 3.3 Elevation view diagram demonstrating the proximity of each victim to the other with the location of hand bones circled

associated with respective victims. Again, if the excavation had simply entailed uncovering the remains and pulling them out of the ground without a detailed record of their positions, the relationship of ballistic and other critical evidence may have been lost or confused between individuals. The forensic anthropologist in this case was provided contextual information through notes, three-dimensional diagrams, and photographs. These were then available to be used in concert with the remains themselves toward taphonomic interpretation of perimortem and post-mortem trauma as well as antemortem pathologies. The forensic anthropologist determined that each victim was shot in the head, with the adults suffering additional traumas.

Clearly, the implementation of basic ERT protocols enhanced the ability of each expert involved in this case. The crime scene reconstruction was ultimately found to be consistent with testimony and other evidence used in the trials of each sus-pect. The presentation of crime scene diagrams alongside crime scene photographs allowed the jury to revisit the scene and clearly understand what each medium alone could not completely demonstrate. Both suspects in this case were found guilty.

Recovery of Multiple Victims from an Airplane Crash

The United States is obviously no stranger to mass disasters both accidental and criminal. The smallest of these scenes may involve only a few individuals but can entail hundreds or thousands of pieces dispersed over several acres, or concentrated within the more confined area of a deep-impact crater. An example of the first type of scene resulted from the October 16, 2000, crash of a small aircraft carrying Missouri Governor Melvin Carnahan, his son Roger Carnahan, and the governor's campaign aide, Christopher Sifford (Fig. 3.4).

During the evening of October 16, 2000, weather conditions combined with equipment problems and pilot error to caused the governor's Cessna 335 to barrel into a heavily wooded hillside near Goldman, Missouri. A small impact crater [1.5 meters (5 feet) wide, 3.0 meters (10 feet long), and 1.2 meters (4 feet) deep] and a stand of sheered trees evidenced the point of impact for the fixed-wing aircraft. Approximately 30.5 meters (100 feet) away from the crater, in the apparent direction of travel, were the twisted and abbreviated remnants of the cockpit and fuselage, which came to rest against a group of trees (Fig. 3.5). With the exception of the horizontal stabilizers and the aft upper fuselage skin, the airframe structure separated into small ($6 \times 6 \times 12$ inch) and medium-sized ($12 \times 12 \times 24$ inch) pieces of debris (NTSB 2002). The distance from the farthest piece of wreckage, a right engine crankshaft, was 274.3 meters (900 feet). A small amount of debris landed as far as 30.5 meters (100 feet) behind the impact crater. The maximum width of the debris field was 76.2 meters (250 feet).

An often ignored, or less often considered, dimension of the terrestrial mass disaster site is that of elevation. At the Carnahan crash site, the problems associated with debris and remains landing in the tree canopy were compounded by the area's steep terrain. Another three-dimensional aspect on any wooded crash site is recording evidence that will help to reconstruct flight dynamics before and after impact. Specifically, the height of damaged and undamaged trees, combined with

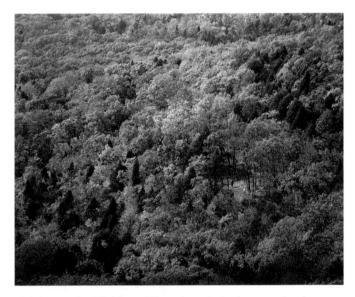

Fig. 3.4 Aerial photograph of Goldman, Missouri, crash site demonstrating the remote and rough terrain (photo by Richard G. Marty Jr.)

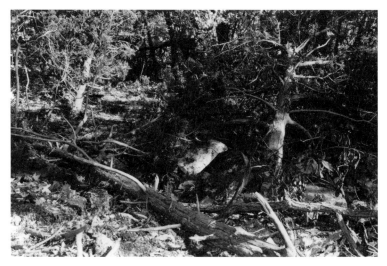

Fig. 3.5 Photograph of the extremely fragmented remains of the cockpit/fuselage (photo by Richard G. Marty Jr.)

the orientation (right and left) of aircraft parts on the ground, helps to determine the attitude at which the aircraft entered the canopy and impacted as well as whether it was right side up or upside down. With information collected by the Missouri State Highway Patrol, as well as the St. Louis and Springfield Division Evidence Response Teams, the National Transportation Safety Board Investigators were able to create a three-dimensional model of the airplane flight path through the trees.

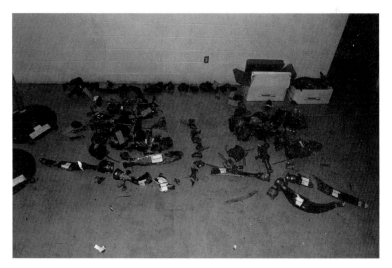

Fig. 3.6 Recovered airplane components laid out for reconstruction and again, demonstrating severe fragmentation (photo by Richard G. Marty Jr.)

They determined the airplane was in a 16° to 18°, right-wing-down attitude during its entry into the trees. Although no computerized video reconstruction of the crash is included in the NTSB's Aircraft Accident Brief for this crash, at least one figure depicts a side view of the broken tree tops left in the aftermath of the crash (NTSB 2002).

The volume of evidence mentioned above as well as that of crash victims, including crew and passenger positions and their proximity to localized aircraft damage (i.e., holes in the fuselage or blast-related evidence), can become overwhelming in any setting, let alone those complicated by rough terrain and thick woods. Without sophisticated mapping technology such as the electronic total station, the collection of spatial data that may reflect patterns in the distribution of otherwise commingled evidence would be difficult and incomplete. Two weeks prior to the crash of Governor Carnahan's airplane, the FBI's St. Louis Division ERT sponsored a medicolegal field school in the recovery of human remains. One of two final practical exercises in that school involved the search, mapping, and recovery of evidence from the simulated crash of a small fixed-wing aircraft using search and recovery protocols described in Dirkmaat et al. (2001). Attendees from across the United States, and especially from the State of Missouri, utilized a combination of mapping techniques from the simplest to the most sophisticated. They recorded the positions of 400 simulated human remains, plane parts, and topography across a debris field encompassing 4,905 square meters (52,800 square feet). The Terrestrial Mass Fatality Scene Protocol introduced in that training includes four steps: (1) search and location effort; (2) total station data collection and assignment of field specimen numbers; (3) photographic documentation; and (4) physical evidence collection and preservation (Dirkmaat et al. 2001). Some of the attendees of that school found themselves as first responders at the scene of their governor's death. Their experience and training in the above-mentioned protocols, in collaboration with the FBI ERT members' familiarity with ERT protocols, as well as the Highway Patrol's expertise in total station mapping caused the joint agency team of responders to realize the efficiency and accuracy of using such methods and technology. As a result, the Terrestrial Mass Fatality Scene Protocol was easily applied in the scheme of the general FBI ERT methods outlined above.

First applied in a commercial air disaster at the crash site of United Flight 427 near Pittsburgh, Pennsylvania, in September 1994 (Dirkmaat et al. 1995), electronic total stations, or laser measuring devices, are now required by the NTSB in the documentation of mass transportation disasters. The Missouri Highway Patrol combined the FBI ERT training they received little more than a week before and their expertise in using multiple total stations for highway accident reconstructions to maximize the information they could get from the Goldman, Missouri, crash site. Shortly after meeting with various investigative teams, two total stations were brought to the crash site. One was devoted to recording the position of human remains marked by search teams, while the second was devoted to mapping the location of diagnostic airplane parts identified by FAA and corporate engineers. The remaining, nondiagnostic airplane debris would be collected using a reference system of 30 sectors established across the scene.

The dedication of two total stations was well conceived and seamlessly applied in the method mentioned above. However, the use of the technology would later reveal another complication that may arise in documenting different categories of commingled evidence. The numbering system used by the total station operators was not mutually exclusive. This meant that a piece of human remains numbered, for example, "1505" corresponded to that shot recorded by one total station, while a piece of aircraft might also be assigned "1505" using the second total station dedicated to aircraft components and other nonhuman remains evidence. A problem occurred in merging the information obtained by the two machines because there was not a mutually exclusive numbering system. This was corrected by the FBI's Investigative and Prosecutive Graphics Unit when each total station's raw data were sent in from the field. However, respective, exclusive numbering systems applied to each type of crash evidence in the field could have saved time devoted toward interpreting the data.

As shown in the first case history, problems are encountered in most scenes of commingled evidence. The formulation, application, and maintenance of appropriate recovery methodologies will lesson the impact of those problems or allow for their correction. The contextual recovery of evidence at the Goldman, Missouri, crash site served as the basis for the NTSB's reconstruction and conclusions regarding this accident (NTSB 2002). The data collected were not only accurate but

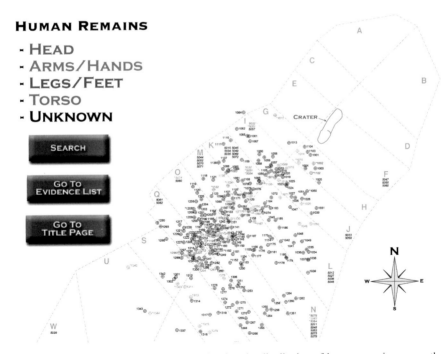

Fig. 3.7 Interactive total station diagram showing the distribution of human remains across the crash site (diagram created by Paula Ernst)

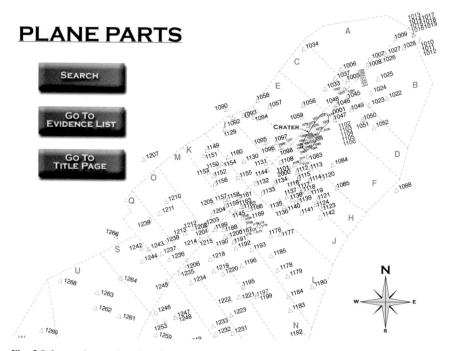

Fig. 3.8 Interactive total station diagram showing the distribution of diagnostic aircraft components across the crash site (diagram created by Paula Ernst)

allowed the FBI's Investigative and Prosecutive Graphics Unit, for the first time in a mass disaster scene, to create an interactive computerized crime scene diagram. Investigators interested in the description of a particular piece of human remains or an aircraft part could simply position the arrow on the computer screen over the item number on a two-dimensional plan view and receive a written description. When the same number or position was double-clicked, a digital image of the fragment would appear. Maps of human remains could be separated from nonhuman evidence and were coded by body part (Figs. 3.7 and 3.8). The impact on future air disaster investigations includes an ability to study potential patterns created by the distribution of human remains and debris in light of recorded and witnessed crash events.

Conclusions

The two cases presented above, as examples of the application of formal protocols by FBI ERTs, demonstrate complications that may arise in dealing with commingled evidence including human remains. More so, however, they demonstrate the value and efficiency of such planned, structured methodologies toward compiling accurate reconstructions of seemingly chaotic collections of evidence. Gone should be the days when medical examiners and the experts they employ are presented with bags of bones simply picked up from a scene. Where investigators once relied on such experts to help solve crimes solely from clues found on the bodies, we can now collect as much, if not more, from subtle clues contained in the recorded contexts of those remains. In cases such as the clandestine mass grave described above, three-dimensional data can offer, among other information, information concerned with (1) the sequence in which victims were deposited, (2) whether or not the victims were shot before deposition or after they were placed in the grave, (3) postburial disturbances such as attempts to relocate or further conceal bodies, and (4) the relocation or absence of evidence due to bioturbation. Similarly, the mass collection of evidence from general areas throughout a crash scene is no longer acceptable in the light of developed protocols and applications of laser technologies, as seen in the aforementioned air crash investigation. The three-dimensional processing of individual items commingled through a crash site may offer insight into (1) flight and impact dynamics, (2) peri- or postimpact explosions versus in flight explosions, (3) passenger and crew positions, and (4) postimpact disturbances via human or nonhuman scavenging. The patterns left in the aftermath of natural and manmade disasters, or criminal conduct, are as unique as the factors that caused them. Only by collecting evidence in a manner that allows us to analyze all of the evidence offered in a scene in context can we begin to accumulate data sets that are comparable between crime scenes or mass disaster scenes. The ability to compare evidence patterns between more and more scenes will lead to an ability to more accurately create interpretive models toward solving crimes and perhaps predictive models for preventing future events.

Acknowledgments The authors would like to thank each and every FBI ERT for their efforts and dedication. Special thanks are offered to members of the Omaha, St. Louis, and Springfield teams. Their efforts contributed to the successful resolution of the cases presented herein. Likewise, the expertise of those who work within the FBI's Investigative and Prosecutive Graphics Unit has helped to continuously advance FBI ERTs in data collection and interpretation.

References Cited

Abarinov, V. 1993 *The Murderers of Katyn*. Hippocrene Books, New York.

Anker, R. and F. Taylor 1989 The Trajectories of Falling Parts Following In-Flight Breakup. Paper presented at the 20th International Society of Air Safety Investigators Forum International Seminar.

Barrie, H. J. and N. Hodson-Walker 1970 Incidence and pathogenesis of fractures of the lumbar transverse processes in air crashes. *Aerosp. Med.* 41(7):805–808.

Bax, M. 1997 Mass graves, stagnating identification and violence: A case study in the local sources of "the war" in Bosnia Herzegovina. *Anthropol. Q.* 70(1):11–19.

Bergen-Henengouwan, S. G. 1973 *Aircraft Wreckage Trajectory Analysis User Manual*. Aeronautical and Mechanical Engineering Department, Southern Alberta Institute of Technology, Calgary, Alberta, Canada.

Binford, L. 1996 *The El Mozote Massacre: Anthropology and Human Rights*. The University of Arizona Press, Tucson.

Briscoe, J. and C. C. Snow 1993 Archaeological report on Koreme, Birjinni and Jeznikam-Beharke cemetery. In *The Anfal Campaign in Iraqi Kurdistan: The Destruction of Koreme.* Human Rights Watch, Washington, DC.

Brooks, P. 1985 Crime scene and profile characteristics of organized and disorganized murderers. *FBI Law Enforcement Bull.* (August).

Burgess, A. W. and R. K. Ressler 1985 *Sexual Homicide Crime Scenes and Patterns of Criminal Behavior: Final Report.* Boston City Health and Hospitals Department, Boston.

Calabrese, C. 1994 Report from the Balkans: Investigating mass graves for the U.N. *Fed. Archaeol.* 7(2):9.

Cigar, N. 1995 *Genocide in Bosnia: The Policy of Ethnic Cleansing.* Texas A&M Press, College Station, TX.

Connor, M. A. 1996a Archaeologists and the United Nation tribunals. *CRM* 19(10):32.

Connor, M. A. 1996b The archaeology of contemporary mass graves. *Soc. Am. Archaeol. Bull.* 14(4):6–31.

Danner, M. 1993 *The Massacre at El Mazote.* Vintage Books, New York.

Dirkmaat, D. C., J. T. Hefner, and M. J. Hochrein 2001 Forensic Processing of the Terrestrial Mass Fatality Scene: Testing New Search, Documentation, and Recovery Methodologies. Paper presented at the 53rd Annual Meeting of the American Academy of Forensic Science, Seattle, WA.

Dirkmaat, D. C., A. Quinn, and J. M. Adovasio 1995 New methodologies for search and recovery. *Disaster Management News* (December):1–2.

Djuric, M. P. 2004 Anthropological data in individualization of skeletal remains from a forensic context in Kosovo—A case history. *J. Forensic Sci.* 49(3):464–468.

Dodd, M. 2000 A report from the killing fields—The East Timor experience. *InForMed* 5(3):21–26.

Doretti, M. and C. C. Snow 2002 Forensic anthropology and human rights: The Argentine experience. In *Hard Evidence: Case Studies in Forensic Anthropology*, D. W. Steadman, ed., pp. 90–310. Prentice Hall, Upper Saddle River, NJ.

Douglas, J. E. and C. Munn 1992a Violent crime scene analysis. *Homic. Invest. J.* (63):69.

Douglas, J. E. and C. Munn 1992b Violent crime scene analysis: Modus operandi, signature and staging. *FBI Law Enforcement Bull.* (61):2.

Douglas, J. E., R. K. Ressler, A. W. Burgess. and C. R. Hartman 1986 Criminal profiling from crime scene analysis. *Behav. Sci. Law* 4(4):401–421.

Gable, W. D. 1968 Pathology patterns in aircraft accident investigation. *Aerosp. Med.* 39(6): 638–640.

Haglund, W. D. 1997 *Report of the Exhumation and Examination of Remains from the Kibuye.* Physicians for Human Rights, Boston.

Hellerich, U. and S. Pollak 1995 Airplane crash. Traumatologic findings in cases of extreme body disintegration. *Am. J. Forensic Med. Pathol.* 16(4):320–324.

Hill, I. R. 1989 Mechanism of injury in aircraft accidents: A theoretical approach. *Aviation, Space, and Envir. Med.* 60(7):A18–25.

Hochrein, M. J. 1997 Buried crime scene evidence: The application of forensic geotaphonomy in forensic archaeology. In *Forensic Dentistry*, P. G. Stimson and C. A. Mertz, eds., pp. 83–99. CRC Press, Boca Raton, FL.

Hochrein, M. J. 2002 An autopsy of the grave: Recognizing, collecting, and preserving forensic geotaphonomic evidence. In *Advances in Forensic Taphonomy: Method, Theory, and Archaeological Perspectives*, W. D. Haglund and M. H. Sorg, eds., pp. 45–70. CRC Press, Boca Raton, FL.

Hochrein, M. J., J. Gabra, and S. P. Nawrocki 1999 The Buried Body Cases Content Analyses Project: Patterns in Buried Body Investigations. Paper presented at the American Academy of Forensic Science, Orlando, FL.

Keppel, R. D. 2005 Serial offenders: Linking cases by modus operandi and signature. In *Forensic Science: An Introduction to Scientific and Investigative Techniques*, 2nd ed., S. H. James and J. J. Norby, eds., pp. 605–614. CRC Press/Taylor and Francis Group, Boca Raton, FL.

Komar, D. 2003 Lessons from Srebrenica: The contributions and limitations of physical anthropology in identifying victims of war crimes. *J. Forensic Sci.* 48(4):713–716.

Kreft, S. 1970 Who was at the aircraft's controls when the fatal accident occurred? In *Aerospace Pathology*, p. 96. College of American Pathologists Foundation, Chicago.

La Fundación de Antropologia Forense de Guatemala 2000 *Informe de las Invetigaciones Antropológico Forenses e Históricas.* Report of Investigations, 1997–1998. Editorial Serviprensa, Guatemala City.

Lundrigan, S. and D. Canter 2001 Spatial patterns of serial murder: An analysis of disposal site location choice. *Behav. Sci. Law* 19(4):595–610.

Manuel, A. and E. Stover 1991 *Guatemala: Getting Away with Murder.* America's Watch and Physicians for Human Rights, Washington, DC.

Matteson, F. H. 1974 Analysis of wreckage patterns from in-flight disintegrations. *J. Safety Res.* (6):60–71.

McCleskey, K. 1983 Medical mission to El Salvador investigates cases of "disappeared." *Science* (219):1209–1210.

Min, J. X. and M. Z. Jia 1992 Correlation of trauma and cause of death to accident reconstruction: A case of a flight accident report. *J. Forensic Sci.* 37(2):585–589.

NTSB 2002 *Aircraft Accident Brief: Accident Number CHI01MA011, Cessna 335, N8354N, Hillsboro, Missouri, October 16, 2000.* http://www.ntsb.gov/publictn/2002/AAB0202.pdf.

Outram, A. K., C. J. Knüsel, S. Knight, and A. F. Harding 2005 Understanding complex fragmented assemblages of human and animal remains: A fully integrated approach. *J. Archaeol. Sci.* 32(12):1699–1710.

Outram, A. K., C. J. Knüsel, S. Knight, and A. F. Harding PHR 1992 *Unquiet Graves: The Search for the Disappeared in Iraqi, Kurdistan.* Physicians for Human Rights and Middle East Watch,.

1996 *PHR Investigates Mass Graves in Rwanda.* Physicians for Human Rights, .

Primorac, D., S. Andelinovic, M. Definis-Gojanovic, I. Drmic, B. Rezic, M. M. Baden, M. A. Kennedy, M. S. Schanfield, S. B. Skakel, and H. C. Lee 1996 Identification of war victims from mass graves in Croatia, Bosnia, and Herzegovina by use of standard forensic methods and DNA typing. *J. Forensic Sci.* 41(5):891–894.

Rajs, J., M. Lundstrom, M. Broberg, L. Lidberg, and O. Lindquist 1998 Criminal mutilation of the human body in Sweden—A thirty-year medico-legal and forensic psychiatric study. *J. Forensic Sci.* 43(3):563–580.

Ressler, R. K., A. W. Burgess, R. L. DePue, J. E. Douglas, R. R. Hazelwood, K. V. Lanning, and C. Lent 1985 Crime scene and profile characteristics of organized and disorganized murderers. *FBI Law Enforcement Bull,* (54):18–25.

Rossi, D. 1982 Crime scene behavioral analysis: Another tool for the law enforcement investigator. *The Police Chief* (January):152–155.

Scott, D. D. and M. Connor 1997 The Koreme execution site: A modern crime scene investigation using archaeological techniques. In *Forensic Taphonomy: The Postmortem Fate of Human Remains*, W. D. Haglund and M. H. Sorg, eds. CRC Press, Boca Raton, FL.

Skinner, M., D. Alempijevic, and M. Djuric-Srejic 2003 Guidelines for international forensic bio-archaeology monitors of mass grave exhumations. *Forensic Sci. Int.* 134(2–3):81–92.

Snow, C. C. 1994 *Observations on Human Skeletal Remains Excavated from Grave 1 Kotebe, Ethiopia.* Special Prosecutor's Office.

Steele, R. M. G. 1983 Trajectory plots of aircraft debris following in-flight break-up. Unpublished Master's of Science Thesis, Cranfield Institute of Technology, England.

Stover, E., W. D. Haglund, and M. Samuels 2003 Exhumation of mass graves in Iraq: Considerations for forensic investigations, humanitarian needs, and the demands of justice. *JAMA* 290(5):663–666.

Swegennis, R. W. 1987 Impact angles and velocities. In *Safety Investigation: Investigative Techniques*, B. Carver, ed., pp. 1–16. Department of the Air Force, Washington, DC.

Chapter 4
Commingled Remains and Human Rights Investigations

Sofía Egaña, Silvana Turner, Mercedes Doretti, Patricia Bernardi,
and Anahí Ginarte

Introduction

The investigation of human rights violations presents a number of difficulties that usually result from limited access to different types of data. The complexity of a case is increased when the evidence consists of commingled skeletonized remains. In fact, the management of large concentrations of such remains for their reassociation, identification, and return to the victims' families, as well as the determination of the cause and manner of death, presents a number of stage-specific challenges that deserve revisiting.

EAAF (*Equipo Argentino de Antropología Forense*/Argentine Forensic Anthropology Team) is a nonprofit scientific NGO that applies forensic sciences—mainly forensic anthropology and archaeology—to the investigation of human rights violations in Argentina and worldwide.[1] The team was founded in 1984 in response to the need to investigate the disappearance of at least 10,000 people by the military regime that ruled Argentina between 1976 and 1983 (Fig. 4.1). In close collaboration with victims and their relatives, we seek to shed light on human rights violations, thus contributing to the search for truth, justice, reparation, and the prevention of future violations. EAAF members also serve as expert witnesses and advisors for local and international human rights organizations, national judiciaries, international tribunals, and special commissions of inquiry, such as Truth Commissions. EAAF has worked in over 30 countries throughout the Americas, Asia, Africa, and Europe to identify victims of disappearances and extrajudicial killings; return their remains to their relatives; present evidence of violations and patterns of abuse to relevant judicial and nonjudicial bodies; and train local professionals to continue this work at a local level. EAAF's guiding principle is to maintain the highest respect for the

---

[1] EAAF's experience has expanded significantly during the past 20 years, although the team remains a small group of committed professionals, including most of its founding members and a small support staff. Headquarters are in Buenos Aires, Argentina; a New York satellite office was opened in 1992. The Board of Directors depends mostly on international funds, both public and private, for the financial support of the organization. Additionally, EAAF receives funding from the UN for participation in field missions.

From: *Recovery, Analysis, and Identification of Commingled Human Remains*
Edited by: B. Adams and J. Byrd © Humana Press, Totowa, NJ

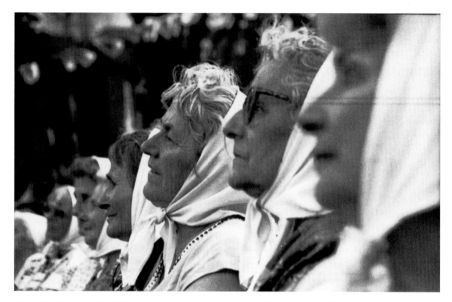

Fig. 4.1 Since April 1977, the mothers of many of the kidnapped and disappeared have been gathering at Plaza de Mayo in Buenos Aires to demand information on the whereabouts of their loved ones (photo by Viviana D'Amelia)

perspective and concerns of victims' relatives and communities and to work closely with them through all stages of the investigation process.

This chapter will present three examples from investigations that EAAF has conducted in El Salvador, Zimbabwe, and Argentina. Our goal is to contribute our experience to a discussion of the best forensic anthropological practices for the treatment of these particularly complex cases. We will further offer some considerations relative to recovery procedures, osteological analysis, and the use of background information as well as the limitations of these methods when working with commingled remains.

Skeletonized Remains and Standards of Practice

There exist at present a handful of international recommendations establishing basic procedures for investigations involving corpses at different stages of decay, particularly in the context of mass disasters and human rights violations. Most important among these are the "United Nations' Manual on the effective prevention and investigation of extra-legal, arbitrary and summary executions," Interpol's Disaster Victim Identification (DVI) autopsy protocol, and relevant sections of the International Committee of the Red Cross's (ICRC) document "The Missing—The Right to Know." These protocols, among others, testify to the growing acknowledgment of forensic anthropologists as necessary experts in the field and stress the need for basic acceptable standards of practice. However, none of them touches upon the particular difficulties involving the recovery and analysis of commingled remains.

The challenge for the forensic investigator is greater when cases involve the large-scale analysis of bones that are difficult to associate with a given individual. The specifics of such an investigation are not addressed by the general protocols. These cases pose a number of practical questions to be addressed by all those experts involved in the investigation, e.g., how to proceed when DNA testing is not operationally feasible, or how to manage bones that cannot be assigned to any one individual.

Proposed methods for the management of commingled skeletonized remains have their origin mainly in archeology and physical anthropology; in fact, it is only in recent years that protocol proposals have involved the application of these methods to forensic science. Among the scientific tools available are morphological techniques (Adams and Byrd 2006; Kerley 1972); osteometrics (Byrd and Adams 2003); mathematical models; statistical methods (Adams and Konigsberg 2004; Rösing and Pischtschan 1995; Snow and Folk 1965); and X-ray, fluorescence, chemical, and molecular analysis. An overview of these methods and useful summaries of the literature related to these issues can be found in Ubelaker's contribution to this volume (See Chapter 1) and his chapter in Haglund and Sorg's *Advances in Forensic Taphonomy* (2002). Every case under investigation is unique to some extent and will call for one or more of these approaches. However, we consider it possible to add a number of recommendations toward a general systematic management of large-scale commingled remains. We have derived these considerations mainly from our forensic investigation of human rights violations in El Salvador, Zimbabwe, and Argentina.

El Salvador

Historical Background

On January 16, 1992, after 12 years of civil war in which an estimated 75,000 people died, the *Frente Martí de Liberación Nacional* (Farabundi Martí National Liberation Front—FMLN) and the Salvadorian government signed a Peace Agreement mediated by the United Nations. The agreement included the establishment of a UN Truth Commission to investigate gross human rights violations committed by both the armed forces and the guerrillas.

The Truth Commission conducted its investigation during 1992 and published its findings on March 15, 1993 in a report titled "From Madness to Hope." The report included recommendations for removing a number of individuals from their positions of power, providing reparation to victims and their families, creating monuments and holidays to commemorate victims, and implementing various judicial and institutional reforms. The report did not recommend prosecution since, in the Commission's opinion, the judiciary at the time could not guarantee a fair trial.

Instead, it provided extensive recommendations for judicial reform.[2] Five days later, on March 20, 1993, the Legislative Assembly passed a general amnesty provision—Legislative Decree 486—for all those involved in human rights violations.

The amnesty law was interpreted as not only foreclosing the possibility of bringing perpetrators to trial but also halting all investigations into human rights violations. Several petitions challenging the constitutionality of the amnesty law were submitted to the Salvadorian courts, but none succeeded.[3]

To date, no judge has suspended enforcement of the amnesty law for a human rights case. Moreover, most cases relative to the civil war have been abandoned by judges or prosecutors. However, trials have continued before U.S. courts and the Inter-American Commission on Human Rights[4] (Doretti and Carson 2003).

The Massacre at "El Mozote"

Between December 6 and 16, 1981, the Salvadorian armed forces initiated a major offensive, "Operation Rescue," in Morazán, a province in the northeast of El Salvador. The purpose of this operation, led by the elite U.S.-trained Atlacatl counterinsurgency battalion, was to force the guerillas from the area, destroy their clandestine radio station, and eliminate any support for them among the civilian population. After several confrontations in hamlets near El Mozote, the FMLN guerillas left the area on December 9, and the army established a base camp in El Mozote. Over the next few days, government troops conducted daytime attacks on the nearby villages of La Joya, Jocote Amarillo, Ranchería, Los Toriles, and Cerro Pando. In each of them, as part of their scorched-earth policy of overwhelming retaliation against FMLN sympathizers, the Army reportedly murdered residents, burned houses and fields, and slaughtered livestock (United Nations 1993).

Soldiers remained in the area for two weeks. When they went back to their camp in El Mozote every evening, survivors from other villages returned to the massacre sites under the cover of darkness and buried as many of the dead as possible. These victims were buried in common graves close to where their bodies were found. However, many bodies remained unburied for fear of army reprisal and were left

---

[2] "From Madness to Hope," United Nations Truth Commission Report, March 1993, pp. 114–119.

[3] CEJIL 11/16/01. www.cejil.org/comunicados.cfm?id=263.

[4] In 2005, the Organization of American States (OAS) decided to reopen the investigation into Salvadorian government complicity in or approval of the massacre at El Mozote. This decision came in March 2005 when the Center for Justice and International Law (CEJIL) and *Tutela Legal*—the legal office of the Archbishop of San Salvador—presented a petition before the Inter-American Commission on Human Rights (IACHR), an organ of the OAS that sees to the promotion and protection of human rights, with additional forensic information. The case was originally at the OAS, but was shelved by the IACHR in 2000. Initially, the IACHR rejected the petition as a result of arguments presented by the Salvadorian government. CEJIL and *Tutela Legal* responded by sending additional observations and urging the IACHR to admit the report of admissibility in order for proceedings to begin before the Inter-American Court. The IACHR then decided to compile and review the new forensic evidence collected by EAAF and determine whether the Salvadorian government was aware of the massacre and permitted it.

where they had fallen. During this period, the Salvadorian army allegedly killed approximately 800 civilians in 6 neighboring villages. The villages in this region were mostly abandoned until 1989, when survivors began to return. El Mozote itself remained deserted until several years later (Doretti et al. 2005).

On October 26, 1990, survivors represented by *Tutela Legal*[5] opened criminal proceedings at a court in San Francisco Gotera, Morazán, to investigate and prosecute those responsible for the massacre. Also, in 1992, the mandate of the UN Truth Commission—created as part of the Peace Agreement—conferred the capacity to investigate major crimes, including ordering exhumations and conducting a thorough investigation of the massacre at El Mozote, one of several emblematic Salvadorian civil war cases. In 1991 and 1992, at the request of *Tutela Legal* and acting as expert witnesses in the local court case and as technical consultants for the UN Truth Commission, EAAF conducted an initial assessment of the case and proceeded to exhume and analyze evidence from one massacre site. Released in March 1993, the UN Truth Commission report cites evidence from the forensic work at El Mozote and concludes that government forces were responsible for the massacre of several hundred civilians, mostly women and children, who were victims of a planned mass extrajudicial execution. However, because of the passage of the amnesty law that followed the release of the Truth Commission's report, the work on the massacre at El Mozote was halted for 6 years. In 1999, *Tutela Legal* successfully appealed to the Supreme Court for the resumption of exhumations on humanitarian grounds to return the remains to the families of the victims.

To date, EAAF has conducted forensic investigations related to the case—specifically in 1992 and from 1999 to 2004—under the authority of the same court where the process began in 1990. The investigation involved the entire area affected, i.e., the hamlets at El Mozote, Jocote Amarillo, Ranchería, Los Toriles, Cerro Pando, and La Joya.

Some burial sites were initially marked by *Tutela Legal* and EAAF in 1992 according to indications from witnesses and people who had helped to bury the bodies. However, the bodies of many of the people killed in the fields had been left where they fell. Burials also took place three weeks after the incidents, once the army had withdrawn from the area. According to the people who buried these remains, they were eaten and dismembered by animals and were highly skeletonized. Thus, remains were gathered from the surface for burial, with the consequent commingling of body parts of different individuals in the same mass grave. The investigation conducted by *Tutela Legal* and expanded by EAAF revealed that the Salvadorian army allegedly killed an estimated 811 civilians in these 6 neighboring hamlets during the operation. According to interviews with surviving relatives, over 40% of the reported victims were children under the age of 10.[6]

EAAF has worked at a total of 27 burial sites containing abundant ballistic

---

[5] *Tutela Legal*, the legal office of the Archbishop of San Salvador, serves as the legal representative for the victims and their family members.

[6] "From Madness to Hope," United Nations Truth Commission Report, March 1993.

Table 4.1 Burial Sites and Graves Related to the Massacre at "El Mozote" at Which EAAF Worked: Characteristics and Minimum Number of Individuals (MNI)

EAAF Missions	1992	2000	2001	2003	2004
Graves containing articulated remains		La Joya 1, 2B, 4, 5, 16, and 17 Jocote Amarillo 1, 2, 3A, 3B, 3C, 4	Los Toriles 1, 2, 3	Cerro Pando 1A and B	
Graves containing commingled remains			Los Toriles 4	Ranchería 2A, 2B, and 3 Mozote 3 Los Toriles 5	
Interior of houses containing commingled remains	Mozote 1		Mozote 2	Ranchería 1 and 2	Mozote 5 and 6
MNI	**143**	**37**	**29**	**57**	**3**

evidence and personal effects associated with the remains. Of these, 12 were mass graves containing articulated remains, 10 were graves with commingled remains, and 5 were houses containing commingled remains (Table 4.1). Especially when victims were killed inside their houses, their remains were severely damaged when the houses were set on fire by the soldiers and the roofs and adobe walls collapsed over them, resulting in the recovery of extensively fragmented commingled human bones (Fig. 4.2).

EAAF recovered the remains of a minimum of 269 individuals. At least 40 of them were identified as female, 26 as male, and 203 as of undetermined sex, mostly children, from newborns to age 12.

As regards the recovery of nonbiological evidence, with the help of a metal detector, ballistic evidence was found in most of the burial sites and adjacent areas. All ballistic evidence was analyzed by ballistic experts, who classified it as either bullets (whole or fragmented) or cartridge cases. In most cases, we found clothing associated with the remains, and personal effects such as belt buckles, combs, mirrors, barrettes, coins, etc. In the graves containing the skeletons of children, several toys were found. Inside the houses, household items such as plates, boxes, plastic containers, etc. were mixed with the remains and clothing.

The communities in northern Morazán built a monument in El Mozote's new plaza, and most of the recovered remains were reburied there after the forensic examination. In some cases, the tentative identification and circumstantial evidence were sufficient for a judge to issue death certificates for victims. Considering the difficulty of re-individualizing part of the exhumed remains and getting the final

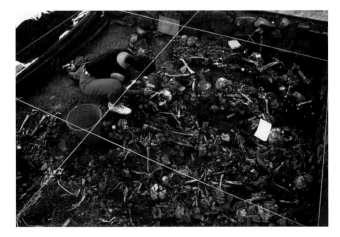

Fig. 4.2 Ruins of a 4.63-meter × 6.94-meter adobe structure adjacent to a church where a minimum of 143 individuals, most of them children, were exhumed. A total of 263 M16-rifle bullet fragments and 245 spent cartridges was found. The majority of the bullets were in direct relation to the concentration of skeletons. (Photo: Mercedes Doretti, EAAF)

positive identifications for each and every victim, the community decided to place the fragmented remains in boxes identified according to the exhumation place, i.e., "human remains recovered at the Arguetas' house." Apart from this, memorial plaques with the names of the victims surround the area of exhumation.

Zimbabwe

Historical Background

Between 1970 and 1987, thousands of Zimbabweans died amidst political violence, first during the war against the white-settler Rhodesian government (1970–1980) and then during a period of internal conflict (1981–1987) following liberation. The suffering inflicted upon black Africans during the colonial period and the war for liberation is well recognized and documented, and the government of Zimbabwe has made major efforts to assist the survivors. In contrast, most of the massive human rights violations that occurred after 1980 were neither investigated nor even officially recognized by the Zimbabwean government. Nationally and internationally their existence remained virtually unknown except to those who suffered them, until 1997 when the Catholic Commission for Justice and Peace (CCJP) and the Legal Resources Foundation in Zimbabwe published a detailed report on human rights abuses in Matabeleland and the Midlands during the 1980s.

The war of independence against the white-settler Rhodesian government (1970–1980) was waged by two separate forces. The larger of these was the Zimbabwean African National Union (ZANU) and its armed wing, the Zimbabwean African National Liberation Army (ZANLA). The other was the Zimbabwean

African People's Union (ZAPU) and its armed wing, the Zimbabwean People's Revolutionary Army (ZIPRA). While the two forces cooperated in the struggle against the white-settler government, there was also considerable animosity between them. ZANU-ZANLA came to be associated with Zimbabwe's Shona-speaking majority and ZAPU-ZIPRA with the Ndebele-speaking minority, although each force included large numbers of members from both ethnic groups. In some cases, the tensions arising from these differences led to clashes between the two armies. By April 1980 the liberation armies had defeated the white-settler government. In the subsequent national elections, ZANU gained a large parliamentary majority in a national vote that fell predominately along ethnic lines. ZANU and ZAPU entered into a coalition government, and efforts were made to combine their armed forces into a single national army.

Relations between the two groups rapidly deteriorated, however, and the political situation in the country became increasingly tense. In 1982, so-called dissidents began staging attacks and robberies in a number of areas in the country. There is no conclusive evidence suggesting that the rebel groups were part of an organized large-scale plot to overthrow the Zimbabwean government. Nor were the rebels numerous; according to the CCJP's report, probably no more than 400 of them were active at any one time. The ZANU-dominated Zimbabwean government, however, responded as though the rebels were mounting a major insurrection. State security forces were directed to take counterinsurgency measures and to repress the Ndebele-speaking civilian population in the Matabeleland and Midlands regions of the country, where the armed dissidents were most active. The government justified the repression of civilians on the grounds that the Ndebele-speaking population supported the rebels, although there was very little substantial evidence to support this claim.

Various dissident groups allegedly committed a number of serious human rights violations, including the rapes and murders of civilians. According to the CCJP's report, however, the human rights violations committed by the state security forces vastly exceeded those committed by the dissidents. Security forces, particularly the notorious Fifth Brigade, reportedly carried out arbitrary executions, forced disappearances, beatings, rapes, and the torture of thousands of civilians. Zimbabwean and international human rights organizations estimate that between 3,000 and 5,000 persons were killed or "disappeared" by state security forces during this period. Zimbabwean human rights organizations have compiled two databases, one with the names of nearly 1,800 victims known to have been killed or "disappeared" during the 1980s conflict and a second, larger database of unidentified victims. They have also identified the sites of a number of mass graves that allegedly contain the remains of victims of human rights violations. The period of massive violence finally ended in 1987 with a general amnesty and the signing of a "unity accord" between ZANU and ZAPU leaders. The Zimbabwean government, however, has never officially recognized the crimes committed by state security forces during this period. One of the most significant consequences of the violence of the 1980s for the surviving residents of Matabeleland and the Midlands was that they could not find their dead to properly mourn and bury them. In some cases this happened because the victims were buried in unofficial mass graves. In other cases the victims were "disappeared," and the survivors never learned their fates, or state security forces killed victims in the presence of their relatives or neighbors and then refused to allow the survivors to bury or even mourn the dead.

In 1999, EAAF conducted the first forensic anthropology work in the region of Matabeleland South on a mission involving both teaching and research. This mission was conducted at the request of the Amani Trust,[7] and one of the five cases we worked on was that in Sitezi (Doretti 1999).

Sitezi

A Fifth Brigade unit was based at Sitezi A1 Rest Camp in the district of North Gwanda during the 1984 curfew and turned the rest camp into a detention center. Amani has had many accounts of torture and murder that took place there during this time. Once the Fifth Brigade moved out, the camp was left derelict and has remained deserted to this day. The only additions that have been made are graffiti on the walls of buildings saying that the Fifth Brigade came and murdered the children of the region. Amani became involved when a person in Mapane revealed that he had climbed alive out of a mass grave in Sitezi. He reported that he and many others had been held and tortured at Sitezi Camp.

The next testimonial in connection with the site came from a woman who said that her father had been murdered and lay in a mass grave in Sitezi. She was disturbed by the fact her father's grave had never been honored and wanted to know if there was any chance of recovering his remains. A Gwanda informant was finally able to locate the site, which was then immediately confirmed by others as the mass grave.

The archaeological exhumation began on August 4, 1999, and members of the victims' families as well as community representatives were present during the two days that the work demanded. The bones were disarticulated, burned, and blackened, and, except for a few phalanges, all of them were fragmented as a result of fire. The extensive damage limited our ability to keep all but the largest bone fragment remains in place. All bone remains were mixed with fragments of charcoal, indicating that logs and firewood had been used to start the fire and to keep it alive. Some of the bones and charcoal had the brightness associated with the use of accelerant. Due to the burning, fragmentation, and mixing of bone remains, it was not possible to individualize them, i.e., to assign bones to a specific skeleton or to a larger body part. However, we conducted a thorough study on them, from which we obtained the following results:

1. All of the recovered bone remains were human.

---

[7] Amani Trust is a Zimbabwean-registered NGO headquartered in Bulayo and established in 1993 for the purpose of providing rehabilitation services to victims of human rights violations, particularly torture, repressive violence, and institutionalized violence. Amani (Swahili for "peace") operates on a nonprofit basis, and its services are free of charge.

2. Most of them were completely burned and blackened (Fig. 4.3).
3. A chemical fuel was used to accelerate the destruction of the corpses.
4. Based on the quantity and estimated ages of proximal epiphyses of right ulnae
   (6) and of proximal epiphyses of left ulnae (6), we determined an MNI of six
   adults of undetermined sex. Due to the extensive fragmentation of the bones, it
   was impossible to proceed to individualization.
5. The condition of the site and remains was consistent with the intentional destruction of evidence.
6. Ballistic evidence (a gun cartridge and a bullet), personal effects, and an identification card were also recovered.

The Sitezi case is one typical scenario of remains found in mass graves where
some major bones are recovered; experts should be able to decide what procedure
to follow in the face of such a situation. Since extreme burning destroys the potential for DNA analysis, the only available techniques for identification are usually
anthropological in nature.

Despite the challenges, even limited anthropological findings have in this case
yielded important benefits to victims' families. The existence of the grave itself was
established, a fundamental element for the historical record as well as for possible
future legal actions. Because it was impossible to individualize the remains of victims at Sitezi, the families agreed to have a common inhumation performed. The
funeral was attended by over 500 people (Doretti 1999).

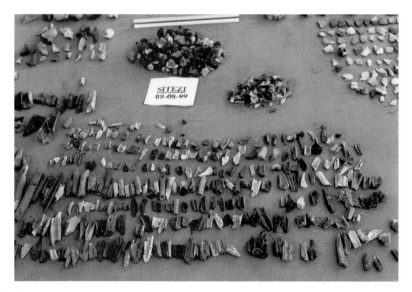

Fig. 4.3 Burned remains at Sitezi during the sorting procedure (photo by Anahí Ginarte, EAAF)

Argentina

Historical Background

During the 1970s, a number of South American countries, particularly Argentina, Bolivia, Brazil, and Chile, were shaken by periods of intense violence and repression. During that decade, severe human rights violations were committed, primarily by military governments (CONADEP 1986).

In the early 1980s, these countries began to move toward reinstating democracy. With the establishment of democracy came the immediate need to investigate the human rights violations of the recent past. In these cases, the role of the judiciary, which had been extremely limited or complicit with the authoritarian regimes, was questioned and in some cases redefined. It became clear that improvements to the administration of justice were crucial to reinforcement of the new democracies. However, while these investigations led to the conviction of guilty parties in some countries, in others various amnesty proclamations allowed those responsible for the crimes to avoid prosecution, even when investigations are ongoing.

Argentina returned to democracy in December 1983. The newly elected president, Dr. Raúl Alfonsín, created the *Comisión Nacional sobre la Desaparición de Personas* (National Commission on the Disappearance of Persons; CONADEP). The commission documented around 10,000 cases of people who had been "disappeared" under the previous military regime (1976–1983), although, according to independent human rights groups, the figure is much higher. The vast majority were abducted, taken to illegal detention centers, tortured, and killed by security forces between 1976 and 1978.

In Argentina, an abductee was typically taken to a clandestine detention center (CDC) where he or she was subjected to interrogation under torture for several weeks or months before being released, held as a legal prisoner, or executed extrajudicially. Some CDCs dumped their victims, bound and sedated, from military aircraft flying over the Argentine Sea; others buried them under the notation NN (for "No Name") in municipal cemeteries. In the latter case, shortly after the killings the bodies were typically deposited in public places, and an "anonymous" call would be made to the local police precinct. The police, sometimes accompanied by local judges, would go to the site and recover the bodies. Prior to anonymous burial in local cemeteries, the bodies were often photographed, fingerprinted, and given a perfunctory examination by a police or judiciary forensic doctor who issued a death certificate, and the registry office would provide a burial certificate. Such thorough official documentation is unusual for bodies that were intended to be buried in anonymous graves. These records have been vital to the identification of victims in EAAF investigations. In 1984, before CONADEP issued its report on the inquiry, judges began to order exhumations in cemeteries known to contain the remains of disappeared persons. The exhumations were attended by relatives of the disappeared desperate to find out what had happened to their loved ones and hoping to recover their remains. However, the process was complicated by a variety of factors.

First, official medical doctors in charge of the work had little experience in the exhumation and analysis of skeletal remains; in their daily professional experience they generally worked only with cadavers. Thus, exhumations were carried out by cemetery workers in a completely unscientific manner (Fig. 4.4). In particular, when bulldozers were used, the bones were broken, lost, commingled, or left inside the graves. As a result, much of the evidence that would have served to identify the remains and support legal cases against those responsible for these crimes was destroyed. In addition, some forensic doctors had been complicit, either by omission or commission, with the crimes of the previous regime. In Argentina, as in most Latin American countries, forensic experts are part of the police and/or the judiciary. During nondemocratic periods their independence is severely limited.

Because most of these initial unscientific exhumations took place in the Province of Buenos Aires, many of the remains were under the jurisdiction of *Asesoría Pericial de La Plata* (the Medical Legal Institute belonging to the judiciary of the Province of Buenos Aires). In 1984, a group of U.S. forensic scientists visited Argentina at the request of CONADEP and *Abuelas de Plaza de Mayo* (Grandmothers of the Plaza de Mayo), a local human rights organization that had requested their help with the identification of disappeared people and the search for disappeared children. The scientists visited *Asesoría Pericial*, saw the bags of remains that had come from the poorly executed exhumations, and made an immediate call to stop the destructive practice so that archaeological and forensic anthropological methods could be used to recover and analyze the skeletal remains. Among these scientists

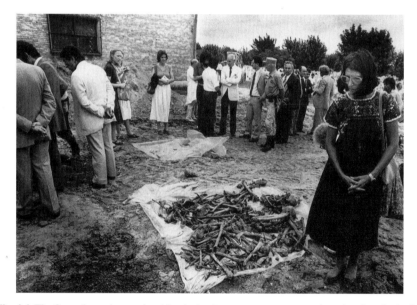

Fig. 4.4 The first exhumations ordered by the justice system were not conducted archaeologically, by as a result of which most of the remains were damaged, commingled, or left in the graves. Mothers of the victims view the remains recovered as a result of these exhumations. Avellaneda, Buenos Aires, 1984. (Photo: Roberto Pera.)

was U.S. forensic anthropologist Dr. Clyde Snow, who, at the request of judges and families of victims, organized the first investigations using archaeological and forensic anthropology techniques to exhume and analyze the remains of disappeared people. He trained EAAF members over the next 5 years.

The bags of remains from these initial exhumations were kept in precarious storage conditions at *Asesoría Pericial*. In time, institutional interest in these cases deteriorated and most judges stopped working on them, abandoning the remains in the storage facility. Requests for information about the remains were met with an inadequate response and eventually led to the conclusion that the information was inaccessible.

At the same time, the results of the historical investigation conducted by EAAF through interviews with survivors of the CDCs and relatives of disappeared people, cemetery and judicial records, fingerprints, and other sources led us to believe that the remains of some disappeared persons could be found and identified from the boxes stored at *Asesoría Pericial*. *Asesoría* agreed to work with EAAF to produce a detailed inventory of the skeletons in the depository and their origin, which was then given to the Buenos Aires Federal Court (*Cámara Federal*). The Court in turn ordered that the remains be entrusted to EAAF for laboratory study with the hope of identifying them.

In December 2002, under the authority of the Buenos Aires Federal Court, 91 significantly deteriorated bags and boxes containing bone material, clothes, ballistic evidence, and labels with partially legible references were transferred from *Asesoría Pericial* to EAAF custody for analysis. These skeletal remains and their associated evidence were severely commingled when we retrieved them (Doretti and Carson 2003).

The bags and boxes received came from at least 10 cemeteries in the provine of Buenos Aires, according to the labels on most of the boxes. These labels indicate the cemetery where the remains were recovered[8] and/or the corresponding judicial file. We also received eight boxes of remains bearing no labels or other indication regarding where they had been exhumed. The skeletal remains in each of these boxes often belonged to more than one individual and were commingled and incomplete.

In the context of the historical and documentary investigation relative to the cases coming from *Asesoría Pericial*, EAAF drafted a spreadsheet showing which box or bag of remains corresponded or might have been related to judicial files about the "discovery" of bodies in wastelands and the exhumation of cadavers. These files often contain information about where the bodies were found, autopsy reports, fingerprints and photos of the cadavers, etc. Similarly, the files relative to the 1984 exhumations also contained information about the date when the exhumation took place, the graves that were exhumed, how the exhumations were conducted, any examination performed, etc. The study of this information yielded results that

---

[8] Moreno, Boulogne, Rafael Calzada, General Madariaga, Lomas de Zamora, Campana, Vicente López, Morón, Mercedes, and Isidro Casanova.

became one more variable to be considered for bone reassociation and the subsequent formulation of identification hypotheses (Fig. 4.5).

In this way, it was possible to cluster most containers—but not all—as corresponding to a given cemetery or judicial case. An assessment of the degree of commingling and a decision regarding the most convenient reassociation procedure then ensued, attending to

- First, the container the remains came from
- Then, all containers coming from the same cemetery
- Finally, all the containers received

For each container, a dated record was made of the existence of ballistic evidence, labels, and clothing.

To date, we have conducted laboratory analysis of 54 of the 91 containers and have obtained the following results:

- Twenty containers (37%) held the remains of only one individual each.
- The Minimum Number of Individuals (MNI) for these 54 boxes has been established as 78, 74 of which were represented by the right tibia and estimated to be adults, while 4 were estimated to be subadults.
- The Most Likely Number of Individuals, MLNI (Adams and Konigsberg 2004), obtained by adult femur pair-matching, was 87 individuals, with a 96% CI of 85–93 individuals (MLNI total: 87; 74 right, 69 left, 58 pairs). Note that the MNI estimate for adults was 74.
- Twenty-three skeletons have been morphologically reassociated.[9] When this total is combined with the 20 containers containing only one individual each, the result is 43 associated individuals from Asesoría. Fourteen of them were determined to be female and 29 male. Thirty of them (19 males and 11 females) presented perimortem injuries consistent with gunshot wounds, mainly to the skull.
- Of the total number of containers, 131 body parts[10] have been morphologically reassociated. One hundred twenty-seven belonged to adults and four to subadults and children. Forty-eight were determined to be male, 8 probably male, 22 female, 3 probably female, and 50 of undetermined sex. A considerable number among these presented perimortem injuries consistent with gunshot wounds, mainly to the skull.

---

[9] The sorting of the remains is based on such morphological techniques as joint match, age and sex similarities, visual pair-matching, process of elimination, and taphonomic appearance.

[10] In this study, body parts refer to groups of bones from the same anatomical part of a skeleton (e.g., lower limbs and pelvis) that are formed by bones that articulate with each other (such as the right femur, the right coxae, and the sacrum) and/or are visually similar (with right and left sides of bilateral bones matching, e.g., the right and left humeri). Those pieces that did not articulate with any other bones and could not be associated with other bones in any way were classified as "isolated."

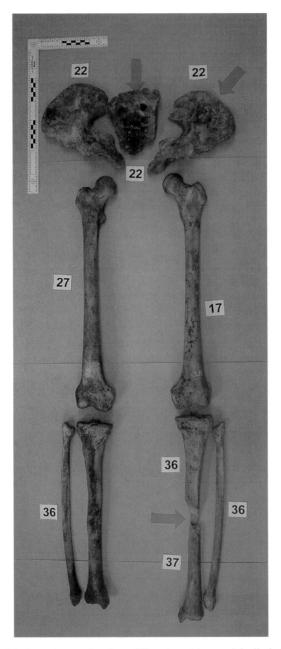

Fig. 4.5 Reasssociated remains coming from different containers originally in the storeroom of Asesoría Pericial de la Plata and exhumed in 1984 at the Cemetery of Lomas de Zamora, Province of Buenos Aires. The numbers correspond to the containers originally holding them. Arrows indicate the presence of perimortem injuries. (Photo: Sofia Egaña, EAAF)

In general terms, the characteristics of remains coming from *Asesoría Pericial* strongly correlated with those of the disappeared at large (Snow and Bihurriet 1984) both biologically (sex and age) and pathologically (perimortem trauma). DNA analysis will further assist in the sorting process and the identification effort.

General Discussion

In all three cases (El Salvador, Zimbabwe, and Argentina), our team implemented a basic research methodology consisting of the following three stages:

1. **Research.** EAAF began by collecting extensive background information on the cases. Techniques included thorough historical research; interviewing relatives, witnesses, and survivors; reviewing military, police, and other official archives; gathering antemortem information about the victims; studying NGO, UN, and other human rights reports; and analyzing hospital and cemetery records, among others. We correlated this information in order to formulate hypotheses about the location of clandestine or anonymous burial sites, the possible name and number of the victims, their biological profile, and the alleged cause of their death. All of this information is instrumental toward planning the strategy for their recovery.
2. **Scene investigation and recovery.** Once the site was located and appropriate permits were obtained, archaeological and forensic techniques were applied to investigate suspected killing and burial sites, analyze the terrain, excavate and carefully recover such evidence as skeletal remains, bullets, clothes, personal belongings, etc. We made a point of documenting every stage of the process by means of written records, video, and photography.
3. **Laboratory analysis.** The recovered remains were then analyzed in a laboratory according to current standards of forensic practice for the management of skeletal remains. In cases in which the remains corresponded to one individual, we conducted routine anthropological analyses, including an estimation of sex, age, height, and laterality as well as a description of antemortem pathologies and old lesions, perimortem trauma, dental information, postmortem alterations, clothing, and nonbiological evidence associated with the remains. We applied the knowledge and techniques of forensic anthropology, pathology, radiology, odontology, and genetic analysis, among others, in an attempt to establish the identity of the victim and to provide information about the cause and manner of death. In cases in which the remains were mixed, we analyzed them as an assemblage or a concentration of commingled skeletal remains. The analysis aimed to reassociate the largest possible number of individual skeletons from the mixed remains in order to conduct individualized studies leading to their identification. We also established an MNI for the entire set of remains under consideration. Where possible, the remains of identified victims were then returned to the relatives or communities, and the evidence was submitted to all pertinent institutions.

The results of the analysis were charted and added to EAAF's Forensic Anthropology Database (FAD) with the purpose of enabling further consultation, searches, and/or matches.

Our experience indicates that the application of this standard procedure for the management of large-scale analysis of commingled skeletonized remains has a number of advantages and limitations that deserve further discussion.

Recovery and Recording of Findings

The results demonstrate that the choice of strategy in initial intervention for recovery and recording of findings has a dramatic impact on the success of subsequent stages. This is particularly true in cases in which the complete, articulated skeleton is not the unit of exhumation and analysis.

The use of archeological methods maximizes the quality and quantity of data obtained, which in turn contribute reliable evidence both for laboratory analysis and for the comparison and matching of forensic records with data obtained from the preliminary investigation. Our experience in La Plata's mortuary facility case also demonstrates that an archeological recovery procedure conducted by trained personnel is needed even in simple cases involving clearly marked individual graves in a cemetery.

The choice of a single technique for recording and recovering remains in all cases is unfeasible. A decision in this regard must be made on the basis of site features. However, adequate recording and description in the field will indicate the level of reliability for the association of commingled remains and can make an enormous difference, as expected, when they are later studied at the laboratory.

As an example, at El Mozote strategies varied according to whether the remains were found in graves or homes, their state of articulation, their spatial distribution, and their state of preservation (Figs. 4.6 and 4.7). Thus, the type or features of each site led to our choice of technique for the recording, lifting, and bagging of the bones. In each case, then, the remains—both biological and nonbiological—were recovered according to level, square, assemblage, or anatomical section/body part.

Osteological Analysis

One of the main objectives of osteological analysis of commingled remains in forensic contexts—and that which presents the greatest difficulties—is the reassociation of bones for the purpose of identifying and restoring the remains to the families.

In Argentina and in El Salvador, our strategy for the reassociation of remains considered a variety of data sources: archeological, biological, and taphonomic, as well as that resulting from the preliminary investigation, all of which contributed to the degree of reliability of reassociation, whether on the basis of body parts or of complete skeletons.

Our criteria to associate bones were

- Archeological information about the arrangement of the remains at exhumation
- Preliminary investigation results (documental and testimonial sources)
- Age and sex
- Joint match
- General morphology
- Continuity in the pattern of traumatic injury
- Consistency of specific antemortem features
- Consistency of postmortem changes

Our results indicated that, for cases that involve large bone concentrations, the sorting of the remains made on the basis of gross morphological techniques presents some limitations that reduce its reliability.

Contributing factors could be summarized as follows:

- Estimations and reassociations were made on the basis of qualitative methods of analysis involving the visual inspection of features (general morphology, joint match, continuity of the traumatic or pathological pattern, etc.); thus, intra- and inter-observer variability increased the probability of bias.
- Reassociation was limited by the extent of preservation of the remains. In El Mozote, the poor state of preservation of the bones and the postmortem loss of a large number of pieces while they were on the surface led to reduced reassociation, limited to very few clear cases. In Sitezi, the degree of fragmentation of

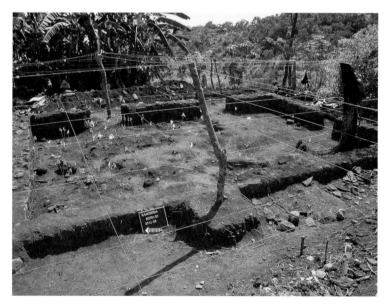

Fig. 4.6 General plan of the exhumation strategy in a case involving remains deposited inside a house at El Mozote. The archeological strategies of square, assemblage, and anatomical section were used simultaneously. (Photo: Mercedes Doretti, EAAF)

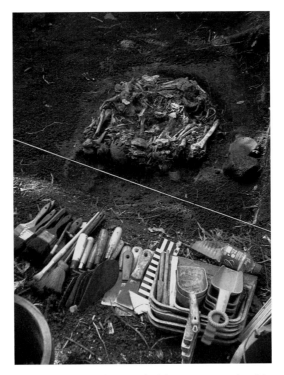

Fig. 4.7 Burial site at El Mozote showing a typical bone concentration (photo: Silvana Turner, EAAF)

bones due to intentional burning of the corpses did not permit any reassociation of identifiable bone elements.

- For homogeneous bone concentrations, i.e., those composed of remains estimated to belong to a group of like-aged, same-sex individuals of the same ethnicity (mostly young adult Caucasian males, for instance), potential morphological similarities among bones belonging to different individuals neither confirmed nor excluded reassociation with only one individual among the group. On the other hand, it was possible to exclude two individuals who were morphologically incompatible because of their different age ranges. We can confirm that an adult pelvis and a child's lower limbs do not yield a morphological match, but in many cases we cannot visually confirm or exclude a match with a morphologically similar adult lower limb. This said, in cases of obvious morphological differences (e.g., a very robust femur and a very gracile humerus), it is possible to sort by exclusion.

These limitations led to the necessary conclusion that reliability of association will be greater as the number of variables contributing to positive association increases. The larger the number of features in common, the higher the likelihood that two bones will belong to the same individual.

The standard procedure for the analysis of commingled skeletonized remains also involves a determination of the MNI, the Lincoln Index (LI), and/or the Most Likely Number of Individuals (MLNI) (Adams and Konigsberg 2004) for the bone concentration as well as a determination of the biological profile, i.e., the represented age range and sex. (See Chapter 12 for more detail on quantification methods of determining number of individuals.)

To determine the MNI, we considered in the first place the duplication of bone type, side, and likely age range at death. Particularly for large-scale cases, our results offer pointers toward a reliable, feasible characterization of sites. However, in some cases—especially when recovery of major elements is nowhere near 100%—it is possible to use the alternative techniques derived from pair-matching mentioned above, i.e., the LI or the MLNI. This information may not be directly instrumental in the formulation of identification hypotheses but serves to correlate with the information resulting from the preliminary investigation.

For biological profiling purposes, for every assemblage we took into account (1) each and every bone element in the concentration presenting significant features to that end (e.g., skull, pelvis) and (2) morphologically reassociated units (skeletons).

It is evident that the value of the information obtained from biological profiling depends on the extent of survival of bone elements. When the skeleton is well-preserved, the determination of sex and age is clearly instrumental in the formulation of identification hypotheses. In any case, this information is significant for correlation with that provided by witnesses or documentary sources.

Another objective of the forensic management of commingled skeletonized remains is to provide information on the cause and manner of death of the exhumed individuals by recording, among other factors, the existence of perimortem injuries. For the three cases described above, such injuries were recorded according to which bones presented trauma within the total assemblage and/or reassociated large units (skeleton or anatomical sections). In Argentina and in El Salvador, the existence of perimortem injuries and their type as well as the associated ballistic evidence, when it existed, correlated with the information yielded by the preliminary investigation and testimonial records. Nevertheless, observations relative to cause and manner of death of a given individual are limited by the possibility and reliability of reassociations.

Our results strongly indicate the value of a thorough preliminary investigation, including witness testimony as well as the examination of cemetery, morgue, judicial, and police records, among others.

The Argentine case provides an example in this regard. Some of the containers at La Plata's mortuary facilities had labels on them bearing the judicial record number of their exhumation orders from 1984. Those judicial records included both police autopsy reports and photos of the remains at the time of their exhumation and/or first examination by facility staff members. Analysis led to a confirmation of either consistency or variability in the number of remains and their condition both at the time of their first autopsy and 20 years after exhumation.

In El Salvador, the information collected during the preliminary investigation also permitted drawing up a database for possible victims that included name, sex, age, and dental data among other antemortem information, as well as any existing relationships between victims and their potential burial site.

The Use of DNA Analysis in a Context Involving Commingled Skeletonized Remains

Discovering the identity of victims from their skeletal remains involves comparing physical data obtained from the study of the remains (postmortem) with physical information about victims such as age at death, sex, height, dental records, and others (antemortem), usually obtained from victims' families and friends. Unfortunately, in many of our investigations antemortem information is frequently unavailable or insufficient for a positive identification. However, since the late 1980s, when it became possible to recover DNA from bones, genetic testing has become a key tool in investigations. In association with genetic laboratories, EAAF has already made identifications using genetic testing for individual cases of disappearances in Argentina, Haiti, and Ethiopia.

In a number of cases, we can formulate a strong hypothesis on the identity of remains and only need confirmation through genetic testing. However, DNA analysis is still expensive, and few genetic laboratories work on the extraction of DNA from bone remains. Another element presenting further complexity in cases involving the large-scale analysis of commingled skeletonized remains is the sampling strategy for genetic analysis. Ideally, genetic confirmation or exclusion of the possibility that a particular person's remains will be present in a given concentration should take place only after each and every bone element has been analyzed. Unsurprisingly, in addition to the prohibitive cost of extensive DNA testing, cases involving large concentrations of incomplete, disarticulated remains have presented a number of technical limitations, such as the state of preservation of the DNA (which may vary with the type of bone recovered) and the laboratory's technical capacity, among others. It is in these cases that morphological reassociation plays a particularly significant role by contributing to a reduction in the number of samples to be sent for genetic processing. In this sense, DNA testing can indeed contribute to confirming the morphological reassociation of anatomical sections. Likewise, when an individual's skeleton is poorly represented—by only one bone, for instance, typically the cranium, jaw, or pelvis—genetic testing can contribute to confirming or excluding the presence of a given person in the concentration, even when it will be impossible to restore the complete skeleton to the family.

In the case of Argentina, EAAF has a blood bank of relatives of the disappeared, but mass DNA testing is not readily accessible. Therefore, cases are processed according to the following priority:

1. Reassociated skeletons or anatomical sections with highly reliable association and presumptive identification, the result of matching ante- and postmortem data and background investigation

2. Single skeletal elements permitting preliminary anthropological identification, e.g., jaw and/or maxillae with significant dental features

Conclusions

When following the aforementioned standards for recovery and analysis of large concentrations of commingled skeletonized remains, we can expect reliable results in the following areas:

- A record of conditions in which the remains and associated nonbiological evidence were found
- A determination of the MNI for the total assemblage on the basis of bone inventorying and additional analyses available (such as LI and MLNI) that may be appropriate in certain scenarios
- A biological profile for the assemblage based on skeletal elements or reassociated skeletal units
- A preliminary morphological reassociation of complete or partial remains
- A record of perimortem injuries for the assemblage or for reassociated units

These results are instrumental for comparisons with the information derived from the preliminary investigation and for the formulation of identification hypotheses.

On the other hand, limitations on the analysis of commingled skeletonized remains mainly relate to identification and to the determination of the cause and manner of death. Given the limitations of morphological reassociation, identification based on osteo-anthropological data must be considered preliminary in most cases and necessarily followed up with DNA testing. This is particularly true in cases involving (1) a large number of commingled remains resulting in a high MNI, (2) "open" or virtually open cases with a large potential list of candidates for those remains, and (3) poor or nonexistent antemortem information. Positive identification will ultimately result from the combined evaluation of osteo-anthropological data and DNA testing results. Additionally, circumstantial evidence—i.e., burial site, body-part–associated personal effects, clothing, etc.—as well as documentary and witness testimony information must also be considered toward identification.

Our ethical, legal, and scientific mandate is to consider a corpse identified only when sufficient reliable evidence has been collected in accordance with national and international protocols and recommendations. To this end, our observations confirm the need for specific standardized guidelines within the framework of forensic protocols for the anthropological management of commingled skeletonized remains that should include consideration of a variety of both biological and nonbiological data sources.

In many cases, it may prove technically impossible to reassociate the whole of the concentration or to genetically test a large number of bone samples in order to maximize the potential for identification of all the persons present in the assemblage. It is important that participating anthropologists provide information to the authorities and the victims' families on the condition of the remains and on the technical difficulties hindering their identification so that their final disposition may be determined on that basis.

References Cited

Adams, B. J. and J. E. Byrd 2006 Resolution of small-scale commingling: A case report from the Vietnam War. *Forensic Sci. Int.* 156(1):63–69.

Adams, B. J. and L. W. Konigsberg 2004 Estimation of the most likely number of individuals from commingled human skeletal remains. *Am. J. Phys. Anthropol.* 125(2):138–151.

Byrd, J. E. and B. J. Adams 2003 Osteometric sorting of commingled human remains. *J. Forensic Sci.* 48(4):717–724.

CONADEP 1986 *Nunca Más*. EUDEBA, Buenos Aires.

Doretti, M. (editor) 1999 *EAAF Annual Report*, New York.

Doretti, M. and L. Carson (editors) 2003 *EAAF Annual Report*, New York.

Doretti, M., L. Carson, and D. Kerr (editors) 2005 *EAAF Annual Report*, New York.

Kerley, E. R. 1972 Special observations in skeletal identification. *J. Forensic Sci.* 17(3):349–357.

Rösing, F. W. and E. Pischtschan 1995 Re-individualisation of commingled skeletal remains. In *Advances in Forensic Sciences*, B. Jacob and W. Bonte, eds. Verlag, Berlin.

Snow, C. and M. J. Bihurriet 1984 Tumbas NN en la provincia de Buenos Aires de 1970 a 1984. In *Informe de la Subsecretaria de Derechos Humanos*. Buenos Aires, Argentina.

Snow, C. and E. D. Folk 1965 Statistical assessment of commingled skeletal remains. *Am. J. Phys. Anthropol.* 32:423–427.

Ubelaker, D. H. 2002 Approaches to the study of commingling in human skeletal biology. In *Advances in Forensic Taphonomy: Method, Theory, and Archaeological Perspectives*, W. D. Haglund and M. H. Sorg, eds. CRC Press, Boca Raton, FL.

United Nations 1993 *From Madness to Hope*. United Nations Truth Commission Report.

United Nations Manual on the Effective Prevention and Investigation of Extra-Legal, Arbitrary and Summary Executions 1991 U.N. Doc E/ST/CSDHA/.12.

Chapter 5
Anthropological Investigations of the Tri-State Crematorium Incident

Dawnie Wolfe Steadman, Kris Sperry, Frederick Snow, Laura Fulginiti, and Emily Craig

On February 15, 2002, a woman was walking her dog in the woods of the small, unincorporated town of Noble in Walker County, Georgia, and discovered a human skull. She called the authorities, who confirmed the skull was human and launched a pedestrian survey of the area. Unfortunately, the skull was just a portent of the macabre scenes awaiting investigators as they walked onto the 16 acres of property owned by the Marsh family, who were, at that time, one of the most prominent African-American families in the county. Three houses, including two inhabited by the Marshes, a spring-fed lake, a crematorium, an adjacent large metal building, and a large storage shed filled a 6-acre section of the property. The rest of the property was wooded (Fig. 5.1). The Marsh family business was the Tri-State Crematorium, which served dozens of funeral homes in Georgia, Tennessee, and Alabama.

An incredible stench drew investigators to the crematorium and adjacent structures, where they found bodies littering the floors. While some were in body bags or cremation boxes, many were uncontained and in various stages of decomposition. As the investigators expanded their search outside the buildings, more bodies were found in abandoned vehicles, open vaults, and coffins scattered across the landscape. Human skeletal remains seemed to be everywhere. The great number of human remains as well as the tremendous variation in decomposition indicated that the process of abandoning bodies on the property had been going on for some time, but for how long and why?

While little of this surreal scene made any sense, it was quite clear that the medicolegal infrastructure in this very rural part of northwestern Georgia was about to be overrun by unidentified human remains, international press, and hundreds of betrayed families demanding to know the disposition of their loved ones. The recovery and identification process would require a multidisciplinary team of criminal investigators, identification specialists, and forensic anthropologists.

The Investigation

Four goals were defined as the investigation began: (1) Recover every body, body part, and bone that could be located on the property; (2) identify as many of the

From: *Recovery, Analysis, and Identification of Commingled Human Remains*
Edited by: B. Adams and J. Byrd © Humana Press, Totowa, NJ

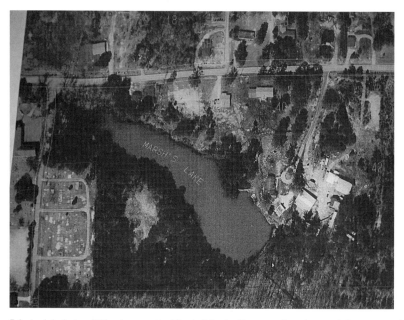

Fig. 5.1 Aerial photo of Marsh property. Most of the bodies were found around the crematorium and storage buildings in the lower right portion of the photo

recovered remains as possible; (3) return the identified remains to families for final disposition; and (4) document all findings for potential legal proceedings.

The Georgia Bureau of Investigation (GBI) was the primary investigative body and requested that the Federal Disaster Mortuary Operational Response Team (DMORT) provide assistance with body recovery and processing. There are 10 regional DMORTs around the country; each consists of identification specialists, including forensic pathologists, odontologists, anthropologists, X-ray technicians and radiologists, as well as funeral directors who work with the families concerning the final disposition of identified remains (Sledzik and Wilcox 2003). Local X-ray technicians, fingerprint experts, and law enforcement officers, as well as personnel from the Armed Forces DNA Identification Laboratory (AFDIL), joined the effort. The anthropologists were divided into three investigative areas—scene recovery, processing and identification of bodies in the morgue, and assessment of urn contents that had been returned to families but may not contain human remains.

Processing the Scene

Forensic anthropologists worked alongside GBI investigators and Walker County Sheriff's deputies in locating and documenting human remains around the property. The crematorium housed the retort, a very small anteroom, and an apparent waiting room or office that had obviously not been used for years, as it was covered with dust and suffered water damage from a leaky roof. The concrete floor in front of the retort was filthy and coated with greasy fluid. A hole had been cut in the baseboard on the opposite wall to allow bodily fluids to drain across the floor to the outside. The retort itself contained a body within a cardboard cremation box (Fig. 5.2), and six other decomposing bodies were on the floor nearby. Over 20 individuals were located in the metal storage building, some mixed with Christmas decorations and refuse and others stacked within large metal burial vaults. The five sealed metal vaults within this building were opened and discovered to contain stacks of bodies as well. Two mummified bodies were found under debris in the storage shed. Several inoperative vehicles, including a hearse, were lined up nearby. A casket containing the mummified body of a man in his burial suit was still in the hearse. The plaque on the casket identified the man and his date of death in 1998. It appeared that the body and hearse had been driven from the funeral home, parked on the Marsh property in 1998, and never attended to again.

As the brush and woods around the buildings were explored, caskets with decaying bodies were discovered in multiple random locations, and human skeletal remains littered the ground underfoot and beneath the underbrush (Figs. 5.3 and 5.4). Further, bones, caskets, and body bags were protruding from gaping holes in the ground. Investigation of trash heaps determined that these overlaid pits contained human remains as well (Fig. 5.5). Thus, anthropologists had to conduct both surface recoveries and excavation of clandestine mass graves, and commingling was an ongoing issue.

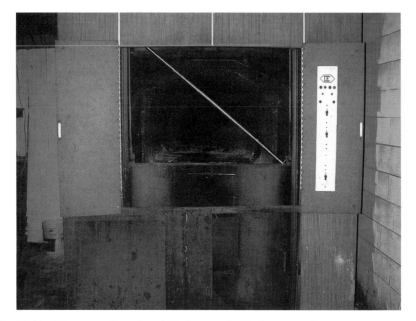

Fig. 5.2 Partially cremated remains within the retort inside the crematorium

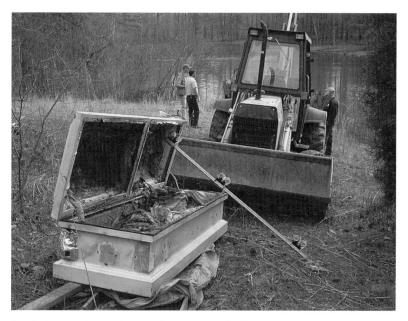

Fig. 5.3 Casket containing a decomposing body near the lake

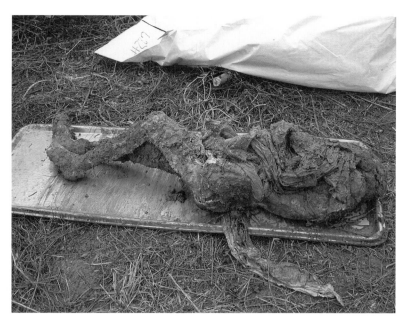

Fig. 5.4 Decomposing body recovered from Site 9

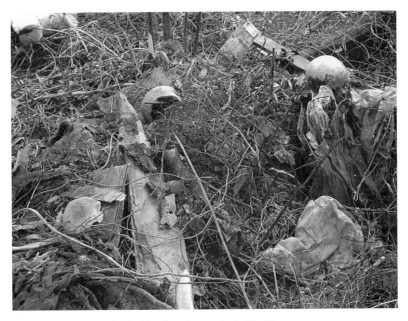

Fig. 5.5 Human remains mixed with refuge in a trash pit (Site 3)

The remains of 75 individuals were found on the first full day of investigation alone, and it was clear that this was just the beginning. One problem that soon arose concerned the methodology by which to address commingled and isolated bones recovered from the site. Individual numbers were assigned to each skull. In addition, isolated long bones were also given individual numbers and sampled for DNA with the hopes that eventually they may be reassociated with the rest of the remains, which may have been located some distance away. Early on investigators decided that DNA sampling all of the recovered bones would be cost-prohibitive and that testing of unassociated remains would be limited to the long bones. As a result, unassociated bones other than the long bones were not given individual case numbers since they were not going to be tested and successful reassociation at a later date was unlikely. Individual bones that could not be reassociated with a specific individual were later buried in a separate vault.

Surface Recoveries

The nature of the remains recovered from the ground-surface contexts ranged from intact bodies in various stages of decay to individual scattered bones. Some of the bodies were inside caskets and body bags, some were skeletonized but intact and relatively complete, some were in total commingled disarray, and at least one skeleton was packed into the ground under one of the small dirt roads that snaked around the buildings. Isolated individual bones were scattered across the entire area. There were also several large circumscribed collections of skeletal remains where it appeared as if numerous bodies had been deposited over time. In one of these, Site 1, the skeletal remains of 23 individuals were on and around the remnants of an overturned pool table. The vast majority of the remains were directly on top of the slate slabs that, in turn, rested on the ground, creating a definite stratigraphy in the central mound of bones. Around the periphery of the central mound of remains, and outside the upturned legs of the pool table, were decomposing remnants of some tarpaulins tied together. The wooden legs and the pool table frame were in an advanced stage of deterioration and infested with termites, but it appeared as if there might have been an attempt to create a makeshift basket using the pool table slate as the bottom and the legs as the side supports. Around the outermost fringes of this pile of bone, skeletal remains were more diffuse, scattered, and commingled. Skeletonization of the remains in this complex pile was complete. Fortunately, some bodies had been wrapped in sheets or had been wearing durable articles of clothing that served as dividers between individuals, but most bodies were neither wrapped nor clothed. Seasonal collections of pine needles and leaves also served as rough indicators of divisions between individuals, but the pile of bones was several feet high, and as the bodies decomposed the uppermost bones had apparently filtered to the bottom. Animal scavenging was also evident and, in addition to damaging the bones, their activity also played a role in the scattering and commingling of the remains.

Several yards away, one of two large refuse piles (Site 2) contained the bones of numerous individuals commingled with trash items and each other. Although there was not as much commingling as in the first assemblage, the matrix of trash and bones created a complex mess. The trash included rotten foodstuffs, logs, leaves, clothing, large appliances, fencing, tires, and other debitage. Once the bottom of the trash pile was excavated, it became clear that there had been some attempt to bury the lowest matrix of individual bodies in shallow trenches covered with a thin layer of hand-shoveled dirt, requiring some excavation of each shallow grave.

Excavations

A total of eight burial pits were found on the property. All except one were in the vicinity of the structures, and it appeared as if all had been dug by a small backhoe, which was stored nearby. Several pits were closely aligned, separated by only a few feet. The exception was a pit near the lakeshore, less than 90 feet from Brent Marsh's residence.

The burial sites were relatively easy to locate, as the disturbed soil was distinct in color and topography from the surrounding undisturbed soil. Whenever a disturbed area was discovered, the initial excavation was carried out by hand. Once the boundaries were discerned, a backhoe was used to enlarge the perimeter of the excavation in order to provide working room and reduce the risk of wall collapse. The pits were relatively deep, averaging around 5 feet (though one was nearly 7 feet deep), and contained between 2 and 23 individuals (Table 5.1). Many of the bodies had started decomposing prior to burial, and the pits were filled with decomposition fluid, which made recovery difficult. Some of the bodies were inside body bags such that even with advanced decomposition all of the remains were contained.

Table 5.1 Remains Recovered from Features

Site	Number of Individuals Recovered	Date of Deposition
Site 1	23	October–November 1999
Site 2	10	September 1997–May 1998
Site 3	17	April 1999
Site 4	10	December 1999–May 2000
Site 5	10	May–June 2000
Site 6	12	August–September 2001
Site 7	19	December 2000–February 2001
Site 8	2	Cannot be reliably dated
Site 9	23	July–August 2000
Site 10	6	October 2000
Site 11	8	Cannot be reliably dated

Unfortunately, some body bags were open, and other individuals were placed in the pit without any container, contributing to the significant commingling within each pit (Fig. 5.6). When present, intact clothing helped separate the individuals. However, some individuals were nearly skeletonized, suggesting that most decomposition occurred before burial and that body parts could have been missing prior to internment. The field conditions were not conducive to conducting large-scale reassociation of commingled remains from these pits. If a relatively intact body was missing a left leg and a left leg was found in the pit, the parts were placed in separate body bags and a note was placed on each telling the morgue personnel they may be associated. The bottom of each pit contained unassociated body parts that were bagged individually and sent to the morgue.

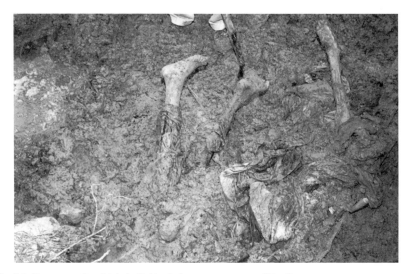

Fig. 5.6 Recovery of multiple individuals from a mass grave (Site 6)

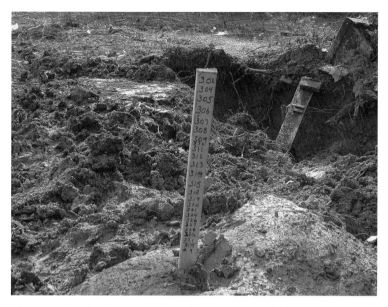

Fig. 5.7 Marker delineating the case numbers of remains recovered from a mass grave (Site 9)

The remains were removed from the pit, photographed, and sequentially numbered from top to bottom such that a stratigraphy of sorts could be established (Fig. 5.7). The numbering system followed the same protocol as that for surface remains and allowed a temporal component of the pit to be assessed as individuals were identified and the dates of death were established. Assuming that the bodies were buried in a single episode and died at approximately the same time, the possibilities could be narrowed for when the as-yet unidentified bodies had been placed within the pits. Each pit was mapped using a total station computerized mapping system, and each set of remains was photographed extensively *in situ* using multiple cameras.

Identification Efforts

Recovered remains were transported to DMORT's Disaster Portable Morgue Unit (DPMU) for processing and identification (Saul and Saul 2003). The morgue setup consisted of an admitting desk and six stations, each of which contained identification specialists and their equipment (Fig. 5.8). A case file was provided for each set of remains as they entered the morgue, and a mortuary officer escorted the remains to every station, beginning with pathology. The chief medical examiner for the State of Georgia determined that since cause of death was not an issue in this incident, full autopsies were not required. The pathologists performed external examinations, noting and photographing tattoos, surgical scars, and other physical variations, and then the remains were radiographed. Each set of remains then went to fingerprinting,

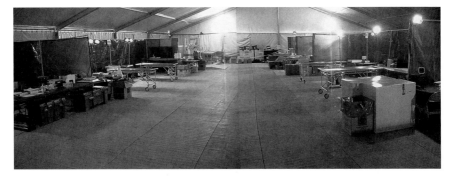

Fig. 5.8 DMORT Portable Morgue Unit. Identification stations included pathology, radiology, fingerprints, odontology, anthropology, and DNA (DMORT 2002)

odontology, anthropology, and ultimately the DNA station, where a section of the right femur was retained for DNA analysis. DNA samples were also taken from some unassociated body parts and isolated bones.

The anthropologist's role varied depending upon the condition of the remains. Whole, fresh bodies received little anthropological attention as identification was likely made via visual or molecular means. The anthropologists were mainly tasked with assessing the biological profile of decomposed, skeletal, fragmentary, and commingled remains. A biological profile consists of age, sex, ancestry, stature, and antemortem pathologies and anomalies that could be used for identification. The completeness of the profile depended upon the amount of material and its state of preservation. Ancestry, typically the most difficult parameter of the biological profile to estimate, was a key variable as individuals of both European and African-American ancestries were abandoned together on the property. The anthropologists and pathologists also reviewed the postmortem radiographs to ensure that all surgical interventions were detected and recorded. Not surprisingly, the majority of the individuals sent to the crematorium were elderly, and many exhibited evidence of surgical intervention, such as amputations, prosthetic joints, and other orthopedic devices (e.g., plates, pins, and screws), pacemakers, prosthetic arterial structures, false teeth, dental implants and restorations, and metal sutures (Fig. 5.9). Any implants or pacemakers were removed by the pathologists, and GBI agents used the manufacturer serial numbers to track down information concerning where the items had been sold and in whom they had been implanted. In addition, some bodies had hospital and nursing home identification bands on their wrists or funeral home tags around the ankles. A few bodies exhibited autopsy incisions, which meant hospital and/or medical examiner's offices would have records and possibly biological specimens that could be used for DNA comparisons.

One significant question early in the investigation was just how long the bodies had been accumulating and, hence, how many families had to be contacted to supply antemortem information. Ray Marsh established the Tri-State Crematorium in 1981 but, after suffering a stroke, handed the business to his son, Ray Brent Marsh, in 1997. As the investigation progressed, it became clear that Brent Marsh did not

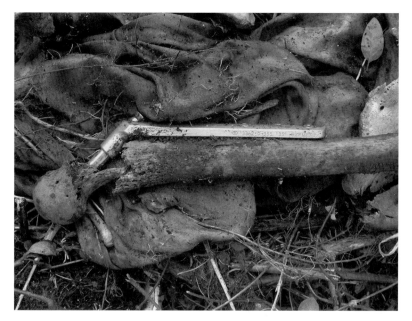

Fig. 5.9 Femur with prosthetic

keep any records of the number or identity of those brought to the crematorium, from what funeral home they originated, which bodies had been cremated and which had not, or when the failure to cremate had begun. Based on the first identifications, it appeared that the bodies began to accumulate in 1997, corresponding to when Brent Marsh took over operations from his father. The GBI had contacted directors of over 30 funeral homes who first furnished lists of all individuals ever sent to the Tri-State Crematorium, but then narrowed the list to those sent between 1997 and 2002. Unfortunately, the GBI found that in addition to receiving bodies from the funeral homes, Brent Marsh had also conducted unauthorized and illegal removals from private residences, nursing homes, and hospitals. Since none of these individuals had been processed through funeral homes and because Marsh kept no records himself, the number and identity of these individuals were unknown. This meant that everyone in the tri-state area who lost a family member since at least 1997 could possibly be affected by Marsh's actions and inactions, yet there was no way to know whose loved ones were cremated and whose were not.

GBI and DMORT personnel interviewed family members to obtain antemortem information that could be compared with the postmortem data collected in the morgue to enable identification. Approximately 80% of the contacted families participated in the identification process. Many of the deceased were elderly and had no living relatives, while some families simply did not wish to revisit the grief over the loss of their loved one. Family members that did come forward provided information concerning age at death, sex, height, handedness, surgical history, tattoos, scars, and other physical features of their loved ones. One of the most basic and reliable forms of identifying antemortem information comes from medical records, but few complete records were available since hospitals, dentists, and physicians destroyed the files following the death of their patient. Further, many of the bodies could simply not be identified by radiographic, dental, or skeletal means, so appropriate family members provided blood samples for nuclear DNA analysis.

While some presumptive sorting of commingled bones had been attempted in the field, all associations of isolated and commingled remains were confirmed by anthropologists in the morgue based on a variety of techniques, including anthropometrics, fracture margins, and joint articulations. For example, the presence of diffuse idiopathic skeletal hyperostosis (DISH) and ankylosing spondylitis helped to reassociate segments of the spinal column by matching fracture margins between bony osteophytes. Eburnation of adjacent joint surfaces was helpful in reassociating limbs in some cases. Also, in at least one amputee, reassociation was possible using hypertrophic development of the other leg.

Following reassociation, 339 individuals were represented as well as over 200 disassociated bones or body parts. The investigation revealed that 999 bodies had been sent to the Tri-State Crematorium from January 1, 1997, through February 15, 2002, when the conditions of the site were discovered. It appears that the remaining 660 individuals were likely cremated. One thing is certain: Additional bodies were not located on the site. The lake was drained and the entire site was searched by cadaver dogs, ground-penetrating radar, infrared imaging, and pedestrian line search. A final check was made by heavy equipment excavation to a depth of 4 feet. Another piece of property owned by the Marshes was also searched, and no remains were found.

Assessment of Cremains

On the first night of the investigation it became clear that the scope of the problem extended beyond the remains found at the scene. That evening a man approached the Chief Medical Examiner and stated that his wife had been contacted earlier in the day and told that her mother's remains had been recovered from the grounds. However, he continued, they had an urn at home on the fireplace mantle that they were told held the ashes of his mother-in-law. A cursory examination revealed that the contents of the submitted urn were not ashes at all but rather cement. When this information became public, hundreds of families brought their urns to the Family Assistance Center (FAC) established by DMORT and the GBI at the local community center. A forensic anthropologist was then assigned to the FAC for the sole purpose of examining submitted urn contents (Fig. 5.10).

Cremains analysis is an exacting and tedious process, so a decision was made early on that the preliminary examination would make a determination of "bone" or "not bone" only. This decision was made to avoid misleading families about the contents of their urns, because at the time they could only be examined under the most primitive of conditions. As the process moved forward, the anthropologist

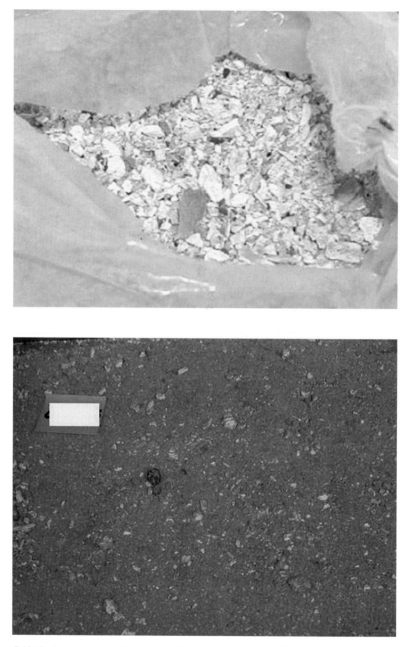

Fig. 5.10 Typical example of commercially cremated bone before (above) and after (below) pulverization. The pictured cremains are not from the Tri-State Incident. (Photo courtesy of Laura Fulginiti)

could sometimes demonstrate that the contents of the urns were "suspicious," usually because they contained items that were inconsistent with the family memory of their loved one.

The urns were brought by the families to the FAC and were examined by the anthropologist while the GBI agents interviewed the members about their loved one. A table was set up behind the stage in the community center, affording privacy for the forensic anthropologist and some measure of respect for the decedent. The urn and the plastic bag inside were opened to reveal the contents. If necessary, the remains were spread on a plastic tray for examination. Items such as dental appliances, tooth roots, and surgical interventions (usually open heart surgery staples) were identified. The family was consulted about the condition of the loved one and any medical history. If the cremains were determined to be bone (there was no good way to say human/nonhuman given the rudimentary facility), the cremains were returned immediately to the family.

In the event that there were suspicions about the cremains, i.e., that they were either "not bone" or that they contained inconsistent evidence, they were impounded and the family was immediately informed and given a release slip. During the course of the deployment, hundreds of sets of cremains were examined in this fashion. Some families even went to the cemetery and brought in urns covered in wet mud from burial plots and from mausoleums as well as urns that had places of pride in their homes.

Some family members refused to allow the urns out of their sight for the examination. In those cases, the GBI agent, the forensic anthropologist, and the family would go into a private room behind the stage and the remains would be viewed in that setting. These instances were rare (perhaps 10 times out of several hundred) but were very emotional for all parties. The GBI agents were uncomfortable, as was the forensic anthropologist performing the examinations. DMORT has a policy of not allowing the family members to have access to the morgue or morgue personnel, but the circumstances in this instance precluded that policy from being enforced. In the end, the grief of the family and the need for resolution outweighed any discomfort on the part of the individuals involved.

When an urn was discovered to be "suspicious," it would be taken into evidence and one of the Georgia medical examiners would be tasked for additional analysis. The most common reason for impounding would be because the remains in the urn consisted of something other than bone. In the majority of cases, the substance was a white powder, thought by most to be some form of lime such as what comes with concrete. The powder had the consistency of talcum powder and, upon opening the bag, could sting the nasal passages and eyes. Such cases were suspicious because the amount and weight of the contents were less than expected for a cremated body and the powder was finer than that of cremated bone. The GBI agents learned to expect that during and after the year 2000, nearly all of the purported cremains would contain no bone. Cremains from 1998 and 1999 were highly variable. Some of the cremains looked like bone, some had a mix of bone and powder, and some had a majority of powder with a few bones thrown in. Cremains from 1997 and earlier were nearly all bone, although they were not always consistent with the decedent.

When the contents of the urn were spread on the plastic tray, certain items would stand out. These included surgical clips, staples, and other medical interventions, dental appliances, and tooth roots. Depending on the quality of the mechanical pulverization, large portions of bone would occasionally be present as well. These bits of bone could be cursorily examined for indications of sex, although, given the primitive nature of the examination, no definitive statements were made. When a dental appliance or other type of nonbone item was discovered, the GBI agent would reinterview the family in an attempt to verify that the decedent allegedly represented by the cremation did in fact have such a procedure. Depending upon the answer, the cremains were either retained or returned immediately. At one point during the height of the cremains submissions, the retention rate reached about 25%. After DMORT ended their deployment in Noble, Georgia, cremations continued to be submitted. Other forensic anthropologists were retained both on behalf of the State and on behalf of the funeral homes involved in the litigation.

Identifications

Of the 339 individuals recovered, 225 (66%) were ultimately identified. Understanding the stratigraphy of the bodies in the pits as related to time of death was helpful, but it was still not possible to identify some of the bodies in the pits, even if they were stacked between identified bodies from known time periods. Further, approximately half of the bodies had been embalmed, which severely hampered DNA recovery from tissues, including bone. Sixty-three (28%) of the 225 identifications were accomplished through DNA comparisons. When the DNA efforts were exhausted, information concerning age, sex, ancestry, clothing, personal effects, and identifying characteristics were placed on a special page of the GBI Website that was available to the public. A handful of additional identifications were made as people recognized the described clothing or physical features of their loved ones. The 114 unidentified bodies and unassociated remains were interred in a cemetery in North Georgia, which had donated the space and burial vaults. A monument marks the burial site.

Legal Ramifications

One of the perplexing questions stemming from this incident is how the disposal of bodies could have continued for 4 years without detection. At the time of the incident, Georgia required that funeral homes containing a crematorium adhere to specific funerary laws and be inspected annually. However, freestanding crematoria, such as that owned by the Marshes, slipped through a loophole that made them exempt from state inspections. In addition, Brent Marsh traveled to funeral homes to pick up bodies with his own van, so funeral home personnel rarely came to his property. This service, as well as the low rate of $225 per body for cremation, was attractive to funeral directors and they consulted him often. Given that the family compound was shielded from the roads by dense woods and only a small sign indicated the presence of the business, few local residents knew of the existence of the crematorium. Thus, Brent Marsh carried out his activities quietly and without detection from either the state or the local community.

Another question is, quite simply, why? Ray Brent Marsh was a deacon in his church and a star football player in college. Despite early rumors, it was determined that there was no evidence that Marsh had altered or abused the bodies in any way other than dumping them on his property. It appears that the retort was ill-maintained and, although investigators were able to start it up, the amount of soot likely precluded efficient cremation and Marsh simply abandoned the process while still accepting bodies. Regardless of the wide range of deposition locations on the property, none required much effort. Even the burial pits, which were dug by a small backhoe, were very close to each other and to the structures. Given the remote location of the property, little energy was expended to hide the bodies.

Ray Brent Marsh was charged with 787 felony counts, which included theft by deception and abuse of a corpse. Marsh had received money from the funeral homes and others for services not rendered, and he had returned adulterated cremains to families. It was estimated that the fraudulent activities totaled $60,000. On January 31, 2005, Marsh pled guilty to the charges and was sentenced to 75 years in prison. He will be eligible for parole in 2009.

The investigation of this incident was the most expensive in Georgia's history, exceeding over $10 million. There have been a number of civil suits filed against Ray Brent Marsh and the Marsh family as well as 39 funeral homes that used his services. The family plaintiffs argued that the funeral homes should have been aware of the problem, especially since they received adulterated cremains from Marsh and passed them on to the families in urns. The judgments called for over $84 million to be paid to the plaintiffs, making this one of the largest civil verdicts in Georgia's history.

Conclusions

The Tri-State Crematorium case is not unique for the need to identify a number of individuals who died prior to the incident. DMORT has responded to several incidents in which floodwaters had opened vaults and displaced coffins (Sledzik and Wilcox 2003). However, the incident in Noble was exceptional in that the accumulation of bodies was due to deliberate acts of abuse and neglect rather than natural events. The human toll of this incident was indeed tragic as families had to endure the grieving process yet again and absorb the emotional trauma of anger and betrayal. The families and the community at large needed a rapid response as well as careful and compassionate resolution. In spite of the time required to extensively document and excavate the area, the entire site was cleared within two weeks and the bodies were processed within three weeks. In this instance, interagency and interdisciplinary cooperation were essential to a successful resolution for a community exposed to a complex and emotional incident.

References Cited

Saul, F. P. and J. M. Saul 2003 Planes, trains and fireworks: The evolving role of the forensic anthropologist in mass fatality incidents. In *Hard Evidence: Case Studies in Forensic Anthropology*, D. W. Steadman, ed., pp. 266–277. Prentice Hall, Upper Saddle River, NJ.

Sledzik, P. S. and A. W. Wilcox 2003 Corpi aquaticus: The Hardin cemetery flood of 1993. In *Hard Evidence: Case Studies in Forensic Anthropology*, D. W. Steadman, ed., pp. 256–265. Prentice Hall, Upper Saddle River, NJ.

Chapter 6
Approaches to Commingling Issues in Archeological Samples: A Case Study from Roman Era Tombs in Greece

Douglas H. Ubelaker and Joseph L. Rife

Human remains in archeological contexts frequently present the problem of commingling, especially when they are secondary deposits and involve multiple phases of funerary treatment and postdepositional disturbance. These problems are often compounded with incidents of recent looting and the prior undocumented removal of remains. Fortunately, the problems of interpreting such assemblages can be ameliorated with careful excavation and skeletal analysis related to context. As a case in point, this chapter focuses on the interpretation of evidence from chamber tombs of the Roman Empire at the site of Kenchreai in southern Greece. The systematic recovery and analysis of the commingled human remains from these tombs has contributed to a better understanding of local mortuary behavior and paleodemography. The study of this complex evidence presents an effective approach to samples of this kind, which are not uncommon in Mediterranean archaeological contexts.

Kenchreai and the Koutsongila Cemetery

Kenchreai is located on the eastern shore of the Isthmus of Corinth, facing the Saronic Gulf of the Aegean Sea (Fig. 6.1). This sizable settlement was the eastern port of the major city of Corinth throughout classical antiquity, but the harbor was especially prosperous during the Roman Empire (1st–7th centuries A.D.). Since 2002, Joseph L. Rife has directed the Kenchreai Cemetery Project (KCP), an interdisciplinary program of archaeological study and conservation sponsored by Macalester College under the auspices of the American School of Classical Studies at Athens (Rife 2003, 2004, 2005; Rife et al. in press). KCP has concentrated on the port town's primary cemetery, located immediately north of the harbor on a coastal ridge called Koutsongila. Although the Koutsongila Cemetery has been studied sporadically by Greek and American archaeologists since 1907, it has also attracted the attention of looters in recent years. So far KCP has documented 30 subterranean chamber tombs and 28 individual cist graves cut into the bedrock in more or less even

From: *Recovery, Analysis, and Identification of Commingled Human Remains*
Edited by: B. Adams and J. Byrd © Humana Press, Totowa, NJ

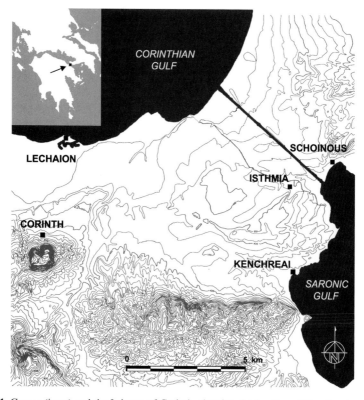

Fig. 6.1 Greece (inset) and the Isthmus of Corinth, showing the location of Kenchreai and other major sites of the Roman Empire (photo courtesy of J. L. Rife)

rows along the seaward slope of the ridge and the adjacent area to the north (Figure 6.2).

The well-preserved chamber tombs are particularly interesting, because they were large structures used over a long span of time for the burial of numerous persons (Rife in press-a). In each tomb, a stairway leads from the surface down into a rectangular chamber area carved from the bedrock measuring on average ca. 3.7 meters long by ca. 3.3 meters wide by ca. 2.5 meters high (Figs. 6.2 and 6.3). Several tombs were marked at ground level by a rectangular structure with a monumental façade, which both protected the entranceway and displayed the epitaph. The few preserved epitaphs reveal that the tombs were constructed and first used by parents and children, and then by their descendents and freedpersons. The interiors of the tombs were finished in white or painted plaster and equipped with benches and altars. Each tomb was designed to accommodate two different modes of corporeal disposal (Fig. 6.3). Some bodies were inhumed in long, narrow compartments (loculi) in the lower zone of the chamber walls. Others were cremated elsewhere, and a selection of incinerated bone was

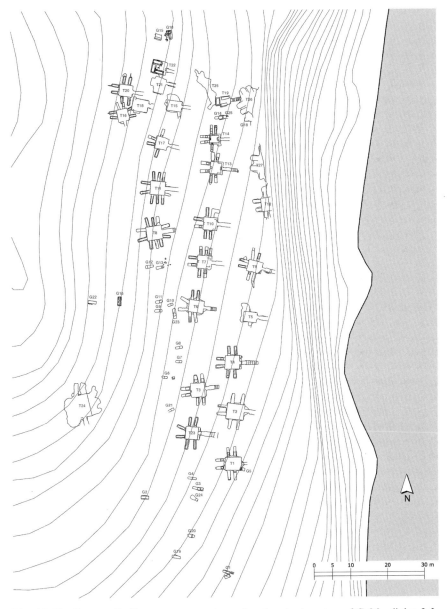

Fig. 6.2 The Koutsongila Cemetery, contour interval = 1 meter (courtesy of C. Mundigler, J. L. Rife, D. Edwards, and M. C. Nelson)

collected in urns, which were deposited in niches in the upper zone of the chamber walls.

The epitaphs and the objects buried with the dead and left by mourners after the funeral indicate that the tombs were primarily used for several generations during

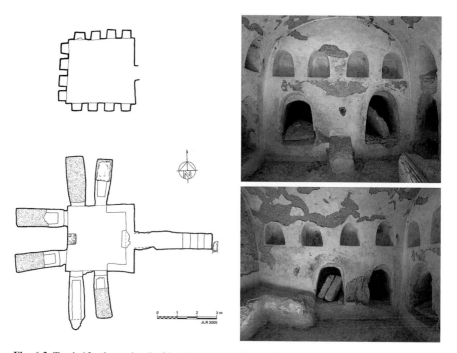

Fig. 6.3 Tomb 13, plan at level of loculi (below left) and niches (above right) and views of west (above right) and south walls (below right) (photo courtesy of J. L. Rife)

the Early Roman period (middle 1st–middle or late 3rd centuries A.D.) There is some evidence that the tombs were subsequently reopened for the continued inhumation of corpses in the loculi during the Late Roman period (ca. 4th–7th centuries A.D.) The monumental scale, rich decoration, and prominent location of these tombs indicate that they originally belonged to a group of elite families in the local community. The identity of later occupants of the tombs is uncertain, but there is no indication that they were either elites or relatives of the earlier occupants.

The Skeletal Assemblage and Its Depositional Context

The development of the skeletal assemblage in the Koutsongila Cemetery from ancient burial until modern study involved several stages of funerary activities and postdepositional disturbance. The initial burials in both the loculi and the niches represent multiple individuals with diverse mortuary treatments during the Early Roman period. Bodies were placed in the loculi, they were covered with a shallow layer of dirt, and the compartments were sealed with large terracotta tiles or limestone slabs, which were removed for the addition of corpses.

Cremated remains were placed in heavy, cylindrical urns, which were then deposited in the niches, though over time the urns were filled with the remains of several individuals. The next stage in the ancient use of the tombs for burial was the addition of corpses during the Late Roman period. Mourners at this time placed bodies over the tiles or slabs covering the loculi, but they might have also displaced, removed, or destroyed the long-since skeletonized remains of individuals interred during the Early Roman period. Thus, when the tombs were last used for burial in Late Antiquity (ca. 6th–7th centuries A.D.), they contained numerous individuals buried in separate periods, and the skeletal remains that had accumulated in confined burial spaces were already commingled and fragmentary.

Over the centuries following these funerary activities, both environmental and anthropogenic processes have affected the state of the skeletal assemblage. Water has continuously entered the chambers, loculi, and niches through the porous calcareous strata into which the tombs were cut, sometimes transporting fine sediment into burial contexts and stimulating the invasive growth of sinuous pine roots. Small rodents (mostly mice and rats) and terrestrial snails (mostly turriculate and discoid species) have also burrowed into burial contexts and nested there. These persistent natural conditions have encrustated bones and teeth with clay, caused superficial deformation and structural decay, and moved bones from their original locations.

Clandestine activity has had a greater impact on the skeletal assemblage. Looters have been active in the Koutsongila Cemetery probably since antiquity, but they have been especially active since the 1960s. Because they are chiefly seeking intact pottery and jewelry, the looters enter loculi, sometimes dislodge or remove covering tiles or slabs, and move the skeletal remains to the side. In this hasty and random operation, they use their hands, small picks, or trowels to dig through and scour the fill. As a result, the bones in the lower compartments have become well-mixed, cancellous tissues, and thin regions have broken down, and large elements, such as innominates and long bones, have repeatedly fragmented. Looters have had a lesser impact on the remains in the upper compartments, which they tend to avoid, because cremation burials at Kenchreai seldom (if ever) contain funerary artifacts. Few niches, however, have been found to contain either cremated bones or urns. This is apparently because the sturdy urns were often removed for secondary use elsewhere, and their contents were either poured out in the niches or onto the chamber floors. Cremated remains left in the niches often ended up on the chamber floors in any event, because they were either swept there by looters or thrown there during seismic ground shaking. Despite the anthropogenic disturbance of both niches and loculi, it seems that the commingling of human remains has occurred only within burial compartments. Looters have not moved remains from one loculus to another, or from the niches to the loculi. Thus, all bones and teeth found in single niches and loculi were deposited in those compartments during the Early or Late Roman period.

Analysis of the Commingled Human Remains

On account of their complexity and history, the tombs in the Koutsongila Cemetery present interesting challenges for the assessment of commingled human remains. In 2004 and 2005, the authors examined the spatial distribution of commingled bones *in situ* in one tomb (no. 13) and identified the skeletal remains recovered from an adjacent tomb (no. 14) with an identical history of use and a comparable depositional environment. These studies were particularly challenging, because of the narrowness of the burial compartments, the density of the commingled deposits, and the fragmentary state of the skeletal remains. The research objectives were to reconstruct the arrangement of the bodies when deposited; to understand better the activities surrounding the deposition of bodies; and to trace the demographic structure of the skeletal assemblage both within a tomb's individual compartments and within the entire tomb.

Spatial and Skeletal Analysis in Tomb 13

The close investigation of the distribution and character of commingled bone found in the loculi of Tomb 13 has shed light on mortuary behavior at Roman Kenchreai. J. L. Rife and Dhruva Jaishankar have studied the spatial distribution of separate anatomical elements among the human remains found over the stone coverings of two loculi, numbers I and V, which appeared most suitable for analysis (Jaishankar and Rife 2004). The deposits were comprised of thinly spread strata of highly fragmentary bone with almost no intervening soil matrix (Figs. 6.4 and 6.5). The commingled remains over the cover in Loculus I included 10,260 fragments weighing 2,250 grams (locus T13-033), while those over the cover in Loculus V included 8,302 fragments weighing 1,690 grams (locus T13-039). Each deposit was divided into 18 roughly square grids that filled the irregular interior space of the loculus. Then the skeletal remains were collected and identified by grid. The locations and dimensions of these grids (25 by 25 centimeters in Loculus I; 25 by ca. 35 centimeters in Loculus V) permitted a high degree of spatial control in tracking the distribution of anatomical elements within each burial context. A large majority of the fragments in each case were too small to identify with precision, but most of these fragments represented long bones and ribs. Numerous fragments from the axial and appendicular skeleton were, however, identifiable.

When the commingled remains from the two contexts were identified and plotted, several noteworthy patterns emerged. First, numerous bones from the hands and feet were found in both loculi. This demonstrates that the commingled remains were not secondary deposits, in which case one would expect a high frequency of major skeletal elements but a low frequency of minor ones. Second, both graves contained the remains of multiple individuals, at least three adults and one subadult in Loculus I and at least one adult in Loculus V. All of these individuals might have been placed in the compartments over the covers during the Late Roman period, well after the

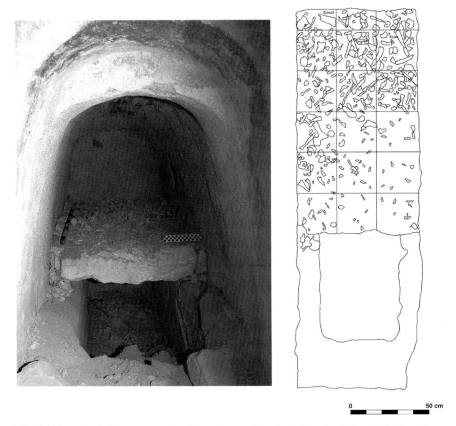

Fig. 6.4 Commingled human remains above the covering tiles in Loculus I, Tomb 13: photo from south and plan showing grids (photo courtesy of D. Jaishankar and J. L. Rife)

initial use and final closure of the cists in the loculi during the Early Roman period. Third, the distribution of anatomical elements across the loculus broadly indicated the original position of the corpses in Loculus V. Almost all fragments of the cranial vault and teeth were located near the back, which suggests that bodies were interred head first, probably supine and extended, according to conventional practice at the time. While natural processes and looting have broken bones and moved them, here the commingled remains seem to have migrated only short distances from their original positions. Loculus V also contained a substantial amount of cremated bone (852 fragments weighing 1,010 grams), which was scattered across the cover slabs. Since cremation was not practiced in Late Roman Greece, these remains might well represent a final deposit of incinerated matter over the covering in the Early Roman period. This deposit was then disturbed and spread out when bodies were deposited on the same slabs at a later date.

Finally, it is striking that 21 permanent teeth and scattered fragments of cranial vaults but no facial or mandibular remains were found among the identifiable

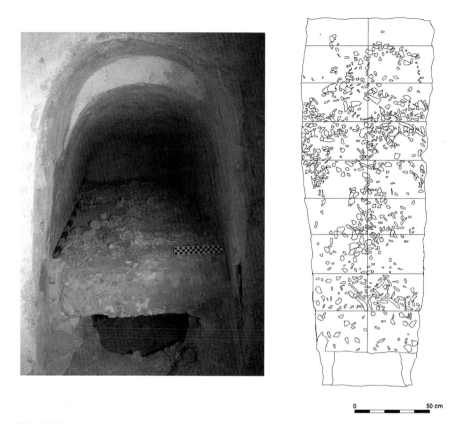

0   50 cm

Fig. 6.5 Commingled human remains above the covering tiles in Loculus V, Tomb 13: photo from north and plan showing grids (photo courtesy of D. Jaishankar and J. L. Rife)

remains in Loculus I which represent all other parts of the human anatomy with relatively high frequency. Considering the durability of several osseous structures in the facial and mandibular regions, it seems unlikely that their absence is attributable to decay by environmental agents. One explanation is that the remains of skulls were preferentially removed from the loculi by mourners during the Late Roman period or the subsequent Byzantine era (ca. 7th–15th centuries A.D.). The handling and selective extraction of skeletonized bones from earlier burials was a widespread practice in the region during Late Antiquity and the Byzantine Middle Ages (Rife in press-b). Greeks during this time removed tractable bones, especially long bones and skulls, from preexisting burials for reburial or storage, because they considered them to be inherently valuable possessions that could preserve the memory or power of the deceased. This mortuary behavior seems to have been a popular corollary to the preservation of saints' relics, particularly bones, by the Greek ecclesiastical community (Meinardus 1970).

Skeletal Analysis in Tomb 14

The identification of all commingled remains from one typical chamber tomb (no. 14) has provided a more complete picture of the demographic profile and skeletal biology of several individuals representing subsequent generations of use. This study by Douglas H. Ubelaker shows how skeletal analysis can be coupled with careful archeological excavation to maximize the information derived regarding the number of individuals and their demographic structure. All commingled remains from Tomb 14 were recovered and studied as total samples of the surviving remains from the individual niches, from the individual loculi, from one anomalous burial compartment in the southeast corner of the chamber, and from stratified contexts on the chamber floor associated with neither niches nor loculi. Few bones in this tomb escaped disturbance by looters, who caused extensive commingling of remains within burial compartments. Therefore, the grid system and spatial analysis used in Tomb 13 was not applicable to Tomb 14. Instead, the human remains within separate loculi were collected in two samples, one representing everything inside the cist and the other representing everything above the cover. The following results of the skeletal analysis first retain this division of samples within the tomb and then combine data for overall tomb interpretations and comparisons of the contents of niches and loculi.

T14-046: Niche A

Only 5 grams of adult size bone fragments are present. Recognizable bone fragments include those from an innominate and long bone diaphysis. Age at death can only be estimated generally from bone size at greater than 6 years. No reliable estimate of sex can be made. Evidence of burning is confined to one cortical long bone fragment, which displays slight calcination and transverse fracturing, suggestive of burning in the flesh (Ubelaker 1999).

T14-047: Niche B

The sample weighs 205 grams. Adult-size bone fragments originate from long bones and the following others that could be recognized: scapula, left temporal, mandible, innominate, thoracic vertebra, right fifth metacarpal, one proximal hand phalanx, one middle hand phalanx, one first metatarsal, two proximal foot phalanges, one distal foot phalanx, and two left ribs.

Two subadult bones are also present: an unburned complete left clavicle and the sternal end of a rib. These likely originate from a child between the ages of 3 and 8 years.

Both burned and nonburned bones are present. The nonburned adult bones include the metacarpal and ribs. Calcined bones include the thoracic vertebrae, mandible, and most of the other fragments.

A lower left rib fragment displays evidence of healed fracture. The fracture is located on the lateral side of the rib, not on the head, neck, or sternal extremity.

T14-049: Niche D

Only one bone fragment is present, weighing less than 5 grams. No heat-related alterations are present, but due to fragmentation and small size it is not clear if it originates from human or nonhuman animal.

T14-050: Niche E

The sample weighs approximately 10 grams. The adult-size fragments originate from long bone diaphysis, a distal ulna, and ribs. A general age at death of 18 years or greater is likely. No reliable estimate of sex can be made. Calcination is confined to one long bone cortical fragment.

T14-051: Niche G

This 5-gram sample consists of one fragment of nonbone material, small cortical diaphysis fragments, and some fragments of cancellous bone. No reliable estimate of sex can be made. Bone morphology suggests the fragments originate from an individual of age 6 years or greater. No diagnostic evidence of burning is present.

T14-052: Niche H

This 25-gram sample contains one nonbone fragment and additional fragments of human origin. Recognizable bones include a cervical vertebra, distal ulna, ribs, and cranium. No reliable estimate of sex can be made. The extent of bone formation, bone morphology, and osteophytosis suggest an age at death between 18 and 35 years.

Fragments of a long bone diaphysis, a probable ulna, and a probable malar show evidence of calcination in the flesh (warping, transverse fracture patterns, etc.). All other fragments show no evidence of heat-related changes.

T14-053: Niche I

Only six fragments weighing approximately 5 grams are present. Of these, five represent nonbone material. One fragment represents bone, but of undetermined species.

T14-054: Niche J

This sample weighs approximately 80 grams. Recognizable adult bone fragments originate from the right clavicle, an innominate, a proximal hand phalanx, capitate, a right third metatarsal, a first metatarsal, and a coccygeal vertebra. The bones appear to be of adult origin (greater than 18 years), but no reliable estimate of sex can be made.

Two bone fragments are present originating from a child likely between the ages of 3 and 6 years. These fragments originate from a second cervical vertebra and a left rib.

Although most of the fragments are not burned, some evidence of heat exposure is present. Three cranial fragments and two long bone fragments are calcined. In addition, a capitate, two long bone fragments, and the two fragments from the immature individual show evidence of charring.

One fragment from the posterior aspect of a first metatarsal displays two areas of alterations consistent with sharp force trauma. No evidence of antemortem bone response in association with the linear cuts is present. The internal cut surface is slightly lighter in color than the unaffected external bone surfaces, suggesting the alteration has considerable antiquity but was made postmortem (Ubelaker and Adams 1995).

T14-055: Niche K

This sample weighs approximately 50 grams. Fragments of adult morphology are present representing the cranium, innominate, long bones, ribs, mandible, a middle hand phalanx, and a right fifth metatarsal. No reliable estimate of sex can be made. Age at death was likely 20 years or greater.

Fragments originating from a subadult are also present. Recognizable bones include a distal humerus, rib, and tarsal bone. An age at death of about 2 years is suggested by bone morphology.

Evidence of calcination is apparent on fragments originating from the cranium, innominate, long bones, ribs, and mandible. Charred fragments include those from a rib and middle hand phalanx. Other fragments lack evidence of burning including those originating from the cranium, long bones, ribs, and the fifth metatarsal.

T14-035: Burial in the Southeast Corner

Weight of this sample is only 10 grams. The six fragments present are calcined and originate from both cranial and long bones. No reliable estimate of sex is possible. Bone morphology suggests an age at death likely greater than 8 years.

T14-036: Loculus I Cover

The sample recovered from above the cover weighs 20 grams and shows no evidence of calcination. Adult bones (fragments) present include an innominate, two middle hand phalanges, a first, second, and third cuneiform, the left and right fifth metatarsals, two proximal foot phalanges, four middle foot phalanges, four distal foot phalanges, and one rib. Bone morphology suggests an age at death of 20 years or greater.

Also present is one subadult tooth. The permanent mandibular first or second molar displays one third crown formation, which suggests an age at death of either 1 year (if it represents a first molar) or about 5 years (if it represents a second molar).

T14-037: Loculus I, Cist

The sample weighs 1,820 grams. Fragments from the following bones were recognized: two left and two right humeri, two left and one right radius, two femora,
two tibiae, two right fibulae, one left and one right clavicle, one left and one right
scapula, one left and one right temporal, one left and two right sides of the mandible,
one left and one right innominate, one left and three right patellae, two first cervical
vertebrae, three other cervical vertebrae, six thoracic vertebrae, one lumbar vertebra,
one coccyx fragment, one left and one right navicular, one left and one right lunate,
one left and one right triquetral, one pisiform, two left and one right greater multangular, one right lesser multangular, two left and two right capitates, one left and
two right hamates, two left and two right first metacarpals, two left and three right
second metacarpals, three left and two right third metacarpals, one left and three
right fourth metacarpals, one left and one right fifth metacarpal, 20 proximal hand
phalanges, 21 middle hand phalanges, 15 distal hand phalanges, two left and two
right calcanei, two left and two right tali, one left and one right cuboid, two left and
one right navicular, one left and three right first cuneiforms, two left and one right
second cuneiforms, two left and one right third cuneiforms, one left first metatarsal,
three left and two right second metatarsals, two left and one right third metatarsals,
one left and three right fifth metatarsals, five proximal first foot phalanges, 22 other
proximal foot phalanges, five middle foot phalanges, six distal first foot phalanges,
two other distal foot phalanges, six left and six right ribs, and other bones of the
cranium.

Thirty-seven permanent teeth are present. Of these, nine (eight molars and one
premolar) indicate the presence of at least two adults.

At least two subadults are present in the remains recovered from the cist. The
bones presented include a left radius, left and right tibia, one fibula, right clavicle, right temporal, right maxilla, left and right mandible, left ilium, two left and
one right ischium, one left and two right pubic bones, five ribs, 30 carpals and
tarsals, and 14 vertebrae. Seven deciduous teeth and two forming permanent teeth
are also present. The long bone lengths suggest a slightly younger individual (about
1.5 years) than the two developing permanent teeth (about 3.5 years). Since two
subadults are indicated by duplication of the left ischium and right pubis, perhaps
both ages are distinct and correct.

Of the adults, three individuals are suggested by the right patella, some
metacarpals, the first right cuneiform, and the right fifth metatarsal. Additional
bones suggest the presence of two individuals.

Analysis suggests that at least one of the adults is a female, likely between the
ages of 25 and 40 years. A second adult is also likely of similar age at death, but sex
is not apparent.

Some of the adult fragments show evidence of heat exposure. Calcined remains
are represented by a left ischium, two cranial fragments, a femoral head, and a vertebra. Charred remains consist of two permanent mandibular molars, a calcaneus,
and one vertebra.

Three of the deciduous maxillary incisors display a green color, possibly indicating contact with copper or a similar metal that can produce such stains.

Observations on bone pathology are confined to one healed fracture on the distal end of a proximal hand phalanx.

Loculus I Summary

Total sample weight from the loculus is 1,840 grams. In consideration of the bone representation and age and sex information, the individuals represented in the cover sample could also be represented within the cist. The subadult ages at death are slightly different, but these differences could fall within the range of variation of the timing of tooth development.

Remains from the cover lacked evidence of heat-related alterations, whereas such evidence was present within the cist. However, unburned bone was present within the cist as well, and the sample from the cover was comparatively small.

T-14-038: Loculus II Cover

The total sample weighs 10,035 grams. Most adult bones are represented. The presence of five individuals is suggested by left fifth metacarpals, left calcanea, second metatarsals, right third metatarsals, and right fifth metatarsals. Multiple adult individuals are indicated by most other bones as well. The detailed inventory of adult bones is as follows: three left and four right humeri, two left and two right radii, two left and two right ulnae, four left and four right femora, three left and two right tibiae, two left and two right fibulae, two left and three right clavicles, two left and two right scapulae, one maxilla, one left and two right mandibles, three gladiolus segments of the sternum, three left and three right innominates, four left and four right patella, two first cervical vertebrae, four second cervical vertebrae, 11 other cervical vertebrae, 28 thoracic vertebrae, 14 lumbar vertebrae, 4 sacra, six coccygeal vertebrae, three left and three right hand naviculars, two left and three right lunates, one pisiform, three left and three right greater multangulars, one left and two right lesser multangulars, three left and four right capitates, three left and four right hamates, three left and three right first metacarpals, four left and four right second metacarpals, three left and four right third metacarpals, four left and three right fourth metacarpals, five left and three right fifth metacarpals, 44 proximal hand phalanges, 43 middle hand phalanges, 42 distal hand phalanges, five left and three right calcanea, three left and three right tali, two left and two right cuboids, three left and three right foot naviculars, three left and two right first cuneiforms, four left and one right second cuneiforms, two left and one right third cuneiforms, three left and four right first metatarsals, five left and five right second metatarsals, four left and five right third metatarsals, four left and four right fourth metatarsals, three left and five right fifth metatarsals, 11 first foot phalanges, 43 other proximal foot phalanges, 10 middle foot phalanges, seven distal first foot phalanges, one other distal foot phalanx, three left and two right first ribs, seven left and four right other ribs, and two hyoid bones. Thirty-seven permanent fully formed teeth are present, representing at least two adults.

Subadult bones present consist of the following: left humerus, a femur, one left tibia, two fibulae, two left clavicles, one right scapula, one left temporal, one left and two right mandible halves, one left and one right ilium, one left and one right ischium, two right pubic bones, seven ribs, 71 carpals and tarsals, and 34 vertebrae. Eleven deciduous teeth and eight forming permanent teeth are present.

Adult bone morphology suggests that of the five adults present, at least one male and two females are present and that both young (18 to 35) and older (35 and older) adults are represented.

The bone inventory summarized above suggests that at least two immature individuals are present. Those bones complete enough to allow length estimates suggesting ages at death between 6 months and about 3.5 years. The immature dental evidence all indicates an age at death of approximately 9 years. Thus, the bone inventory considered with the evidence for subadult age indicates at least three subadult individuals are present: one between 6 months and 2 years of age, one about 3.5 years of age, and one about 9 years of age.

The subadult and adult analysis indicates that at least eight individuals are present in the cover sample, five adults and three subadults.

Both burned and unburned remains are present. Approximately 300 grams (3% of the total sample) of bones and teeth were calcined. These included the following bones: scapula, lumbar vertebra, iliac crest area of the ilium, long bone diaphysis, distal fibula, proximal femur, sciatic notch area of a likely male ilium, other pelvic fragments, cranium, distal humerus, and three tooth roots.

Approximately 40 grams (0.4% of total sample) of fragments showed evidence of charring. These fragments included a distal foot phalanx, long bone diaphysis, vertebrae, subadult ribs, and carpals.

The following pathological conditions were noted.

An adult fibula diaphyseal fragment approximately 205 mm in length displays irregular, well-remodeled enlargement of most of its surface, likely indicating antemortem infection.

The lateral aspect of a right clavicle displays extensive well-remodeled abnormal bone deposits on its anterior surface, likely produced by antemortem fracture.

One lumbar vertebra presents extensive osteophytosis, with extreme development on the right inferior surface near the midline.

A left second cuneiform displays irregular bone formation on the posterior aspect of the superior surface, probably representing healed antemortem trauma.

An apparent healed fracture is present on the superior third of a proximal hand phalanx with slight misalignment of the affected segments.

Extensive well-remodeled new bone formation is present on the lateral side of the articular surface of the distal first foot phalanx.

A first rib displays extensive cartilage ossification on its sternal end.

Four rib segments present evidence for antemortem healed fractures; all are well remodeled with extensive new bone formation.

T14-039: Loculus II Cist

This sample weighs approximately 2,710 grams. At least two adults are present as indicated by the following bone inventory: one left radius, two femora, one right tibia, one left and one right fibula, one left and one right scapula, one left and one right temporal, one mandible, one sternum, one right patella, one first cervical vertebra, two other cervical vertebrae, 10 thoracic vertebrae, three lumbar vertebrae, one sacrum, one coccyx, one right navicular, one left lunate, one left lesser multangular, one left hamate, one left and one right first metacarpal, one right fourth metacarpal, 20 proximal hand phalanges, 10 middle hand phalanges, eight distal hand phalanges, one left and two right calcanea, two left and one right talus, two right cuboids, two left and one right navicular, one left and one right first cuneiform, one left second cuneiform, two left and two right third cuneiforms, one left and two right first metatarsals, one left and one right second metatarsal, one left third metatarsal, one left and one right fourth metatarsal, one left and one right fifth metatarsal, one proximal first foot phalanx, six other proximal foot phalanges, one middle foot phalanx, two first distal foot phalanges, one other distal foot phalanx, five left and three right ribs, three hyoid cornu, and cranial fragments.

Twenty-three permanent teeth are present. Two duplicate mandibular first and second molars indicate the presence of two individuals.

All subadult bones present are those of an adolescent. Bones present consist of a right humerus, right femur, two ribs, 30 carpals and tarsals, and four vertebrae.

No reliable estimate of sex can be made due to the fragmentary and incomplete nature of the remains.

An age of death of between 25 and 40 years is suggested for at least one adult by bone formation and the extent of vertebral osteophytosis. The subadult age at death is likely between 12 and 16 years based on the extent of bone formation and epiphysis fusion. One forming permanent third molar is also present with 50% root formation, suggesting an age at death of about 15 years.

The remains are fragmentary but well preserved. Light brown soil is present on most bone surfaces. Some periosteal surfaces display slight erosion reflecting taphonomic influences.

Twelve fragments weighing approximately 20 grams are calcined. The color range of these fragments varies from gray to white, suggesting exposure to extreme heat.

Loculus II Summary

The total Loculus II sample weighs 12,745 grams. The ages at death and the general bone inventories of the adults recovered from the cist and the cover are similar and thus cannot rule out the possibility that some adults may be represented in both samples. Careful comparison of the detailed bone inventories for both samples reveals that at least six individuals are represented in the total sample by the presence of six left calcanea (five in the cover sample and one in the cist sample), six right first metatarsals (four in the cover sample and two in the cist sample), six left and right second metatarsals (five in the cover sample and one in the cist sample), and six right fifth metatarsals (five in the cover sample and one in the cist sample).

Four subadults were detected in the total sample: three (ages 6 months, 3.5 years, and 9 years) in the cover sample and one (age about 15 years) in the cist. The subadult bone inventories for the cover and cist overlap, but the individual ages at death of each of the four subadults present in the total sample are sufficiently distinct to indicate that a minimum of four subadults is present in the total sample.

Remains in both the cover and cist sample show some evidence of burning. Remains showing evidence of heat exposure (calcination and charring) constitute 3.4% of the cover sample and only 0.7% of the cist remains. The higher percentage of heat-altered remains in the cover sample argues against the possibility of past random mixing of the two samples.

T14-040: Loculus III Cover

The cover sample (Fig. 6.6) weighs 5,170 grams. Bones of adult morphology suggest the presence of at least four individuals. The detailed inventory is as follows: two left and two right humeri, one left and two right radii, one left and three right ulnae, two left and three right femora, two left and two right tibiae, one left, one right, and three other fibulae, one left and one right clavicle, two right scapulae, one left temporal, one left maxilla, two mandibles, one sternum, two right innominates, three left and four right patellae, two first cervical vertebrae, eight other cervical vertebrae, 32 thoracic vertebrae, 13 lumbar vertebrae, two sacra, two coccyx bones, two left and three right hand naviculars, three left and four right lunates, two left and two right greater and lesser multangulars, four left and three right capitates, one left and one right hamate, three left and three right first metacarpals, three left and two right second metacarpals, two left and two right third metacarpals, two left and three right fourth metacarpals, two left and one right fifth metacarpals, 33 proximal hand phalanges, 22 middle hand phalanges, nine distal hand phalanges, one left calcaneus, three left and two right tali, two left and two right cuboids, three left and two right foot naviculars, three left and three right fist cuneiforms, two left and two right second cuneiforms, one right third cuneiform, one left and two right first metatarsals, three left and three right second metatarsals, three left and two right third metatarsals, two left and three right fourth metatarsals, one left and one right fifth metatarsal, four proximal first foot phalanges, 14 other proximal foot phalanges, four distal first foot phalanges, four other distal foot phalanges, 13 left and 13 right ribs, and cranial fragments. Thirteen permanent teeth are also present.

Subadult bones present consist of the following: two left and one right humerus, two right radii, one left and one right ulna, two left and one right femur, one left tibia, one right clavicle, one left and one right scapula, one left temporal, one right mandible, one left and one right ilium, one left and one right ischium, two left pubic bones, five left and five right ribs, 37 carpal or tarsal bones, 29 vertebrae, and cranial fragments. Seven deciduous teeth and two forming permanent teeth are also present.

Adult bone morphology suggests the likely presence of one male and two females. Morphological features on two preserved female left pubic bones, in con-

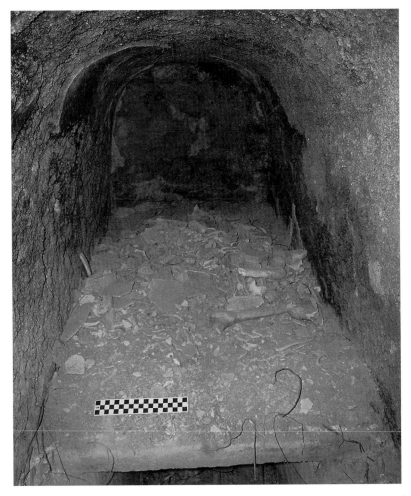

Fig. 6.6 Commingled human remains above the covering tiles in Loculus III, Tomb 14: photo from east (photo courtesy of J. L. Rife)

sideration of other age indicators, suggest ages at death of between 35 and 45 years for one female and 45 to 55 years for the other female. Other age indicators in the adult sample suggest a younger age at death, likely 20 to 30 years for a third individual, sex unknown.

Within the subadult sample, most of the bone and dental evidence is consistent with origin from an individual of about 2 years of age. Some evidence is also present of an older individual likely between the ages of 13 and 20 years. Note that the patellae and carpal bones of this older subadult would appear mature and may be represented as the fourth individual on the adult bone inventory.

Consideration of the detailed bone and dental inventories, as well as the assessments of age and sex, suggests that at least five individuals are represented in the cover sample: three adults (two females ages 35 to 45 and 45 to 55) and one male (probably age 20 to 30) and two subadults, ages 2 years and about 16 years.

Light brown soil is adhering to many bone surfaces, in some cases forming a uniform layer over the periosteal surface. Exfoliation of the periosteal bone surface is apparent on some fragments. No evidence of burning was noted.

One adult proximal hand phalanx displays extensive remodeled bone on the proximal end, likely suggesting antemortem trauma and/or infection.

T14-041: Loculus III Cist

The cist sample weighs approximately 2,800 grams. Adult bones present consist of the left and right humerus, radius, femur, tibia, temporal, innominate, patella, third metacarpal, calcaneus, talus, cuboid, foot navicular, and first metatarsal, three left and two right ulnae, two fibulae, one clavicle, one left scapula, one cervical vertebra, seven thoracic vertebrae, four lumbar vertebrae, one sacrum, three coccygeal vertebrae, one left hand navicular, one right lunate, one right capitate and hamate, two left and two right first metacarpals, one left second metacarpal, two left and one right fourth metacarpals, one right fifth metacarpal, seven proximal hand phalanges, four middle hand phalanges, two distal hand phalanges, one left second cuneiform, one left third cuneiform, one right fourth metatarsal, one proximal first foot phalanx, one other proximal foot phalanx, two middle foot phalanges, four rib fragments, and cranial fragments. Nine fully formed permanent teeth are also present.

The following subadult bones are present: left and right humerus and femur, right radius, left ulna, a tibia, two fibulae, right clavicle, scapula, mandible, ilium, sternum, left ischium, two patellae, three left and six right ribs, 34 carpal and tarsal bones, 13 vertebrae, and cranial fragments.

Within the adults, the large size and robusticity of some remains suggest male sex for one individual. Morphological features on a left ilium suggest female sex.

Within the adult remains, the extent of cranial suture closure, occlusal dental attrition, and other factors suggest an age at death of between 35 and 45 years. Bone morphology and dental features of the subadult remains are consistent with an age at death of approximately 12 years.

The preponderance of evidence suggests that at least three individuals are present in the cist sample: two adults (one male and one female) and one subadult.

Light brown soil is adhering to many of the remains. No evidence of burning is present.

Loculus III Summary

Total sample weight from the loculus is 7,970 grams. The possibility of mixing of individuals between the cover and cist samples cannot be ruled out from this study due to the similarity of ages and sexes within the two samples. The analysis suggests that at least eight individuals are represented within the loculus: five adults and three subadults. Of the adults, three are female and two are male. Ages of the subadults are approximately 2, 12, and 16 years. No evidence of burning was detected within the loculus samples.

T14-043: Loculus IV Cover

The cover sample weighs 2,380 grams. Adult bones represented include the right humerus, two right ulnae, two left and one right femur, one left and two right tibiae, one left and one right fibula, one right maxilla, a mandible, one left and one right innominate, two left and three right patellae, one first cervical vertebra, two other cervical vertebrae, 10 thoracic vertebrae, six lumbar vertebrae, one sacrum, two left and one right hand navicular, two left lunates, one left greater multangular, one left and one right lesser multangular, two right capitates, two left and two right hamates, one left and one right second metacarpal, two right third metacarpals, one left and one right fourth metacarpal, one right fifth metacarpal, 14 proximal hand phalanges, 19 middle hand phalanges, 10 distal hand phalanges, one left and one right calcaneus, two left and two right tali, one left and one right cuboid, three left and one right navicular, two left and three right first cuneiforms, two left and two right second and third cuneiforms, two left and one right first metatarsal, two left and two right second metatarsals, one left and one right third and fourth metatarsals, two left and one right fifth metatarsals, six proximal first foot phalanges, 15 other proximal foot phalanges, five distal first foot phalanges, and rib and cranial fragments. Eighteen permanent fully formed teeth are present as well.

Subadult bones present consist only of the right humerus, right radius, a femur, fibula, left ischium, left calcaneus, 18 carpals and tarsals, and cranial fragments.

Within the adult sample, no reliable estimates of sex or age at death are available, although there is some evidence for the presence of an elderly individual (greater than 50 years). The bone inventory is highly variable, but at least three adults are indicated by right patellae, left foot naviculars, and right first cuneiforms.

Age at death analysis of the subadult remains suggests the presence of two individuals, one with an age at death of about 6 months and a second with an age at death of about 4.5 years.

Although the remains are relatively clean, some light brown soil is adhering to some fragments. Two fragments show evidence of calcination, one from a thoracic vertebra and one from a long bone diaphysis (probably femur).

T14-042: Loculus IV Cist

The cist sample weighs approximately 3,380 grams. Fragments displaying adult morphology originate from the following bones: one left and one right radius, fibula, clavicle, capitate, second and third metacarpals, second cuneiforms, two left and two right femurs, tibiae, first and fourth metacarpals, calcanea, cuboids and all metatarsals, one left and two right humeri, one left and two right ulnae, one left and two right scapulae, one sternum, one left innominate, one first cervical vertebra, three other cervical vertebrae, 12 thoracic vertebrae, seven lumbar vertebrae, two sacra, one left hand navicular, one right lunate, two right fifth metacarpals, 22 proximal hand phalanges, 15 middle hand phalanges, 11 distal hand phalanges, two left and three right tali, two left and one right foot navicular, two left and one right first cuneiform, two left and one right third cuneiform, three proximal first foot phalanges, 12 other proximal foot phalanges, three distal first foot phalanges, seven left and three right ribs, and cranial fragments. Ten fully formed permanent teeth are also present.

Immature bones present consist only of a clavicle, three ribs, one carpal or tarsal bone, and two vertebrae.

Analysis suggests that at least two females and one male are present. An age likely between 30 and 35 years is suggested for one female and between 33 and 40 for the other. Although relatively few subadult bones are present, their variation in size and formation suggests they originate from four individuals of ages less than 6 months (young infant), about 3 years, about 5 years, and about 15 years. This analysis suggests a minimum number of individuals of six for this sample: the two adult females, an adult-size male, which might be presented by the immature clavicle, and the three young subadults (children and infant).

The remains display a coating of light brown soil. Some of the fragments display a thin sedimentary crust on their exposed surfaces. Some fragments also display a slight green stain. No evidence of burning was noted within the sample.

One left fibula (sex unknown) displays a maximum length of 370 mm. This suggests a living stature of about 171 cm if the individual is male and about 169 cm if the individual is female using the formulae of Trotter for Whites (Ubelaker 1999).

Loculus IV Summary

The total loculus sample weighs 5,760 grams. In consideration of the inventory information and the sex and age distribution, it is possible that some individuals are represented in both the cover and cist samples.

Of concern are the few small bones that represented evidence for the third adult in the cover sample. Although it is unlikely these originated from the young subadults in the cover sample, it is possible they relate to the adolescent in the cist sample if commingling between the samples occurred.

Evidence for burning was confined to the two calcined fragments in the cover sample.

T14-045: Loculus V Cover

This cover sample weighs only 300 grams. Recognizable adult bones include the right temporal, left hand navicular, rib, long bone, and cranial fragments. Subadult remains are limited to two arches from cervical vertebrae. No reliable estimate of sex can be made. The extent of cranial suture closure of the adult remains suggests an age at death likely between 30 and 45 years. The immature remains originate from an infant of about 1.5 years of age.

Approximately 120 grams or 40% of the sample is calcined with transverse fracturing and warping. Affected bones include a temporal, long bone, cranial, and rib fragments. The remaining portion of the sample shows no evidence of heat-related changes.

T14-044: Loculus V Cist

The cist sample weighs 1,960 grams. Although the adult remains are fragmentary, the following bones could be recognized: one left and one right humerus, radius, fibula, hand navicular, lesser multangular, capitate, second and third metacarpals, calcanea, first cuneiforms and all metatarsals, one right ulna, scapula, temporal, lunate and greater multangular, one left mandible, patella, talus and foot navicular, two first cervical vertebrae, one second cervical vertebra, five other cervical vertebrae, 10 thoracic vertebrae, three lumbar vertebrae, one sacrum, one coccyx, two left and one right first and fourth metacarpals, one left and two right fifth metacarpals, 13 proximal hand phalanges, eight middle hand phalanges, three distal hand phalanges, two proximal first foot phalanges, six other proximal foot phalanges, one distal first foot phalanx, and rib and cranial fragments. Twelve fully formed permanent teeth are present.

Subadult remains are limited to the left clavicle and one left and one right rib.

Bone morphology suggests that at least two adults are present: one male and one female. Morphology of the female pubic symphysis suggests an age at death of between 35 and 45 years. The few subadult bones present likely originate from a young child of approximately 3 years of age.

The remains display a coating of light brown soil. Calcination with transverse fracturing is present on approximately 25 grams of the sample. Bones showing calcination include a first cervical vertebra and four long bone fragments.

An adult proximal tibia displays a prominent exostosis on its proximal articular surface, likely reflecting antemortem trauma to the area.

Loculus V Summary

The entire loculus sample weighs approximately 2,260 grams. Given the similarity of the age and sex distribution and limited inventory within the cover sample, the possibility cannot be excluded that some individuals could be represented within both samples. The evidence is strong for at least two adults within the entire loculus sample; the possibility of a third adult is dependent upon the extent (if any) of commingling between samples. Calcined bone is present in both samples but more common in the cover sample (40% of the total weight) than in the cist sample (only 1.3% of the total weight).

T14-010 to T14-034: Tomb Floor Outside Loculi and Niches

Material in this sample weighs at least 3,260 grams and presents a combination of calcined bone with transverse fracturing and warping as well as bone showing no evidence of heat-related changes. The material is quite fragmentary, and relatively few bones could be recognized in the assemblage. Those of adult morphology represented at least one young adult, likely between the ages of 23 and 35 years, as well as an older adult likely of greater than 35 years. Estimated ages of the relatively few subadult remains in this sample were about 6 months, about 3 years, about 5 years, and about 10 years. Individuals matching these demographic profiles are well represented in the other samples from within the tomb. No non-age-related bone pathology was noted in this sample. A small quantity of additional fragments from this area had been recovered but had not been sufficiently processed to allow analysis and inclusion in this report.

Tomb 14 Summary

The total weight of the studied Tomb 14 sample is approximately 34,235 grams. Of this amount, 37.2% originated from Loculus II, 23.3% from Loculus III, 16.8% from Loculus IV, 6.6% from Loculus V, 5.4% from Loculus I, 9.5% from outside the loculi and niches, and only 1.2% from the nine niches and the sample from the southeast corner. Of the 30,575 grams of material recovered from loculi, 17,905 grams (58.6%) were recovered from covers and 12,670 grams (41.4%) were recovered within cists. These proportions reveal that the number of individuals buried in the loculi varied considerably. It is significant that Loculi II and III seem to have been the most frequently used, because they are the most centrally located compartments on the back (west) wall facing the entrance. This focal placement in the plan of the tomb seems to have encouraged their preferential use. Moreover, it is clear that little remains in the niches after the removal of the cinerary urns, perhaps for reuse elsewhere, and the displacement of cremated remains. If bodies deposited inside cists represent Early Roman burials and those deposited above the slabs represent Late Roman burials, then it appears that local residents frequently used the loculi for interment during both periods. However, a low degree of commingling between remains interred above and below the coverings is probable. Presumably this has been caused by the forceful displacement of tiles or slabs during looting.

The minimum number of individuals in Tomb 14 is 52. Of these, 30 are adults, 19 are subadults, and 2 individuals are of very uncertain age. This estimate assumes not only that samples from the niches were not commingled with those from loculi, but also that separate loculi were not commingled with each other, as has been proposed. It also assumes that remains found within the tomb but associated with neither the niches nor the loculi could have originated from them. Adults were detected in all samples except Niche G and the burial in the southeast corner. They might have also been present in these two contexts, because extreme fragmentation allowed age estimates of only greater than 6 and 8 years for these two samples.

Ages at death were assigned for all individuals in Tomb 14. Among individuals for whom age was estimated as a range, the mean value of the range was utilized. Among individuals for whom age was estimated as "greater than" a minimal age, the maximum age for the sample was set at 65 and the mean value was calculated within the range established. This approach established the following age distribution for the entire tomb sample: thirteen between birth and 4; three between 5 and 9; one between 10 and 14; three between 15 and 19; three between 25 and 29; four between 30 and 34; four between 35 and 39; 17 between 40 and 44; two between 50 and 54; and one between 55 and 59. The mean age at death for the entire sample is 26.3 years. Although fragmentation limited the ability to assess sex of the remains, analysis suggested that at least five males and nine females are present, all adults. Males were present in Loculi 2 (cover), 3 (cover and cist), 4 (cist), and 5 (cist). The nine females were found in samples from Loculi 1 (cist), 2 (cover), 3 (cover and cist), 4 (cist), and 5 (cist).

This demographic profile corroborates the interpretation based on epitaphic and artifactual evidence that the tombs were used by several generations of families and their emancipated associates during the Early Roman period and then reused for burial in the Late Roman period. Such a protracted burial chronology would lead to the accumulation of numerous corpses of both sexes and all ages. It seems plausible, but it cannot be proven, that individuals buried together inside loculi were closely related to each other, such as spouses, parents and children, or siblings.

Although all samples contained at least some unburned bone, many presented evidence of heat exposure ranging from slight blackening to complete calcination. In addition, four samples (Niche A, Niche H, and Loculus V both cover and cist) presented not only calcination but the warping and transverse fracture pattern that strongly indicates cremation in the flesh. It is possible, if not likely, that other burned remains also were cremated in the flesh, but without the patterns described above, the evidence is not diagnostic. Some evidence of burning was apparent in all samples except Niche G, Loculus I cover, Loculus III cover and cist, and Loculus IV cist. Burning patterns reflect complex factors, including fire heat and duration, the extent of exposure of the remains to direct heat, the size of the fire, and the condition of the remains at the time of exposure.

Of the remains showing traces of burning, all appeared to originate from adults except for fragments of subadults in the Niche J sample and the Loculus II cover sample. Due to the extreme fragmentation and heat-related alterations in morphology, no more exact estimations of age at death are possible for the individuals represented. One adult pelvic fragment from the Loculus II cover sample with evidence of burning displayed morphological characteristics suggestive of female sex. Assuming that the samples from the niches, the loculi, and the southeast corner burial are not commingled, the evidence suggests that the minimum number of individuals represented by burned remains is 15, including 13 adults (at least one female) and 2 subadults.

As documented in Table 6.1, charred and calcined remains comprised a relatively minor component of the total bone assemblage. Of the 34,235 grams of remains present in the entire sample, only about 7% displayed evidence of heat alteration.

Table 6.1 The Weights of Human Remains from Contexts in Tomb 14 Showing the Relative Amounts of Charred, Calcined, and Unburned Remains

Context	Charred		Calcined		Charred and Calcined		Total Weight
	Grams	%	Grams	%	Grams	%	
A	0	0	1	20	1	20	5
B	0	0	175	85	175	85	205
D	0	0	0	0	0	0	5
E	0	0	1	10	1	10	10
G	0	0	0	0	0	0	5
H	0	0	8	32	8	32	25
I	0	0	0	0	0	0	5
J	5	6	8	10	13	16	80
K	10	20	25	50	35	70	50
SE Corner	0	0	10	100	10	100	10
Loc I Cover	0	0	0	0	0	0	20
Cist	25	1	30	2	55	3	1, 820
Loc II Cover	40	< 1	300	3	340	3	10, 035
Cist	0	0	20	< 1	20	< 1	2, 710
Loc III Cover	0	0	0	0	0	0	5, 170
Cist	0	0	0	0	0	0	2, 800
Loc IV Cover	0	0	15	< 1	15	< 1	2, 380
Cist	0	0	0	0	0	0	3, 380
Loc V Cover	0	0	120	40	120	40	300
Cist	0	0	25	1	25	1	1, 960
Total	80	< 1	738	2	818	3	30, 975
Other	73	2	1, 580	49	1, 653	51	3, 260
Total	153	< 1	2, 318	7	2, 471	7	34, 235

Evidence of heat alteration in individual contexts varied from none in seven samples to 100% in the small sample from the southeast corner. Note that all samples presenting evidence of heat alteration contained calcined remains, whereas evidence of charring was lacking from some of these contexts. While it is uncertain how much cremated material has been removed from the tombs, perhaps in cinerary urns, it appears that mourners invested more effort in inhumation in the loculi than in cremation and deposition in the niches. Those who did cremate the dead seem to have burned the corpse shortly after death at high temperatures for a long period, which caused thorough calcination, and in some cases fracturing and warping.

The distribution of cremated remains throughout the tombs is also noteworthy. Cremated bone occurs in small quantities over several coverings in loculi. The traces of cremated remains inside the cists presumably came to rest there when the coverings were disturbed by looters and contiguous, overlying bones were dispersed. The cremated remains left over the coverings might well have been deposited there during the Early Roman period, as has been suggested in the case of Loculus V in Tomb 13. It is unclear why mourners did not place these cremated remains in niches, unless they meant to express and commemorate a special relationship between the inhumed and cremated individuals deposited in single loculi. The fact that most cremated remains from Tomb 14 were found outside burial compartments on the chamber floor supports the scenario noted above, in which cremated remains have been either swept or ejected from the niches, or dumped there before urns were carried from the chamber.

The major taphonomic observations on the commingled remains in Tomb 14 are general structural degradation and the adherence of brown soil to the surfaces of many fragments. These postmortem alterations were caused by a burial environment exposed to water and roots entering through relatively soft, porous limestone. The encrustation of bones in several contexts points to the pooling of water that had washed in from the surface through crevices. The cuts observed on the metatarsal fragment in Niche J were probably produced after death but long before discovery, perhaps by early looters. Two samples (Loculi I cist and IV cist) presented remains with characteristic green stains suggesting contact with copper or a similar metal capable of producing such stains. The excavation of Loculus I cist produced a bronze coin (KC004) that had been placed in or on the mouth of the deceased after the ancient custom of "Charon's obol," or the final fare for the Stygian ferryman (Stevens 1991). The excavation of Loculus IV cist did not produce metal artifacts, but it is an unusually moist burial environment, in which case any bronze objects would have disintegrated before discovery.

Five samples contained remains with non-age-related pathological conditions. These consisted of the rib fracture from niche B, the phalanx fracture in Loculus I cist, the evidence for trauma and/or infection on the proximal hand phalanx from Loculus III cover, and the tibia displaying trauma from Loculus V cist. The Loculus II cover sample presented the most evidence for pathological conditions: a fibula with evidence of infection, a fractured right clavicle, a fractured left second cuneiform, a fractured hand phalanx, evidence of infection in a first foot phalanx, and four fractured ribs. All these conditions reflect conditions suffered antemortem with evidence of bone response, and they were all sustained months if not years before death.

Conclusion

Careful excavation, systematic recovery, and skeletal analysis have greatly enhanced the interpretation of commingled human remains from chamber tombs dating to the Roman Empire at the port of Kenchreai in Greece. Another crucial component in this study was the evaluation of the environmental and anthropogenic processes that have shaped the skeletal assemblage over time from deposition to discovery. The examination of commingled remains from Tomb 13 involved the spatial analysis of skeletal elements by anatomical region. In the investigation of the much larger skeletal sample from Tomb 14, it was possible to assess the full extent of commingling, to establish the minimum number of total individuals buried over time, and to construct a demographic profile by considering the numbers of individual bones and teeth represented and their side, age at death and sex, bone morphology and pathology, the nature of cremation and taphonomic alterations, and archaeological context. This multifaceted approach has shed light on the complex history of mortuary behavior in the Koutsongila Cemetery, including the use of tombs by familial groups, multiple burial by both inhumation and cremation, the placement of corpses, and, possibly, the extraction of bones for ideological reasons. This study also offers a methodological model for the study of similar burial environments involving the long-term accumulation and disturbance of commingled human remains.

Acknowledgments This research was conducted under the auspices of the American School of Classical Studies and with the permission and direct oversight of the Ministry of Culture of the Greek State, as represented by Alexandros Mandis and the staff of the 37th Ephoreia of Classical and Prehistoric Antiquities at Archaia Korinthos. The authors gratefully acknowledge the generous financial support of the Office of the Provost of Macalester College, Dan Hornbach, and the International Catacomb Society of Boston.

References Cited

Jaishankar, D. and J. L. Rife 2004. The taphonomic processes affecting the skeletal assemblage at the Roman cemetery at Kenchreai, Greece. Unpublished technical report, Classics Department, Macalester College.

Meinardus, O. 1970. A study of the relics of saints of the Greek Orthodox Church. *Oriens Christianus* (54):130–278.

Rife, J. L. 2003 Archaeology in Greece 2002–2003: Kenchreai, Koutsongilla. *Archaeol. Rep.* (49):17–18.

Rife, J. L. 2004 Archaeology in Greece 2003–2004: Kenchreai, Koutsongila. *Archaeol. Rep.* (50):16–17.

Rife, J. L. 2005 Archaeology in Greece 2004–2005: Kenchreai. *Archaeol. Rep.* (51):15–16.

Rife, J. L. in press-a Inhumation and cremation at Early Roman Kenchreai (Corinthia), Greece in local and regional context. In *Inhumations in the Roman Empire from the First Until the End of the Third Century A.D.: Proceedings of an International Colloquium*, A. Faber, P. Fasold, M. Struck, and M. Witteyer, eds. Schriften des Archäologischen Museums Frankfurt, 20. Archäologisches Museum Frankfurt, Frankfurt.

in press-b *Isthmia IX: The Roman and Byzantine Graves and Human Remains*. American School of Classical Studies, Princeton, NJ.

Rife, J. L., M. M. Morison, A. Barbet, R. K. Dunn, D. H. Ubelaker, and F. Monier in press Life and death at a port in Roman Greece: The Kenchreai Cemetery Project 2002–2006. *Hesperia*.

Stevens, S. T. 1991 Charon's obol and other coins in ancient funerary practice. *Phoenix* (45): 215–229.

Ubelaker, D. H. 1999 *Human Skeletal Remains, Excavation, Analysis, Interpretation*, 3rd ed. Manuals on Archeology, 2. Taraxacum, Washington, DC.

Ubelaker, D. H. and B. J. Adams 1995 Differentiation of perimortem and postmortem trauma using taphonomic indicators. *J. Forensic Sci.* 40(3):509–512.

Chapter 7
Anthropologist-Directed Triage: Three Distinct Mass Fatality Events Involving Fragmentation of Human Remains

Amy Z. Mundorff

Introduction

Identifying victims from mass fatality events requires the synchronization of several processes including, but not limited to, recovery, antemortem information collection, mortuary processes, death certification, family assistance, and finally, repatriation. This chapter will discuss one small aspect of the mortuary process, triage, and its interplay with other aspects of the process of identifying highly fragmented remains. Specifically, this paper will focus on anthropologist-directed triage and how it differed during the World Trade Center (WTC) disaster, the crash of American Airlines Flight 587 (Flight 587), and the crash of the Staten Island Ferry. Each of these incidents involved significant variation in the number of victims, the number of recovered human remains, their degree of fragmentation, site characteristics, and recovery processes. Each of these considerations affected the triage teams' composition and duties.

Triage

The Oxford English Dictionary defines triage as "the actions of sorting according to quality", "to pick, cull, ... the assignment of degrees of urgency ... in order to decide the order or suitability of treatment ..." (1989). The term "triage" was commonly used in the early 1700s when describing the sorting of wool in degrees of fineness and quality. The military has also used triage to rank injured personnel in accordance to the seriousness of their injuries, ensuring the most critically injured are treated first. As applied in this chapter, the term "triage" encompasses the first assessment human remains receive once they have been recovered and transported to a mortuary or temporary mortuary facility. Actions performed during the triage examination can differ greatly depending on event characteristics. But the central feature in any mass disaster triage situation involves sorting, or culling, material useful in identification from material that is not.

The triage station is usually the first stage of the mortuary process in high-fragmentation mass fatality events (Mittleman et al. 2000). Traditionally, an

From: *Recovery, Analysis, and Identification of Commingled Human Remains*
Edited by: B. Adams and J. Byrd © Humana Press, Totowa, NJ

anthropologist or pathologist directs triage, depending on the disaster type and the condition of the remains. The triage team is empowered to sort out commingling, identify and discard nonhuman remains, rearticulate or reassociate disparate pieces within a body bag, and anatomically identify fragments for later examination. Because an in-depth understanding of human skeletal anatomy drives all of these activities, triage of fragmented remains is most effective when directed by an anthropologist (Byrd and Adams 2003; Levinson and Granot 2002; MacKinnon and Mundorff 2006; Rodriguez 2005).

Every disaster is unique, and each incident's individual characteristics will determine triage team composition, how it functions, and where it is integrated into the identification process. Characteristics directly influencing the triage process include the number of deceased, degree of fragmentation, and taphonomy of skeletal elements recovered (Alonso et al. 2005; Leclair et al. 2004; Rodriguez 2005). It is well recognized that site characteristics, recovery-induced commingling, trauma inflicted by digging activities, and improper and unscientific recovery techniques complicate mortuary analysis (Egana et al. 2005; Sledzik and Kontanis 2005; Tuller et al. 2005). These are some of the problems that are recognized and addressed during triage.

The Three Disasters

In each of the three disasters, human remains were first collected at the disaster scene and transported to the OCME in Manhattan for processing and identification. Upon reaching the Medical Examiner's Office, remains from all three incidents were examined at a triage station, which was directed by a forensic anthropologist. This was an important first step in the lengthy identification process. Significantly, the unique characteristics of each mass fatality required that the anthropologist's role at triage be tailored to that specific incident (Table 7.1).

World Trade Center

At 7:59 on the morning of September 11, 2001, American Airlines Flight 11 left Boston's Logan International Airport en route for Los Angeles, carrying 81 passengers, 2 pilots, and 9 flight attendants. The aircraft was hijacked shortly after departure, diverted to New York City, and flown into the North Tower of the World Trade Center between the 94th and 98th floors at 8:46 a.m. Hundreds of people were killed immediately and hundreds more remained trapped. At 8:14, United Airlines Flight 175 also left Boston's Logan International Airport bound for Los Angeles, with 56 passengers, 2 pilots, and 7 flight attendants on board. This plane was also hijacked shortly after departure, was also diverted to New York City, and was flown into the South Tower of the World Trade Center between the 77th to 85th floors. Again, hundreds of people were killed instantly and hundreds more remained trapped.

Table 7.1 Factors Influencing Triage Protocol for Each Disaster

World Trade Center	American Airlines Flight 587	Staten Island Ferry
Open population	Closed population	Open population
2,749 Victims	256 Victims	11 Victims
~20,000 Fragments recovered	~2,100 Fragments recovered	~35 Fragments recovered
8 Months recovery duration	Days recovery duration	Hours recovery duration
Recovery personnel untrained in forensic arch/anthro	Recovery personnel mixed with medicolegal trained staff	Recovery personnel directed by medicolegal staff
Buried site, heavy machinery used	Surface recovery	Surface recovery
Unlimited resources	Unlimited resources	Unlimited resources
High Type 1 (recovery) commingling	Medium Type 1 commingling	Low Type 1 commingling
High Type 2 (disaster) commingling	Low Type 2 commingling	No Type 2 commingling

According to *The 9-11 Commission Report*, on September 11, New York City and the Port Authority of New York and New Jersey mobilized the largest rescue operation in the city's history (2004). At 9:58 a.m., less than one hour after impact, the South Tower collapsed in approximately 10 seconds, killing all remaining civilians, first responders, and emergency personnel who were still trapped inside. At 10:28, 102 minutes after impact, the North Tower also collapsed. Again, all remaining individuals in the building, except for 12 firemen, 1 Port Authority police officer, and 3 civilians, were killed.

Two thousand seven hundred and forty-nine victims lost their lives in the September 11, 2001, World Trade Center disaster. Five years later there have been 20,730 fragments of human remains recovered from the disaster site and the landfill operation. Identification efforts with these remains have led to the accounting of 1,598 of the victims, or 58% of the missing. Because many remains were either completely pulverized in the towers' collapse or consumed in the fires that burned at the site, there are victims of whom nothing is likely to be recovered. As of September 11, 2006, 10,933 of the recovered fragments have been identified, approximately 53%, leaving 9,797 fragments unidentified. As of this writing, the identification process continues and these numbers are likely to change.

After recovery, the initial sort of human remains takes place at the triage station. This sorting becomes increasingly complicated as the number of victims and their degree of fragmentation increases (Rodriguez 2005). The World Trade Center disaster is by far the most complicated of the three disasters to be discussed. As previously mentioned, there were 2,749 victims and over 20,000 fragments of human remains. This number does not include thousands of nonhuman remains that were recovered but discarded.

The World Trade Center site characteristics presented unprecedented challenges to recovery personnel. Because the remains were not scattered across the landscape, as often seen with aviation accidents, but were buried within the debris of 7 destroyed buildings covering over 16 acres, Ground Zero might best be analogized to a typical buried archaeological site. The debris mound, often referred to as "the pile," stood 70 feet above ground and was later excavated 70 feet below ground. And like an archaeological site, all of the excavated debris was sifted to recover artifacts, or in this case, human remains. Excavating Ground Zero took approximately 8 months and workers spent an additional month to finish sifting through the debris sent to the Staten Island Landfill.

American Airlines Flight 587

On November 12, 2001, American Airlines Flight 587 crashed into a residential neighborhood in Queens, New York, approximately 90 seconds after takeoff from John F. Kennedy International Airport. The flight, en route to Santo Domingo, Dominican Republic, held 251 passengers, 7 flight attendants, and 2 flight crew members. All were killed, as were an additional five people on the ground. According to the National Transportation Safety Board,

> The probable cause of this accident was the in-flight separation of the vertical stabilizer as a result of the loads beyond ultimate design that were created by the first officer's unnecessary and excessive rudder pedal inputs. Contributing to these rudder pedal inputs were characteristics of the Airbus A300-600 rudder system design and elements of the American Airlines Advanced Aircraft Manoeuvring Program. (NTSB 2004)

The crash of American Airlines Flight 587 occurred 2 months and 1 day after the World Trade Center disaster. Already on high alert for terrorism, the City of New York responded quickly with a wide variety of personnel from the Police Department, Fire Department, Port Authority, FBI, and the Medical Examiner's Office. Initially, the crash was thought to be related to terrorism, and law enforcement personnel were assigned to recover the human remains. The remains and airline wreckage were scattered over several blocks, destroying four homes and damaging six others. Due to the easy accessibility of the crash site, all of the approximately 2,100 fragments of human remains were recovered within days.

Taphonomically, the remains recovered from the crash of American Airlines Flight 587 differed drastically from the WTC remains. American Airlines Flight 587, with 256 victims, involved approximately 2,100 fragments of human remains. Although the victim-to-remains ratios between Flight 587 and the World Trade Center disaster were very close—approximately 7.5 remains recovered for every victim—the disaster sites, recovery periods, and condition of the remains differed substantially (Brondolo 2004). In contrast to the remains at Ground Zero, Flight 587 remains were not buried, but scattered on the surface, destructive machinery was not used in recovery, and the remains suffered little secondary damage. Also, where the WTC excavations lasted months, this collection took days, and the fuel-induced fires at this crash site burned for hours, not months as at Ground Zero. Finally, the short recovery period meant that decomposition did not set in as it did during the prolonged World Trade Center disaster recovery. All of these factors directly affected triage protocols and identification success rates.

The Staten Island Ferry Crash

On October 15, 2003, the Staten Island ferry *Andrew J. Barberi* ploughed into pier B-1 killing 11 passengers. Although this ferry carries up to 6,000 passengers, the accident occurred before evening rush hour and only an estimated 1,500 passengers and 15 crew members were on board. With an annual ridership of 19 million, the Staten Island Ferry is second only to Seattle, Washington, as the largest U.S. urban ferry operation. That day, the ferry made its standard 5.2-mile trip from Manhattan to Staten Island, a trip that usually takes about 21 minutes traveling at approximately 15 knots (NTSB 2005).

The National Transportation Safety Board investigation concluded that the probable cause of this accident was "the assistant captain's unexplained incapacitation and the failure of the New York City Department of Transportation to implement and oversee safe, effective operating procedures for its ferries. Contributing to the cause of the accident was the failure of the captain to exercise his command responsibility over the vessel by ensuring the safety of its operations" (NTSB 2005).

The Staten Island Ferry crash will be the third mass fatality event discussed and contrasted. This incident involved 11 fatalities, approximately 35 fragments, and 10 near-complete bodies. These remains were recovered within a few hours, this time under the direct guidance of medicolegal staff from the Office of Chief Medical Examiner, NYC. This was also a quick recovery of predominantly surface-scattered remains. This incident involved substantially fewer victims and a lower victim-to-remains ratio (approximately 3.5 remains recovered for every victim) than the other two incidents profiled in this chapter. Reflecting this reality, the subsequent triage process was comparatively simple. Unlike the remains from Flight 587, these were not burned. Additionally, because they were relatively recognizable, were not buried or decomposed, and were not as severely fragmented or commingled, they shared more taphonomic similarities with the Flight 587 remains than with those of WTC.

The World Trade Center Disaster

Open vs. Closed Population and DNA Testing Decisions

Often, mass disasters are categorized as either having a closed population, where the number and names of the victims involved are known, or an open population, where this information is not available. The crash of American Airlines Flight 587, with a passenger list, was considered a closed population, while the Staten Island

Ferry crash was considered an open population. The World Trade Center disaster was both. Although investigators were provided passenger manifests for the two planes that hit the buildings, as well as rosters of other probable victims, the actual number and names of the victims in the towers remained unknown. The process of generating an accurate missing persons list with an open population is slow and complicated, and it took nearly 3 years to compile a final fatality list for the WTC disaster (Brondolo 2004). In light of the unknown number of victims and the degree of fragmentation, the Chief Medical Examiner, Dr. Charles Hirsch, decided to DNA-test every piece of human remains no matter how small. Establishing this standard assured that no possible victim profile would be missed. Fulfilling this standard necessitated an exacting triage process, requiring the detection and dissection of small bone fragments that had become embedded in other fragmented remains.

The decision to DNA-test every fragment was unprecedented. Investigators in mass fatality incidents generally do not DNA-test every fragment and criteria, for determining which pieces to test varies from incident to incident (Holland et al. 2003; Hsu et al. 1999; Meyer 2003; Mittleman et al. 2000; Olaisen et al. 1997). In an incident with an open population, such as the London Underground bombings of July 7, 2005, investigators considered both the remains' size and relative identifiability when deciding which fragments to sample. In that incident, if a fragment was less than 5 square centimeters and unrecognizable, it was not tested for DNA (Roberts, personal communication). As a result, approximately half of the recovered remains were sampled. Similarly, investigators of the September 11 crash of United Airlines Flight 93 in Shanksville, Pennsylvania, an incident with a closed population, also decided that about one-third of the recovered remains were suitable for DNA sampling. Factors that may mitigate against sampling include types of remains known to be unsuitable for testing, such as fat, or the condition of remains, such as those that are calcined or soaked in jet fuel. The criteria for determining which remains are suitable for DNA testing will change over time as the science of DNA technology evolves.

WTC Remains Recovery

Human remains were recovered daily from both Ground Zero and the Staten Island landfill operations. Barges transported debris from Ground Zero to the landfill, where large pieces of building material were separated from the debris, which was spread out in open fields to be sorted. The dirt and other small bits were taken to sifters. In a process that is similar to screening the fill from an archaeological site, this material was shaken through industrial-size screens and sifters until the remaining material was carried onto a conveyor belt (Fig. 7.1). This belt was monitored by individuals who collected each item of human tissue or bone fragment (Warren et al. 2003). Each of these items was bagged separately and transported to the Medical Examiner's Office for processing and identification. This methodical sifting process allowed for individual remains collection, nearly eliminating incidents of

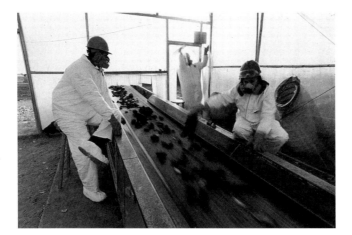

Fig. 7.1 Service members monitoring the conveyor belt for human remains at the Staten Island landfill operation
(*Source*: Rich Press, Copyright © 2001.)

recovery commingling at the landfill. However, the process of excavation, transport, screening, and sifting, along with decomposition, caused articulated elements to become disarticulated from each other. As a result, disparate pieces later had to be reassociated by DNA.

By contrast, the remains received from the disaster site were extremely commingled. Since Ground Zero accounted for most of the recovered remains, this commingling greatly complicated the triage process (MacKinnon and Mundorff 2006).

Commingling from the WTC disaster can be reduced to two primary types. This chapter will refer to Type 1 commingling as that involving remains collected together in one bag, but not attached by hard or soft tissue. Therefore, the commingling is recovery-induced. The potential for this type of commingling has long been recognized, and most recovery operations are equipped to cope with it. An experienced practitioner can easily detect Type 1 commingling by examining the remains to see which pieces are actually attached to each other. When the remains are not attached, the triage team disassociates them. However, another more severe and difficult to recognize type of commingling was also common in the WTC site. Type 2 commingling, which is disaster-induced, was caused by the extreme destructive and explosive nature of the building collapses. The explosive force that blew over fire trucks and peeled stone façades from buildings also disintegrated human bodies, turning bones into flying shrapnel, which became embedded in fragments of soft tissue from other individuals. The tidal wave of debris that carried human remains blocks away, depositing them on top of buildings, also fused soft tissue to bone fragments from multiple individuals so completely that the remains appeared to be from the same individual. This type of commingling is not as easily recognized as the commingling commonly seen in other disaster scenarios. Additionally, the sheer number of fragmented pieces of human remains—nearly 20,000— complicated efforts to resolve both types of commingling.

Site formation processes primarily determined the condition of the remains. These processes include the forces that initially formed the site, manipulation for excavation, as well as transformations over time including decomposition (Schiffer 1987). In the World Trade Center disaster, these initial processes included both primary and secondary events. The primary events that created this "archaeological site" included the impact of the two planes, the collapse of the South Tower, the collapse of the North Tower through the debris of the South Tower, and the subsequent destruction of five additional commercial buildings. Additionally, subterranean fires burned for 12 weeks, water was applied to those fires, and remains decomposed over the 8-month excavation (Fig. 7.2). Often, one or more of these factors are present at a disaster, but rarely, if ever, have they all occurred at one disaster site (Sledzik and Rodriguez 2002). These processes determined the shape and condition of the remains, in turn determining the methods used to process and identify them.

Secondary events also affected the composition of the remains and their condition upon arrival at the Medical Examiner's Office. The site consisted largely of 5,000-pound steel beams mixed with chunks of concrete making a "by hand" deconstruction impossible. Large machinery, including grapplers and cranes, was brought in to assist (Fig. 7.3). In order to place these cranes close enough to "the pile," it was first necessary to create platforms for them, which involved bulldozing and compacting sections of the site. Additionally, as the site was excavated below ground level, a ramp was built to allow excavation equipment to move in and out of "the pit." The material bulldozed for these constructions came from the pile itself and undoubtedly contained human remains. When these platforms and roads were later excavated, human remains were indeed recovered from this debris. This manipulation of decomposing and already fragmented human remains caused further destruction and commingling.

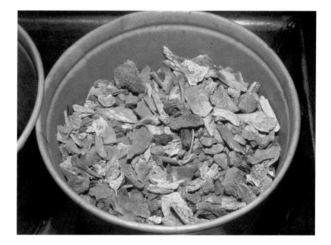

Fig. 7.2 Bucket of completely calcined remains recovered from one of the "hot spots" in Ground Zero that burned for 12 weeks
(*Source*: Office of Chief Medical Examiner, New York City.)

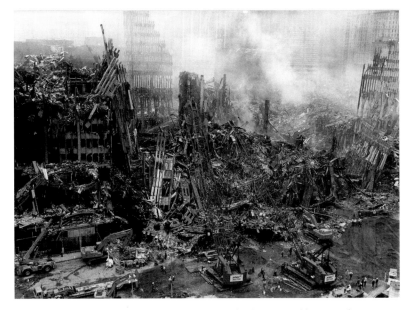

Fig. 7.3 Complicated excavation of Ground Zero showing heavy machinery used (*Source*: Unknown.)

The methods used in recovering individual remains further complicated the identification process and are also characterized as a secondary event. Excavations by untrained personnel and those performed in an unscientific manner affect the recovery process and may cause further commingling (Egana et al. 2005; Sledzik and Kontanis 2005; Tuller et al. 2005). The recovery and excavation of the human remains from Ground Zero was performed predominantly by Fire Department of the City of New York (FDNY) personnel. These individuals are not trained in techniques of forensic archaeology, excavation of human remains, identification or recognition of human remains (especially fragmented ones), or site formation processes. This lack of training complicated the recovery process and allowed for significant additional Type 1 (recovery-induced) commingling. Instead of consigning each piece of remains to a single bag, FDNY personnel filled body bags with potentially unrelated body parts before sending them on to the Medical Examiner's Office. FDNY also lacked knowledge and training on techniques for properly excavating a body found nearly intact yet buried within debris, especially those bodies in an advanced state of decomposition. Once decomposed, the smallest amount of movement or disturbance easily disassociates body parts. These issues can be mitigated with deeper knowledge of human anatomy and the application of forensic archaeological techniques (Blau and Skinner 2005; Skinner and Sterenberg 2005).

Intentional commingling at the site by the recovery personnel also complicated identifications. For instance, upon finding an empty monogrammed fire department bunker jacket during the excavations, FDNY personnel often placed the nearest human remains inside the jacket before transporting it to the Medical Examiner's Office. It seems that in placing these pieces in the bunker gear, FDNY hoped identifications would be accomplished faster and that families would receive "more" of their loved ones because the remains were in a jacket with a name on it. Upon arrival at the mortuary, however, anthropologists immediately detected these reconstructions. Often, these reconstructions were quite obvious, as in leg bones placed in jacket sleeves. In another instance, examination of what appeared to be the nearly complete remains of a fireman fully clothed in bunker gear revealed two left feet, in boots neatly tucked into the bunker pants. The left foot tucked into the right pant leg was clearly not associated with this body yet had been grouped with it at the site during recovery. Although driven by understandable grief and the urge to identify their fallen, reconstruction activities at the site slowed the identification process, causing the triage team to more closely examine, and often separate into multiple cases, body parts found within clothing.

WTC Triage

A temporary mortuary specifically for WTC was set up in the receiving bay of the morgue, allowing regular autopsies to continue in the main autopsy suite. The WTC morgue was constructed to process a high-volume caseload. Two refrigerated tractor-trailer units were placed outside the mortuary, where the remains were held prior to triage, and eight tables were set up in the receiving bay. One table was designated for triage, six were staffed by medical examiners and their examination teams, while one held cases post-triage and awaiting examination. The identification process flowed like an assembly line, from triage to medical examiner to other stations including fingerprint, X-ray, dental, personal effects, and final storage.

Initially, forensic pathologists staffed the triage station. However, within days of the disaster, the management team determined that an anthropologist should direct triage. Two main considerations motivated this change. First, only medical examiners were allowed to fill in death certification forms, and it was important to free them to work the exam tables. Second, the remains were highly fragmented, with soft tissue obscuring obvious anatomic landmarks. This meant it would be advantageous for individuals with a deeper knowledge of osteological detail to identify the elements recovered. Additional factors, such as the substantial amount of nonhuman remains recovered from the destroyed restaurants, also made it advantageous for an anthropologist to direct triage.

The triage team consisted of an anthropologist and up to five assistants. The assistants varied in skills and expertise from OCME employees and medical students, to members of service from the Port Authority Police Department (PAPD), New York Police Department (NYPD), and Federal Bureau of Investigations (FBI) (Fig. 7.4). These law enforcement agencies were incorporated into the identification process both because of the criminal nature of the event as well as the significant number of members of service who had been lost. Their presence during triage allowed them to seize potential items of evidence, collected along with the remains.

Protocols and standards employed in the triage process changed drastically over the eight months of human remains recovery. Initially, the process was as follows:

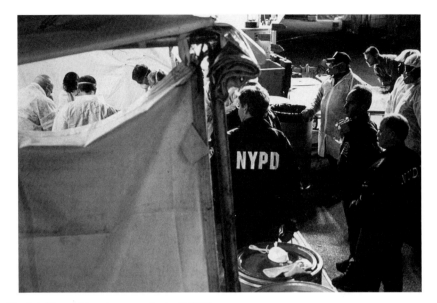

Fig. 7.4 View of the triage team in the OCME mortuary tent
(*Source*: Rich Press, Copyright © 2001.)

A body bag was taken from the refrigerated truck outside the mortuary and brought to the triage table. Before opening a body bag, the triage team located a grid recovery tag, if there was one. After locating the tag, an anthropologist opened the bag and the contents were assessed. Bags from Ground Zero contained a wide variety of material, ranging from a single whole body to dozens of small red biohazard bags each filled with fragments of human remains. Additionally, building material, personal effects, and nonhuman remains were intermingled in these bags. The remains recovered from the Staten Island Landfill operation were bagged individually from the conveyor belt and, therefore, did not require an in-depth triage examination, other than to discard nonhuman remains.

Each bag was examined to eliminate unassociated and unattached parts within the body bag. Every piece·of human remains that was not attached to another by hard or soft tissue was segregated. When such parts were found, they were removed individually, passed to an assistant, and placed in their own bag. Each of these bags became its own case. A case is a single set of human remains that is individually processed for identification and could be as small as a 1-inch bone fragment or as large as an entire body (Fig. 7.5). These new cases, created from the original single body bag they had been recovered with, were also labeled with the accompanying grid location attached to that original bag. These bags were then placed on another table to await medical examiner processing.

Within weeks, a coordination grid was established for Ground Zero, and recovery locations—usually written as a letter and number (e.g., K-10)—were recorded on tags attached to the body bags. If this grid number was attached to a bag, that

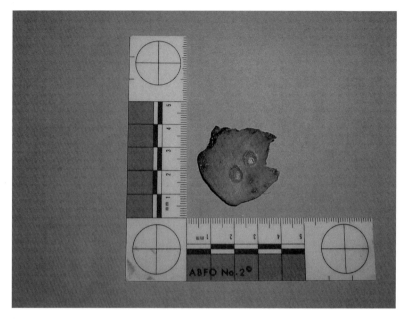

Fig. 7.5 Fragment of distal scapula; one of nearly 5,000 fragments from WTC that were approximately 1 inch or smaller. Note two drilled holes where DNA sample was removed (*Source*: Office of Chief Medical Examiner, New York City.)

locator followed all remains associated with that body bag. Although locator tags indicated from which 75-foot by 75-foot section of Ground Zero the human remains had been recovered, the accuracy and therefore usefulness of that information are uncertain. Depth was not accounted for and a fragment found on the surface of Grid K-12 as well as a fragment found at the bottom of the "pit" in Grid K-12 both received the same location designation, even though there may have been up to 140 feet of variance in depth between the two fragments. Additionally, bulldozing and road construction to assist excavations caused human remains to be moved and deposited outside their original grid location. Triage personnel invested substantial time and effort in transferring this grid locator to all of the bags that were subsequently split out of a single body bag from Ground Zero. Due to the unreliability of the information captured, it is questionable whether this was a good use of time and energy.

Medical Examiner personnel were initially caught off guard by the amount of destruction and fragmentation to the human remains. They simply possessed no theoretical schema to account for the injuries a human body endures in the collapse of a 110-story building. Compounding this, at the beginning of the disaster, the sense of urgency was intense and triage was sometimes bypassed altogether to speed bodies through identification. (Larger body parts that initially bypassed triage in favor of quick identification generally possessed standard identifiers such as fingerprints or dental.) However, within weeks, Medical Examiner personnel came to appreciate the true force of the disaster and the extreme commingling. Because of this, investigators came to believe that small bone fragments were likely embedded in the tissue of body parts that had bypassed triage and that some cases of commingling might have initially gone undetected. The policy of testing each piece of remains made it imperative to retrieve these small fragments, and a secondary review of all of the remains was undertaken by a group of anthropologists. This process, known as the Anthropological Verification Protocol (AVP), detected and corrected instances of commingling that were missed in the initial investigation (Budimlija et al. 2003; MacKinnon and Mundorff 2006). Of the nearly 17,000 cases reexamined, fewer than 100 were found to be commingled, and these were subsequently split into approximately 300 new cases.

In addition to implementing the AVP project, the triage process was strengthened to account for the extensive Type 2 (disaster-induced) commingling. Sorting out this type of commingling is much more complicated than looking for separate pieces within a single body bag. Often pieces of muscle and bone from different individuals can become fused together, mimicking the appearance of a contiguous piece (Rodriguez 2005). During triage it was not uncommon to find skull fragments of one individual deep within another individual's thigh muscle, and rib fragments were frequently found embedded in other body parts. It became clear that bone fragments of multiple individuals could be commingled together into one large tissue mass. Even cases that appeared to be independent body parts frequently had dozens of small bone fragments embedded throughout. This type of commingling also has the potential to bias DNA analysis if the sample taken from the remains inadvertently includes a fragment from a different individual. For this reason, the anthropologist conducting the triage process began sorting out even the smallest fragments of human remains.

Every fragment of bone and tissue was removed and placed in its own bag for individual processing. It was not uncommon for anthropologists to reduce a body bag recovered from Ground Zero into as many as 100 new cases. When the anthropologist believed, based on morphological characteristics, that numerous unattached fragments within a body bag likely belonged to one individual, the new cases triaged out of that bag were grouped together for a single medical examiner to process consecutively and cross-reference. For example, a body bag might contain multiple ribs, all appearing to originate from the same individual—with no overlap in rib number or side—yet unattached by soft tissue because of decomposition. Even if it was thought these all belonged to the same individual, these ribs were not treated as one case and instead each rib was bagged as an individual case. However, all of those case bags were placed into one bin so a single medical examiner could process them consecutively (Fig. 7.6). Upon receiving a grouping of individually bagged remains, thought to be from the same victim, the medical examiner noted a case number cross-reference in the case file of each fragment examined. This notation indicated that, although these were separate case numbers, the anthropologist believed they might belong to the same individual. This information was useful later when some cases that were cross-referenced to each other were identified to the same individual, but other cross-referenced fragments were not. Because there was additional

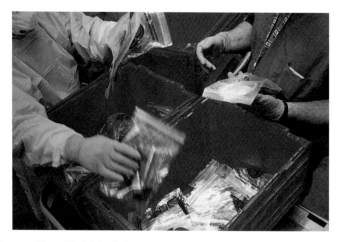

Fig. 7.6 Separate bins of individually bagged remains that will be cross-referenced to each other as groups
(*Source*: Rich Press, Copyright © 2001.)

evidence of association, these fragments could be further targeted for identification. Years later, it appears that many of the cases that were cross-referenced to a primary case have indeed been linked by DNA to that same primary case.

Each of the World Trade Center disaster's individual characteristics shaped the triage protocols established in the mortuary. The number of victims, the number of recovered remains and their degree of fragmentation, and the condition of the remains were all influencing factors. Additionally, the recovery duration, the relative lack of expertise of the recovery personnel, and the recovery techniques demanded a complicated and exacting triage.

Crash of American Airlines Flight 587

The crash of Flight 587 is notable for the relative speed—only 28 days—with which the victims were identified. It is worth noting the factors leading to this rapid identification, especially as contrasted with the lengthy identification process of the World Trade Center disaster. First, this mass fatality incident involved a closed population, meaning a manifest existed documenting each victim's name. (In addition, local residents provided information for those killed on the ground.) This allowed the Medical Examiner's Office to begin collecting antemortem information and facilitated rapid fingerprint and dental identifications. By comparison, it took years to finalize the total number and names of missing persons for the World Trade Center disaster. Second, the remains' size and condition made them easier to identify. Many of the remains from Flight 587 were large enough to autopsy and quickly identify, meaning that some part of the body retained an identification modality that allowed for rapid identification, such as fingerprints or dental. By comparison, the remains from WTC were fragmented into such small pieces (over 5,000 of which were no larger than an inch) that other means of identification were not available, forcing a lengthy DNA identification process. Third, the WTC disaster involved nearly 10 times as many fragments as Flight 587. Finally, because the crash followed closely on the heels of the WTC disaster, the Office of Chief Medical Examiner was already set up to process a major incident.

Victim remains began arriving at the mortuary by late afternoon the day of the crash. Since the cause of the crash was initially unknown, all of the bodies were autopsied. This allowed the FBI to collect evidence to determine if the crash was caused by terrorism and allowed for toxicological testing on the pilot, co-pilot, and passengers. Autopsies were preformed when approximately half of the body was present; of the nearly 2,100 human remains recovered, 305 warranted autopsies. In addition to the fragmentation from impact forces, jet fuel-fed fires caused extensive charring and most of the victims were burned and unrecognizable. However, in contrast to WTC, the Flight 587 fragments were large enough that most were anatomically identifiable. Therefore, identifications relied heavily on fingerprint, dental, and personal effects.

The remains were transported to the Medical Examiner's Office and placed into a refrigerated truck outside the temporary morgue previously constructed to process the World Trade Center remains. Although the same facility was used to triage and process the fragments from Flight 587, the bodies were autopsied in the main autopsy room. The remains were recovered from the crash site in two types of bags. The large body parts—torsos and bodies—were collected in body bags while the fragments were collected in smaller red plastic biohazard bags. Each bag was unloaded individually and brought to the triage station. The triage team consisted of an anthropologist and up to five assistants. The assistants were again personnel from the FBI, PAPD, and NYPD already present at the OCME working on the WTC remains. The anthropologist opened each bag to sort through the contents. Unlike WTC, there were many relatively whole bodies and large body parts with little decomposition. The bodies were given priority over the fragments since they were to be autopsied and were likely to be identified quickly.

Responding to the insight gained from processing the WTC disaster, the OCME had established a strict triage protocol by the time Flight 587 went down. However, this protocol was flexible, allowing modification according to a disaster's characteristics. The Flight 587 triage process was as follows: A single body bag was brought to the triage team and opened. An examination of the remains was performed to determine that everything associated with the body was indeed physically attached by hard or soft tissue. At the crash site, isolated fragments of human remains such as skull fragments, amputated hands and feet, and pieces of fat and soft tissue had been collected along with bodies and grouped into the same recovery body bag (Type 1 recovery-imposed commingling). These additional fragments were removed from the original body bag and placed in their own bags to await processing. If a body bag contained a body lacking a foot due to traumatic amputation and if a foot was also found in the bag, these two items did not automatically remain together. However, if tissue or skin held the remains together, or if the fractured bones conjoined with each other, then the two pieces were kept together. If this standard was not met, the smaller fragment was removed from the body bag, placed into its own bag, and processed with the other fragments after the autopsies were completed.

As compared with WTC, commingling in the Flight 587 remains was easier to recognize and generally resulted from recovery techniques and not the Type 2 explosive commingling discussed above. However, like WTC, rescuers collected multiple unassociated body parts and placed them in the same bag. Type 1 recovery-induced commingling is comparably easy to discern and mitigate during the triage process by separating out unattached and unarticulatable remains. But, unlike WTC, very few nonhuman remains were recovered from the Flight 587 crash site. When it was determined at the triage station that only a single body or body part remained in a body bag, it was zipped shut, the word "triaged" was written on top (Fig. 7.7), and a file containing a case number and all of the paperwork was assigned to the body. A red folder (to differentiate them from the neutral-colored ones used for WTC) in a plastic cover was attached to the top of the body bag, to accompany that body through all of the identification processing stations. As with the World Trade Center, the body part and its corresponding paperwork were then taken through all of the other stations by an escort, usually a member of service. Depending on which part of the body was present, station stops might include X-ray, dental, and fingerprint, all followed by the autopsy.

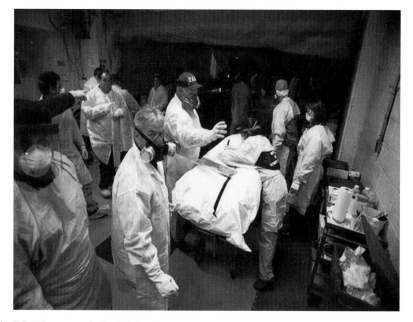

Fig. 7.7 Triage team during Flight 587
(*Source*: Rich Press, Copyright © 2001.)

Once all of the large body bags had been triaged, allowing the autopsies to proceed, the small bags of fragments were triaged under the same protocols. Each bag was opened individually and examined by the anthropologist. Bags containing only a single fragment were closed and placed on the next table to await processing. If the bag being triaged contained multiple fragments, each piece was isolated and placed into its own bag, sealed, and then placed on the next table to await examination and further processing. Dozens of new bags could be created from the contents of a single recovery bag. The anthropologist was empowered to evaluate the fragments for possible reassociation with other fragments within the same recovery bag. However, reassociation of fragments from disparate recovery bags required verification by dental, fingerprint, DNA, or some other means. Since the fragments were processed after the bodies had been autopsied, no attempts were made to physically reassociate fragments to bodies. This would have been logistically impossible, since many of the bodies were identified and released before the fragments were processed. Reassociation of fragmented remains in the Flight 587 and WTC disasters relied primarily on DNA. These reassociation methods differed for the Staten Island Ferry Crash, which will be discussed below.

The autopsies were completed in 7 days, and the approximately 1,800 unassociated fragments were processed in 12 days. Procedures for examination and documentation of these fragments followed protocols developed for WTC, and, as with the WTC disaster, every recovered fragment was sampled for DNA. This is unusual for a plane crash or an incident with a closed population where 100% victim identification can be achieved without testing every fragment. Following triage, each bag was reopened individually and each fragment was assigned its own sequential case number. All of the information relevant to that fragment was documented in the file, including injury patterns, personal effects, a detailed description of the remains, and information about which other stations the fragment visited. For instance, an amputated hand would go to the fingerprint station but not the dental station. The DNA sample was taken during the examination, which enabled the piece to be identified and reassociated to a body if other modalities of identification were lacking, such as dental or fingerprint.

As with every mass disaster, recovery techniques affect how medical personnel process and identify victim remains. This is especially true with fragmented human remains because of the heightened potential for commingling or contamination. As seen with the WTC disaster, the techniques employed in recovering remains increased commingling, which in turn required a very strict triage process, even to the extent of separating remains found within clothing. Remains recovered from Flight 587 endured less Type 1 (recovery-induced) and significantly less Type 2 (disaster-induced) commingling than the remains from the World Trade Center disaster. Additionally, the number of victims, recovery techniques, and characteristics of the site were drastically different and therefore the protocols for triage were modified. The nature of this disaster meant that measures such as cross-referencing and grid locators were not utilized. However, with well-coordinated recovery methods and fewer victims and fragments, the tasks performed during triage again are modified. The crash of the Staten Island Ferry will be the next disaster discussed and will illustrate these differences.

The Staten Island Ferry Crash

The *Andrew J. Barberi* crashed into a concrete maintenance pier south of the docking point at the Staten Island Ferry terminal, which sliced through the front of the vessel (NTSB 2005). Ten people were killed instantly, and one more died later from medical complications. In addition, 70 passengers suffered severe injuries including amputated limbs (NTSB 2005). The vessel's primary impact area was the midship section on the main deck of the New Jersey side. However, as the allision continued, the concrete pier also passed through the passenger cabin. "All of the fatally injured passengers were found on the New Jersey side of the vessel's main deck" (NTSB 2005).

The Staten Island Ferry crash involved relatively few victims and would not normally stress an agency as large as the New York City Medical Examiner's Office. However, several circumstances conspired to dictate that this should be designated as a mass fatality. First, the accident occurred in a public transit area, which meant there was no initial manifest of the victims, making this an open population. Second, because so many of the victims were reasonably identifiable, public and local officials expected speedy identification (Brondolo 2004; NTSB 2005). Third, the ensuing publicity resulted in thousands of inquiries from possible victim families, stressing OCME's internal systems. Finally, a significant number of amputated body parts and unassociated bone and tissue fragments were recovered from the boat and the water. Along with the 10 bodies, approximately 33 bags in total were removed from the site and transported to the Manhattan Office of Chief Medical Examiner. Taken together, these circumstances mitigated in favor of designating this incident as a mass fatality.

Emergency personnel were dispatched to the accident scene within minutes of the event. These included over 300 personnel from New York Police Department (NYPD), 200 from the Fire Department (FDNY), 60 Emergency Medical Service (EMS), 6 Coast Guard vessels, the Army Corps of Engineers, and other rescue and support units. This response even included dive teams, for individuals who might have fallen into the water (NTSB 2005). Along with this massive response, medicolegal investigators (MLIs) from the Medical Examiner's Office arrived on scene to assess the casualties and participate in victim recovery. Following the 9/11 events, OCME MLIs had been working hand in hand with the FDNY and NYPD to streamline the response to mass fatality incidents, and this extensive multi-agency training and communication helped ensure an efficient recovery and identification of the deceased victims.

Emergency personnel recovered several fatalities from the main deck, moving them before the Medical Examiner's team arrived. The rest of the bodies and body parts were recovered over the next few hours by emergency personnel under the guidance of the medicolegal investigators. MLI guidance helped limit the number of fragments placed into a single recovery bag (Type 1 commingling). This reduced commingling and contamination and ensured proper labeling of the recovery location for each individual remain. Even when found in close proximity, fragments that were not physically attached were placed in separate bags. However, this did not negate the need to stringently triage all remains when they reached the mortuary. It is impossible to accurately assess commingling at a disaster site, especially Type 2, or disaster-imposed commingling, which is often deeply embedded into tissue masses and difficult to see. Upon further examination in the mortuary, especially with radiography, fragments thought by recovery personnel at the scene to be intact, comprising only one individual, have been shown to be commingled (Viner et al. 2006).

The victim's bodies and recovered body parts began arriving at the Manhattan mortuary early in the evening on the day of the accident. Because the victims were mostly recognizable (9 of the 10 bodies), the Chief Medical Examiner decided to have the medical examiners perform a preliminary analysis of the victims, that evening, for identification purposes only. The complete autopsy and examination of the bodies and associated fragments took place the following morning.

The following morning, the victims were laid out in the autopsy room, most suffering serious blunt force injuries, traumatically amputated limbs, eviscerated torsos, and massive head trauma. In addition to the 10 bodies receiving autopsies, bags of unassociated body parts including amputated limbs, organs, skull fragments, and pieces of fat and soft tissue were also brought into the autopsy room. Unlike WTC and Flight 587, there were no explosive forces involved with this disaster, minimizing the fragmentation and associated commingling, and limiting the commingling to Type 1. And, as mentioned above, the MLIs' presence at the scene helped ensure that proper recovery techniques were utilized, significantly reducing this commingling as well. As compared with Flight 587 and WTC, the triage process for the Staten Island Ferry crash was less concerned with sorting out commingled remains, focusing on reassociating fragments to nearly complete bodies.

In this incident, the triage team consisted of an anthropologist and an assistant with significant experience in mass fatality work and knowledge of human anatomy. As opposed to WTC and the crash of Flight 587, the triage and autopsy processes were closely integrated and the triage team worked directly with the medical examiners in a concerted effort to reassociate fragments with bodies during autopsy. The limited number of victims and fragments meant that quick reassociation to the bodies was often possible. As autopsies were being conducted, the triage team opened the recovered bags one by one, according to the OCME triage protocol. An initial sort was performed to isolate all of the individual fragments. As before, anything not attached to another fragment by hard or soft tissue was isolated as its own case. However, these cases were not rebagged as in the previous disasters discussed, but instead were laid out on a gurney. At this point, the anthropologist anatomically evaluated all of the displayed body parts and fragments.

Concurrently, the medical examiners conducting the autopsies evaluated the bodies for missing parts. With this information, attempts were made to reassociate isolated body parts with those bodies missing a correlative part.

Many of these reassociations were simple. For instance, an isolated hand could be matched with a body that was missing a hand. For the association to be acceptable, the bones must conclusively conjoin at the fracture site. An exception to this rule would be when process of elimination is valid (Adams and Byrd 2006). When this standard was met, the isolated body part was not given its own case number, but instead was included in the autopsy case number assigned to the body and the separation was noted along with the other injuries documented in the autopsy notes. In another case, a fragment of liver was reassociated to a body that suffered a partial liver avulsion. This is rare, but in some instances it is appropriate to rearticulate soft tissue.

Other cases were more complicated. For instance, multiple skull fragments were recovered from the accident scene. Many of these fragments articulated to each other and were grouped together as a single case. However, because so many of the bodies being autopsied suffered skull trauma, reassociation of skull fragments to a body was quite difficult. Although some skull fragments were reassociated, others could not be assigned to any particular individual. In these instances, each isolated fragment became its own case. Fragments, such as pieces of fat or muscle, that could not be reassociated to any one individual were also assigned their own case number and treated as individual cases. Reassociations during autopsy accelerated the process of identification for unassociated fragments by creating fewer cases, resulting in less DNA testing. In addition, immediately reassociating fragments with bodies during autopsy reduced the likelihood of further parts being identified to that individual weeks or months later. As the above discussion demonstrates, reassociation during the triage process for the Staten Island Ferry crash differed from WTC and Flight 587, where reassociation during triage was only attempted for fragments found within an individual recovery bag.

The paperwork completed for each unassociated fragment was similar to the other disasters discussed. It consisted of a detailed anatomic description of the remains, which other fragments were found in association with that piece, and the location of recovery, if documented on the original recovery bag. Like WTC and Flight 587, a DNA sample was removed from every unassociated fragment, placed in a 50-mL tube, labeled with the same case number, and submitted to the Department of Forensic Biology for analysis. After sampling, the remaining fragment was rebagged, labeled with the case number, and stored within a refrigerated unit until it was identified. A DNA sample was also taken from each body during autopsy, enabling these unassociated fragments of bone and tissue to be identified and reassociated with the correct body.

With little Type 1 (recovery-induced) commingling, and no Type 2 commingling, the triage process for the Staten Island Ferry crash differed significantly from the WTC and Flight 587 disasters. Additional characteristics such as a small victim-to-fragment ratio, little decomposition, and a controlled surface recovery also shaped this triage process. As compared to the other two disasters, the triage process for the Staten Island Ferry crash was still quite valuable but involved more reassociation of fragments to bodies than sorting out commingled remains.

Conclusion

Identifying victims from mass fatality events can be a long and complicated process. Many components including recovery, numbering, mortuary processes, death certification, and antemortem information collection affect the overall success rates. Other important factors affecting the identification process include the number of victims, the degree of fragmentation, the length of the recovery operation, and whether or not it is an open or closed population. This chapter discussed one aspect of the mortuary process, triage, and its interplay with the other aspects of the process of identifying fragmented remains from three distinct mass fatality events in New York City (WTC, Flight 587, and the Staten Island Ferry). Each event differed in the degree of fragmentation, recovery duration, and the number and population characteristics of victims, all of which was reflected in the triage process. Additionally, the methods used to recover the remains varied greatly between the different events, which also shaped triage. Although the lengthy WTC recovery could not have been avoided, changing certain recovery practices could have helped in reducing needless commingling created at the site. This was highlighted by the Staten Island Ferry crash, where Medical Examiner personnel were not only present but were active participants in the organization of the recovery of human remains, greatly reducing commingling. This chapter illustrates the value of using personnel trained in recovering human remains. However, political, social, and cultural factors oftentimes place these decisions beyond the jurisdiction of medicolegal professional, who must be able to adapt and contend with the condition of the remains as they are received.

References Cited

1989 *Oxford English Dictionary*. Oxford University Press, Oxford.

2004 *The 9/11 Commission Report: Final Report of the National Commission on Terrorist Attacks upon the United States*. Government Printing Office, Washington, DC.

Adams, B. J. and J. E. Byrd 2006 Resolution of small-scale commingling: A case report from the Vietnam War. *Forensic Sci. Int.* 156(1):63–69.

Alonso, A., P. Martín, C. Albarrán, P. García, L. Fernández de Simón, M. J. Iturralde, A. Fernández-Rodríguez, I. Atienza, J. Capilla, J. García-Hirschfeld, P. Martínez, G. Vallejo, O. García1, E. García, P. Real, D. Álvarez, A. León, and M. Sancho 2005 Challenges of DNA profiling in mass disaster investigations. *Croat. Med. J.* (46):540–548.

Blau, S. and M. F. Skinner 2005 The use of forensic archaeology in the investigation of human rights abuse: Unearthing the past in East Timor. *Int. J. Hum. Rights* (9):449–463.

Brondolo, T. J. 2004 Resource requirements for medical examiner response to mass fatality incidents. *Medico-Legal J. Ireland* 10(2):91–102.

Budimlija, Z. M., M. K. Prinz, A. Zelson-Mundorff, J. Wiersema, E. Bartelink, G. MacKinnon, B. L. Nazzaruolo, S. M. Estacio, M. J. Hennessey. and R. C. Shaler 2003 World Trade Center human identification project: Experiences with individual body identification cases. *Croat. Med. J.* 44(3):259–263.

Byrd, J. E. and B. J. Adams 2003 Osteometric sorting of commingled human remains. *J. Forensic Sci.* 48(4):717–724.

Egana, S., S. Turner, P. Bernardi, M. Doretti, and M. Nieva 2005 Commingled Skeletonized Remains in Forensic Cases: Considerations for Methodological Treatment. Paper presented at the American Academy of Forensic Science, New Orleans.

Holland, M. M., C. A. Cave, C. A. Holland, and T. W. Bille 2003 Development of a quality, high throughput DNA analysis procedure for skeletal samples to assist with the identification of victims from the World Trade Center attacks. *Croat. Med. J.* (44):264–272.

Hsu, C. M., N. E. Huang, L. C. Tsai, L. G. Kao, C. H. Chao, A. Linacre, and J. C. Lee 1999 Identification of victims of the 1998 Taoyuan Airbus crash accident using DNA analysis. *Int. J. Legal Med.* 113(1):43–46.

Leclair, B., C. J. Fregeau, K. L. Bowen, and R. M. Fourney 2004 Enhanced kinship analysis and STR-based DNA typing for human identification in mass fatality incidents: The Swissair Flight 111 disaster. *J. Forensic Sci.* 49(5):939–953.

Levinson, J. and H. Granot 2002 *Transportation Disaster Response Handbook.* Academic Press, San Diego.

MacKinnon, G. and A. Z. Mundorff 2006 World Trade Center—September 11, 2001. In *Forensic Human Identification: An Introduction,* T. J. U. Thompson and S. M. Black, eds., pp. 485–499. CRC Press, Boca Raton, FL.

Meyer, H. J. 2003 The Kaprun cable car fire disaster—Aspects of forensic organisation following a mass fatality with 155 victims. *Forensic Sci. Int.* 138(1–3):1–7.

Mittleman, R. E., J. S. Barnhart, J. H. Davis, R. Fernandez, B. A. Hyman, R. D. Lengel, E. O. Lew, and V. J. Rao 2000 *The Crash of ValuJet Flight 592: A Forensic Approach to Severe Body Fragmentation.* Miami-Dade County Medical Examiner Department.

NTSB 2004 *In-Flight Separation of Vertical Stabilizer, American Airlines Flight 587, Airbus Industrie A300-605R, N14053, Belle Harbor, New York, November 12, 2001: Aircraft Accident Report NTSB/AAR-04/04.* National Transportation Safety Board, Washington, DC.

2005 *Allision of Staten Island Ferry Andrew J. Barberi, St. George, Staten Island, New York, October 15, 2003: Marine Accident Report NTSB/MAR-05/01.* National Transportation Safety Board, Washington, DC.

Olaisen, B., M. Stenersen, and B. Mevag 1997 Identification by DNA analysis of the victims of the August 1996 Spitsbergen civil aircraft disaster. *Nat, Genet,* 15(4):402–405.

Rodriguez, W. 2005 Methods and Techniques for Sorting Commingled Remains: Anthropological and Physical Attributes. Paper presented at the American Academy of Forensic Science, New Orleans.

Schiffer, M. B. 1987 *Formation Processes of the Archaeological Record.* University of New Mexico Press, Albuquerque.

Skinner, M. and J. Sterenberg 2005 Turf wars: Authority and responsibility for the investigation of mass graves. *Forensic Sci. Int.* 151(2–3):221–232.

Sledzik, P. and E. J. Kontanis 2005 Resolving Commingling Issues in Mass Fatality Incident Investigations. Paper presented at the American Academy of Forensic Science, New Orleans.

Sledzik, P. S. and W. C. Rodriguez 2002 Damnum fatale: The taphonomic fate of human remains in mass disasters. In *Advances in Forensic Taphonomy: Method, Theory, and Archaeological Perspectives,* W. D. Haglund and M. H. Sorg, eds., pp. 321–330. CRC Press, Boca Raton, FL.

Tuller, H., U. Hofmeister, and S. Daley 2005 The Importance of Body Deposition Recording in Event Reconstruction and the Reassociation and Identification of Commingled Remains. Paper presented at the 57th Annual Meeting of American Academy of Forensic Science, New Orleans.

Viner, M. D., C. Rock, N. Hunt, G. MacKinnon, and A. W. Martin 2006 Forensic Radiography: Response to the London Suicide Bombings on 7th July 2005. Paper presented at the American Academy of Forensic Science 58th Scientific Meeting, Seattle, WA.

Warren, M. W., L. E. Eisenberg, H. A. Walsh-Haney, and J. M. Saul 2003 Anthropology at Fresh Kills: Recovery and Identification of the World Trade Center Victims. Paper presented at the American Academy of Forensic Science.

Chapter 8
The Use of Radiology in Mass Fatality Events

Mark D. Viner

History

On December 28, 1895, Wilhelm Conrad Roentgen submitted his manuscript "On a New Kind of Ray" outlining the essential features of X-rays to the Würzburg Physical Medical Institute (Roentgen 1895). The new discovery aroused considerable interest. Roentgen's description of the ability to see through the body was greeted with incredulity by the scientific community, and early descriptions went to great lengths to reassure the public that this was indeed a serious discovery by a respected scientist. Within months of Roentgen's announcement, X-rays were in widespread use for a plethora of medical and scientific applications as well as some more frivolous uses (Burrows 1986).

Roentgenography, or radiography as it is now better known, utilizes the principles of the absorption of X-ray photons to demonstrate differentiations in atomic structure of the subject under examination. To the scientists of the late 19th century, the ability to conduct non-invasive examinations of animate and inanimate objects was nothing short of miraculous and made readily accessible by the fact that such examinations could be achieved with equipment that was relatively simple to assemble from instruments easily available throughout the Western world (Brogdon and Lichtenstein 1998).

It is no surprise then that this new tool was quickly applied to forensic examination and to the examination of the deceased. Within months, X-ray examinations had contributed to the forensic investigation of the cause of death and injury in murder and attempted murder cases in the UK and United States, negligence cases in the UK, United States, and Canada, the examination of suspicious packages, archaeological examination of Egyptian mummies, authentication of oil paintings, and numerous other forensic applications (Eckert and Garland 1984; Evans et al. 1981; Glasser 1931; Halperin 1988).

X-ray imaging techniques are minimally invasive, objective, permanent, and comparatively cost-effective. As a result, radiographic imaging is now in common use throughout many aspects of forensic investigation.

From: *Recovery, Analysis, and Identification of Commingled Human Remains*
Edited by: B. Adams and J. Byrd © Humana Press, Totowa, NJ

Uses of Radiology for Analysis and Human Identification

The possibility of applying this new and exciting tool in the field of human identification was soon under discussion. As early as May 1896, Bordas suggested that X-rays be used "... for identification through the visualisation of old fractures, bullets, or other known peculiarities..." (Brogdon and Lichtenstein 1998). In the same year, Angerer suggested that observation of wrist bone development could be used to measure bone age (Goodman 1995). In 1899, Levinsohn recognized that X-ray images could provide more accurate measurements of the skeleton than the then-popular Bertillon method of anthropological classification, which relied on external measurements and was thus subject to variation (Levinsohn 1899).

Radiology is now widely used to assist in the analysis and identification of human remains, and the applications of the use of X-rays first suggested by Levinsohn, Angerer, and Bordas comprise the main methods by which medical imaging contributes to the identification and investigative process. Radiological imaging has the advantage of enabling the examination of remains in a variety of states of decomposition from fully fleshed to completely skeletonized. As such, it affords the opportunity to obtain a considerable amount of data without the need to clean and completely deflesh the remains. It provides the investigative team with a rapid method of triage and classification by answering a number of fundamental questions:

- Determination of human vs. nonhuman remains
- Recognition of commingling
- Evaluation of the biological profile (age, sex, stature, and ancestry)
- Recognition of embedded/hidden foreign objects
- Interpretation of trauma
- Positive identification of individuals by comparison of antemortem and postmortem radiological data

Human Versus Nonhuman

In most cases involving animal bones that are brought to the attention of forensic investigators, a simple visual examination is all that is necessary for the trained anatomist or osteologist to determine nonhuman characteristics. In some cases, however, the most distinctive parts of the bones, the articular surfaces, may be missing due to fragmentation, decomposition, or animal activity. In such cases, radiographic examination of the bone structure and trabecular pattern can be useful in determining human from nonhuman remains (Brogdon 1998b; Chilvarquer et al.1987).

Recognition of Commingling

In cases involving large amounts of fragmented remains, such as a mass fatality incident, remains may be commingled and mixed with large amounts of debris and artifacts. Physical examination of such remains, particularly in cases of fire damage where there is a uniformity of discoloration of all samples retrieved, is both difficult and time-consuming. In such cases, radiological examination can prove useful in determining the presence of one or more individuals but also in identifying and locating small body parts, especially teeth, which may otherwise be overlooked in the absence of a thorough and time-consuming fingertip search (Goodman and Edelson 2002; Kahana et al. 1997; Viner et al. 1998). The use of radiological methods in this context will be discussed in greater detail later in this chapter.

Age Estimation

The development and maturation of the skeleton from birth through childhood, puberty, adolescence, and early adulthood provides reliable age indicators. The appearance and fusion of primary and secondary ossification centers within the developing skeleton follows a predetermined chronological pattern and, in the same way that a physical examination of the defleshed skeleton can determine age at the time of death, so can skeletal radiography deliver the same information in the case of less decomposed remains. There are a number of radiological standards for determination of bone age throughout the first two decades of life, based upon the appearance and fusion of the secondary ossification centers. The final epiphysis to fuse is the medial end of the clavicle, normally occurring during the mid- to late 20s.

In addition to dental development, one of the most useful examinations in determining the age of children is radiography of the hand and wrist, although examination of the knee, foot, and ankle can also be helpful (Greulich and Pyle 1959; Hansman 1962; Hoerr et al. 1962; Pyle and Hoerr 1955; Scheuer and Black 2004). In the mature skeleton, it is the degenerative changes that begin to appear at the margins of the articular surfaces of major joints at around age 40 that will allow the experienced radiologist to estimate adult age (Brogdon 1998b). Calcification of the costal cartilage associated with the ribs and sternum may be readily visualized in people over 50, although it is sometimes observed in younger subjects (Mora 2001). Although chest radiography demonstrates this calcification, its specificity as an aging method is reduced due to similar amounts of mineralization throughout adulthood (McCormick 1980). It is, however, a quick, inexpensive method to obtain a general age estimate that can be used along with other anthropological examinations (e.g., pubic symphysis morphology).

Sex Determination

Differentiation of sexes by skeletal radiology is unreliable until after puberty, as the features that distinguish male from female are not sufficiently developed until this point (Krogman and Iscan 1986). Although on examination the appearance of the male skeleton is more substantial than the female, being generally heavier and the long bones of greater length, it is the examination of certain specific bones that is most useful in determining the sex of an individual. In particular, the shape, size, and geometry of the pelvis (Kurihara et al. 1996; Rogers and Saunders 1994; Sutherland and Suchey 1991), skull, and mandible (Bass 1990; Kurihara et al. 1996) and patterns of calcification of the costal (Navani et al. 1970), tracheobronchial, thyroid, and arytenoid cartilages (Kurihara et al. 1996) can be used to determine sex from skeletal remains by radiological means (Brogdon 1998b).

Stature Estimation

Physical anthropologists are able to make estimations of stature by direct measurement from unfleshed human remains. The length of the femur is usually used, as this has been shown to be reliable (Trotter and Gleser 1952, 1958). In the case of fleshed remains, the same measurements can be made radiographically, provided that correction for magnification is made. This can be achieved by means of an adapted radiographic technique, applying a simple correction factor, or by utilizing modern imaging techniques.

Adapted Radiographic Techniques

By far the simplest method is to utilize a long focus to object distance (FOD) of 180 centimeters and a minimal object to film distance (OFD), by placing the limb directly on the cassette or nonscreen film packet. This will effectively negate any magnification (Maresh 1943).

Another simple method is to take a series of images of the leg on a single film using a narrow-slit aperture X-ray beam directly above each joint space, so as to use the central ray for each image, avoiding divergence. A ruler with radiopaque markings is positioned adjacent to the leg, and measurements are read directly from the film (Bryan 1979). Alternatively, a scanogram technique can be used. The limb is positioned on the cassette together with the radiopaque ruler, as for the previous method. However, instead of taking a series of images over each joint, the X-ray tube (with narrow-slit aperture X-ray beam) is moved along the length of the limb during a long X-ray exposure (Bryan 1979).

Applying a Correction Factor

By applying a correction factor to the measured size of an object on the film, the actual size of the object can be determined. The correction factor is the distance of the object from the focal spot of the X-ray tube divided by the distance of the film from the focal spot of the X-ray tube (Jenkins 1980). Thus, $CF = (D - d)/D$ (Fig. 8.1).

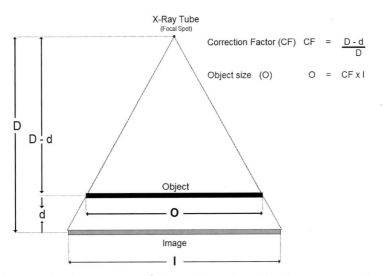

Fig. 8.1 Correction factor to determine the actual size of an object by measurement from the radiographic image

CT Scanning and Digital Radiography

CT scanners and digital X-ray systems can be calibrated to undertake this correction calculation automatically, thus allowing measurements to be made directly from the image. In the case of CT scanning, a scanogram is performed using the scanner to undertake an automated version of the manual process described above (Aitken et al. 1985). Digital X-ray machines using a slit beam can also be used to take direct measurements from the resultant scans, and many other direct digital X-ray machines can be calibrated so as to render accurate anatomical measurements from the resultant images (Beningfield et al. 2003).

Determination of Ancestry

Determination of ancestry is challenging, especially when the remains are badly decomposed or skeletonized. Similar methods to those used by physical anthropologists to determine ancestry from skeletal remains can be applied radiographically with fleshed remains. In particular, examination of the skull and mandible (Bass 1990; Fischman 1985), the distal end of the femur (Craig 1995), and the ratio of long bone length can be useful in determination of population ancestry (Krogman and Iscan 1986).

Recognition of Embedded/Hidden Objects and Interpretation of Trauma

X-ray imaging can be utilized to detect and retrieve hazardous objects, personal effects, projectiles, aircraft parts, and other artifacts and forensic evidence, especially when body fragmentation is extensive (Fig. 8.2). It can assist with determination of the manner of death, document trauma, negate the requirement for invasive autopsy, permit anthropological assessment without the requirement for defleshing, and, of course, establish identification through positive matching of postmortem and antemortem data (Gould 2003; Viner 2001a, b, c). It has proved particularly useful in mass fatality incidents resulting from air disasters (Alexander and Foote 1998; Mulligan et al. 1988; Viner et al. 1998), explosions, and terrorist incidents including suicide attacks (Harcke et al. 2002; Kahana et al. 1997; Nye et al. 1996; Society of Radiographers 2005; Viner et al. 2006). Radiological methods have also been employed extensively in the investigation of war crimes and human rights abuses involving the exhumation of buried human remains (Gould 2003; Tonello 1998; Viner 2001a). In such incidents, the systematic application of radiology has proved essential to the investigation and identification of victims.

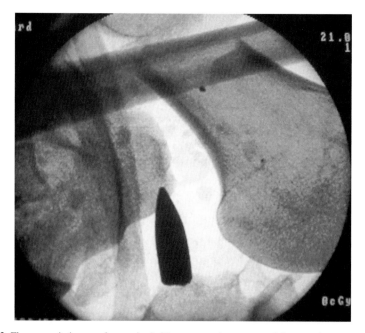

Fig. 8.2 Fluoroscopic image of commingled human remains recovered from a crime scene reveals the presence of ballistic evidence

Positive Identification of Individuals by Comparison of Antemortem and Postmortem Radiological Data

Some of the methods of identification (such as fingerprint analysis) depend upon the integrity of the soft tissues of remains (Brogdon et al. 2003). In some cases involving skeletonization, fragmentation, decomposition, incineration, mutilation, or other disfigurement, identification by means of the skeleton and highly resilient dentition assumes a greater importance; it is here that X-ray imaging comes into its own. Such incidents are often characterized by damage to the soft tissues caused by fire or water or severe disarticulation due to explosion or rapid deceleration injury.

Radiological identification of human remains requires specific and unique findings on postmortem images to be matched exactly with antemortem images of the individual. In some cases, identification can be made from a series of relatively common or nonspecific pathological anatomical changes that appear in identical locations in ante- and postmortem images. In other cases, a single unique feature is sufficient (Brogdon 1998a). In 1927, Culbert and Law (1927) made the first identification of human remains by comparison of antemortem and postmortem radiographs of the frontal sinuses. The degree of human variation in sinus patterns, based on size, asymmetry, outline, partial septa, and supraorbital cells, makes effective comparison for identification possible (Kirk et al. 2002; Marlin et al. 1991; Nambiar et al. 1999).

Medical imaging has long been used for the identification of human remains and is well documented (Binda et al. 1999; Buchner 1985; Craig 1995; Jensen 1991; Kahana and Hiss 1997; Murphy et al. 1980; Sanders et al. 1972; Schwartz and Woolridge 1977). Radiology is used extensively in anthropological and odontological assessment of postmortem and antemortem radiographs, records, or other images for concordance, as they represent an excellent source of data for comparison of anatomical features (Fig. 8.3). Many specific cases have been reported in which radiology has played the leading role in the identification of human remains (Goodman and Edelson 2002; Greulich and Pyle 1959; Kahana et al. 1997; Viner et al. 1998). Binda et al. (1999) even report on a case where radiology proved to be more accurate than DNA

Radiographs taken for medical purposes are often required by statute to be retained for long periods of time. In the UK, for example, the Department of Health requires that radiographs are retained for 8 years, and longer in the case of children (until the patient reaches his 25th year), and 3 years following death (Dimond 2002). In many cases, particularly in privately run clinics, radiographs are routinely given to the patient for safe keeping and thus may be in existence for much longer than the statutory period. With the advent of digital imaging and the decreasing cost of digital storage, many institutions are retaining medical images far beyond their previously applied practice for X-ray film. Records are thus, on the whole, fairly accessible.

The last assessment of the frequency of medical and dental X-ray examinations undertaken by the National Radiological Protection Board (NRPB) in the UK for the year 1997–1998 showed an overall examination rate of 704 examinations per 1,000 head of population per annum. Of this figure, 30% were dental radiography

(a)

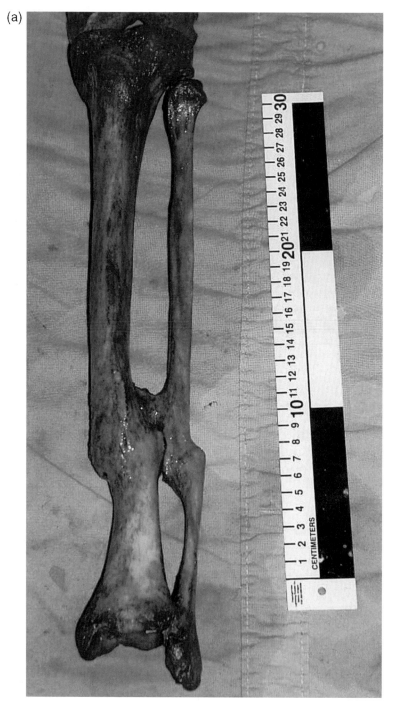

Fig. 8.3 (continued)

(b)

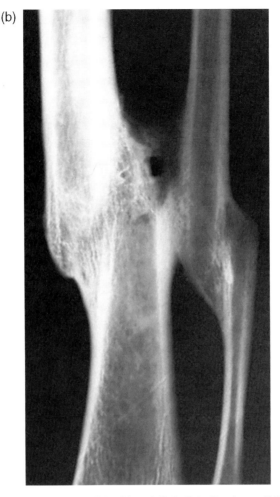

Fig. 8.3 A previously healed fracture of the tibia and fibula (2a) offers the possibility of identification by radiology as such trauma will usually have been well documented at the time of the original injury and throughout the healing process. This subject was later identified by comparison of the postmortem radiograph (2b) with an antemortem film

examinations, with a total of 494 examinations per 1,000 head of population being medical X-ray examinations. This figure was almost exactly half of the rate for medical examinations in the United States. The great majority of examinations were conventional X-ray studies (79%), with the majority of these being teeth, chest, and limb radiographs, which accounted for 75% of all examinations. A further 15% were pelvis, spine, and hip examinations. CT examinations represented 5% of the total (9% in the United States), with 50% of these being head and neck, 30% abdomen and pelvis, and 14% chest (Tanner et al. 2001). This position echoes Brogdon's evaluation of the distribution of radiological examinations by body part and modality in the United States undertaken during the same period. As Brogdon asserts, examinations of the chest demonstrate consistency of bony structures over time, and extremities may contain useful radiographic identifiers due to previous injury, degenerative change, or malformation (Brogdon 1998a). All of the above points to a wealth of useful antemortem data being available to the investigator, with the possibility of obtaining a clear and decisive identification if postmortem and antemortem data can be matched.

As demonstrated by the NRPB study, radiographic examinations of the skull have declined dramatically since the advent of CT scanning, and antemortem radiographic data are thus less likely to be available. However, positive identification can be established by CT by comparison either with other CT scans or with some conventional radiographs (Brogdon 1998a; Reichs and Dorion 1992).

Imaging Modalities

Until recently, much forensic examination of the deceased carried out in the Medical Examiner's office or incident mortuary has relied on traditional X-ray technology, which is little changed from the time of Roentgen. In recent years, however, some of the newer technologies that have been available within hospitals and clinics have been used for the forensic examination of the deceased. Most recently, these have included computed tomography scanning (CT) and magnetic resonance scanning (MR) (Bisset et al. 2002; Brookes et al. 1996; Thali et al. 2003).

All of the imaging modalities described in this chapter rely upon the principles of the absorption of X-ray photons to demonstrate differentiations in atomic structure of the subject under examination. In order to achieve a satisfactory result, it is essential that the operator is conversant with the physical principles of X-ray interaction with matter and has a sound knowledge of human anatomy.

Contrast and density on the resultant image are dependent upon the chemical composition of the subject under examination, the energy of the X-ray photons [determined by the peak kilovoltage (kV) applied across the X-ray tube], and the number of photons reaching the film or digital detector [determined by the milliamperage (mA) applied to the coil of the X-ray tube, the time of the exposure, and the distance of the film or receptor from the X-ray source]. It is essential to match the kV applied to the body part under examination in order to achieve an optimum result. Even small variations can enable visualization of anatomical structures that would otherwise be missed, particularly in the juvenile skeleton.

The examination technique, imaging system (be it either film or digital technology), and a number of other factors, including the structure of the examination table, will introduce a number of additional variables that will all need to be taken into account to produce the optimum result. In the case of the photographic image, these factors are also dependent upon the availability of consistent processing conditions that rely upon accurate temperature control, regular replenishment of appropriate chemicals, and control of development time. For these reasons, it is desirable that examinations are conducted by a trained radiographer and are undertaken on equipment that has been regularly and appropriately maintained and is subject to a regular quality control program. As Brogdon points out,

> ... the person who actually positions and exposes the roentgenograms is absolutely critical to the success of the entire endeavour. The educated, experienced, and sophisticated eye of the radiologist or other professional observer may be required to detect and interpret the subtle nuances recorded on the film, but without adequate technical support, that eye will be blinded. (Brogdon 1998a)

Discussion of all the available imaging modalities is not possible here, and this section will focus on those techniques that may be more commonly used in the examination of commingled human remains resulting from mass fatality incidents.

Film Radiography

The radiograph, as demonstrated by Roentgen, still remains as the method of choice for the examination of the skeleton. It delivers a high-quality image of skeletal structures and can be relatively easily and cheaply acquired and replicated. The radiograph is in essence a "shadow-gram," a still-life image produced by radiation emerging from a subject and striking a sheet of film (Fig. 8.4). The film is developed using a standard photographic process, resulting in a negative image in which the dark areas represent those areas of the subject through which a greater number of X-ray photons have been transmitted.

Since the early days of radiography, it has been common for the majority of the image to be formed, not by radiation, but by light emitted by phosphorescent "intensifying screens" placed on either side of the sheet film in a cassette. These screens emit light in proportion to the number and energy of the X-ray photons absorbed within them. While this considerably reduces the exposure time and thus the radiation dose, it can introduce a degree of unsharpness to the image. For this reason, a wide range of screen types are available, both for general and more detailed skeletal work, where the unsharpness is minimized within the intensifying screens. For optimum trabecular detail, nonscreen film may be used, and this type of examination is favored for the examination of samples in a lead-lined "Faxitron"®machine where such minute detail may prove to be of value. For the majority of examinations, and certainly in the mass casualty situation, the speed and ease of use of a film/screen combination will suffice.

Fluoroscopy

One of Roentgen's earliest observations was that of a fluoroscopic image (Burrows 1986). In fluoroscopy, a continuous "beam" of radiation is directed at and passes through the subject under examination. The emergent rays strike a fluorescent screen that emits light in proportion to the energy of the incident X-ray photons falling upon it. This image, visible to the naked eye, is amplified several thousand times via an "image intensifier" and is recorded and projected onto a computer screen via a closed-circuit TV system (Fig. 8.5).

The resultant image is viewed in "real time." Thus, as the apparatus is moved over the subject, the image seen reflects the movement over the subject, thus allowing rapid coverage of a scene in the same way that a video camera can be panned over a landscape. Alternatively, the apparatus can remain stationary, and any movement of the subject will be detected and demonstrated upon the image.

Fluoroscopy offers significant advantages to the investigator, particularly in the examination of commingled human remains following a mass fatality incident. The real-time nature of the examination makes it particularly suitable for rapid examination of body bags as a triage method. The resultant image, derived from the relative density of objects, rather than their appearance, makes it a simple matter to identify even small fragments of bone and teeth among debris, personal effects, and possible items of evidence from fire, crash, explosion, and other disaster scenes. Employing fluoroscopy as the first stage of the examination process in a mass fatality incident also permits the presence of any hazardous material (sharp objects or unexploded ordnance) to be detected and located, thus reducing the potential hazard at subsequent stages of the process.

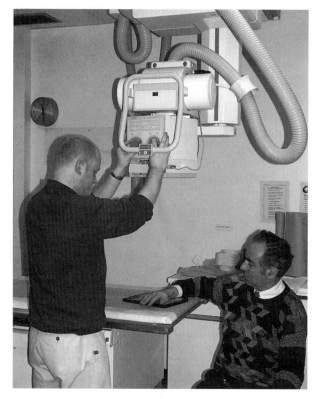

Fig. 8.4 (continued)

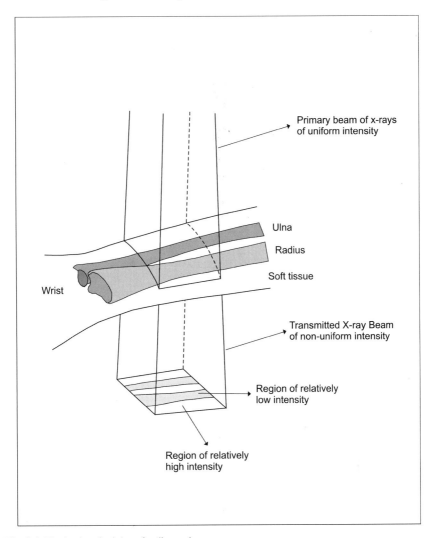

Fig. 8.4 The basic principles of radiography

The use of a mobile C-Arm fluoroscope allows the X-ray tube and detector to be rotated and angled to give better visualization of superimposed structures, which can be particularly useful when examining fragmented, commingled human remains. It is also useful for rapid retrieval of small objects (e.g., ballistic material) under X-ray control. Without fluoroscopy (and appropriate protective equipment), location and removal of these objects would otherwise be difficult and time-consuming (Association of Forensic Radiographers 2004; Tonello 1998; Viner et al. 2003, 2006).

Fluoroscopy does, however, have its limitations in terms of both image quality and the total amount of information that can be permanently recorded on a single image. In this respect, it is best suited for use as an initial triage tool, to be

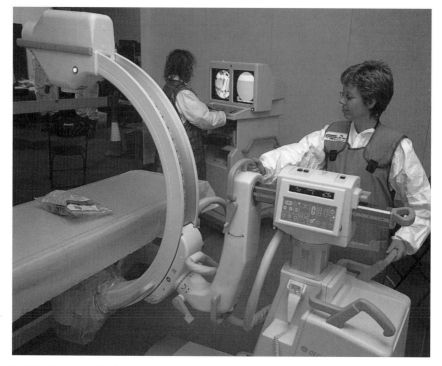

Fig. 8.5 C-Arm mobile fluoroscopy unit

supplemented by further examination by digital radiography (Association of Forensic Radiographers 2004; Viner et al. 2003, 2006).

Digital Radiography

In recent years, technological advances have allowed the traditional film-/screen-
based system to be replaced by digital technology. Digital images offer enormous
benefits to medical and forensic applications. They can be relatively easily acquired
without the need for use of photographic chemicals and equipment. The recording
methods require a decreased radiation dose and have a wider dynamic range than
film, resulting in the ability to demonstrate both soft tissue and bony structures from
the same image data by altering the display factors. This makes digital imaging
an ideal method for detailed examination of fragmented remains with tissue; the
same image data can be used to display soft tissue structures, nonmetallic foreign
bodies, bony detail, and metallic foreign bodies by simple adjustment of the display
parameters.

Digital images can also be superimposed accurately over one another, allowing
accurate comparison of antemortem and postmortem data. The fact that digital
information can be sent electronically speeds up and simplifies this process

dramatically, facilitating rapid identification of the remains of an individual from antemortem data recovered thousands of miles away.

Current systems fall broadly into two categories: computed radiography (CR) and digital radiography (DR). In the process of computed radiography (CR), a photo stimulable phosphor plate replaces the film and screens within the X-ray cassette. The examination is performed in an identical manner to the traditional X-ray examination, and following exposure, the cassette is placed in a CR reader (Fig. 8.6a). The reader withdraws the plate, scans it, and converts the data stored upon it into a digital image. The entire process takes a similar amount of time to the conventional film-based process, but the end result is a digital image (Emerton et al. 2005).

With digital radiography (DR), a flat-panel X-ray detector replaces the X-ray cassette (Fig. 8.6b). The examination is performed in the same way as conventional and CR imaging, but the image appears almost instantly on a monitor following the exposure (Lawinski et al. 2005). Aside from the increase in speed and productivity, this process offers significant advantages for forensic work. First, with DR there is no need to remove the plate following exposure in order to be able to view the image. Thus, with cases that are difficult to position or for commingled remains where structures may overlay one another, making interpretation difficult, the subject can be repositioned immediately, thus improving accuracy and minimizing examination time. Second, where foreign body removal is required (e.g., ballistic material or traces of explosive devices), the same image can be instantly replicated with a radiopaque pointer used to highlight the subject. The item can then be retrieved by the pathologist with the aid of sequential radiographs.

Digital radiography (DR) can successfully be employed as a triage tool in place of fluoroscopy, providing a series of survey radiographs covering an entire body bag. This imaging will allow for the identification of small fragments of bone, teeth, personal effects, and possible items of evidence among debris in the same way as fluoroscopy. However, the static nature of the image and the limitations of the gantry systems currently available reduce its flexibility for identification of superimposed structures and a more complex process for retrieval of items under X-ray control. In cases where it is likely to be a requirement to retrieve small items of evidence from bags containing commingled remains, or when assisting the pathologist to locate and retrieve evidential items from within the soft tissues, a combination of DR and fluoroscopy should be considered to be the gold standard.

Digital X-Ray Scanography

An alternative method, which offers the combined advantages of digital imaging and fluoroscopy, is the use of digital X-ray scanography. The Lodox Statscan® was developed originally for examining suspected diamond smugglers in the mines of South Africa. This machine employs a digital version of the "scanogram" technique described earlier (Fig. 8.7). A narrow-slit beam of radiation passes rapidly over the subject, and the resultant image is recorded using digital technology employing 12 solid-state detectors in a linear array detector. An entire body can be examined from head to toe in approximately 13 seconds, and the gantry can be rotated through 90 degrees (and any angle in between) to give a lateral or oblique image (Beningfield et al. 2003).

The Statscan is a relatively new machine that is currently being employed very successfully for the investigation and management of polytrauma in shock trauma centers in the United States, Europe, and Africa. Due mainly to its high cost, the application of this machine for forensic use is in its infancy but clearly offers significant advantages over conventional X-ray techniques.

Dental Radiography

One of the most useful tools available to the investigator in a mass casualty situation is the use of dental radiography. Identification by odontological means remains one of the major primary methods of identification in mass fatality incidents, despite advances in DNA technology. Comparison of dental radiographs is an important tool for the forensic odontologist. Production of dental X-ray images is rapid, cost-effective, and simple and can be achieved without the need for complex equipment. The principles are identical to those of skeletal radiography and can be accomplished with plain film (without the use of intensifying screens), computed radiography, or direct digital systems.

One of the problems associated with dental comparisons is the postmortem replication of antemortem images. The most common examinations performed by dentists upon their patients are the intra-oral "bite-wing" projections and extra-oral panoramic survey view (Hart and Wall 2002). The bite-wing projection relies on

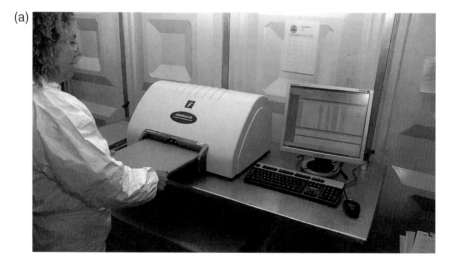

Fig. 8.6 Two options for digital radiography. (a) Computed radiography (CR) and (continued)

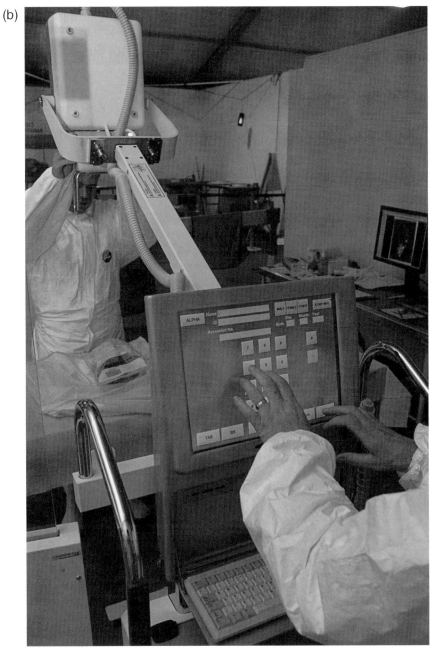

Fig. 8.6 (b) direct digital radiography (DR)

the subject's ability to hold an intra-oral film in position in the mouth by biting upon a card support attached to the film. Achieving an exact replication of this view can be very difficult in postmortem analysis for obvious reasons.

The panoramic or "orthopantomographic" technique produces a single film showing the entire dentition, mandible, maxillae, and maxillary sinuses on the same image (Fig. 8.8). The examination is performed using a technique known as rotational tomography in which the X-ray tube and film rotate around a series of fulcrum points that follow the line of the mandible. Structures that are not in the same plane as the fulcrum are blurred out, so that superimposition of the structures is avoided (Mason and Bourne 1998). Since Siemens plc ceased production of its Zonarc®, all currently available orthopantomography equipment operates on the principle that the patient is able to sit or stand in the erect position. This single factor makes replication of the orthopantomograph image very difficult to undertake postmortem and results in the requirement for a series of intra-oral radiographs to be undertaken. An alternative method for achieving a comparable projection to that obtained using orthopantomography that is currently in use in clinical dentistry and under evaluation for postmortem identification is CT scanning (Jackowski et al. 2006; Rocha Sdos et al. 2003; Thali et al. 2006).

CT Scanning

Computed axial tomography (CAT) scanning was developed in the 1970s by a British scientist, Godfrey Hounsfield, working for the EMI Corporation. Hounsfield applied the physics of rotational tomography, going a stage further so that the tube

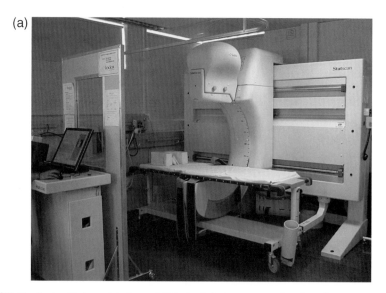

Fig. 8.7 The Lodox Statscan (a) gives a full-body digital scanogram (continued)

(b)

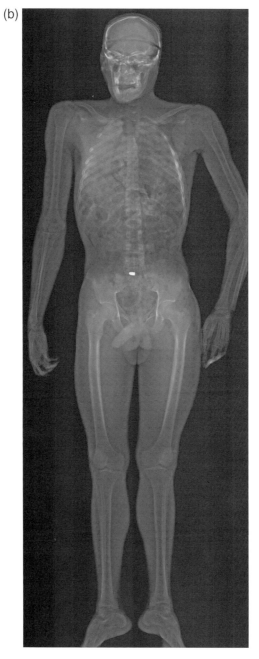

Fig. 8.7 (b) in just 13 seconds.

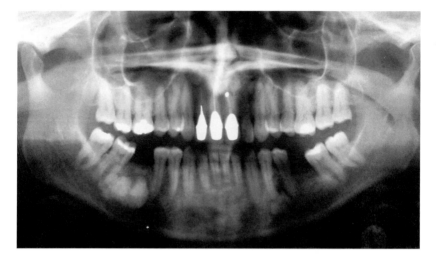

Fig. 8.8 Orthopantomograph: Standard panoramic X-ray view of the dentition routinely performed in general dental practice

and X-ray detector gantry rotate about a single axis in the body. X-ray detectors replaced film and took a series of measurements continuously while the gantry rotated (Fig. 8.9). A computer analyzed the recorded data and reconstructed it as a digital image of an axial "slice" of the subject displayed on an image matrix on a CRT screen. Each pixel was allocated a level on a gray scale that corresponded to the level of radiation transmitted through the body at that location and thus the relative density of the subject. These values are now known as Hounsfield Units and the scale, in which the density level corresponding to 0 is equivalent to water (mid-gray), spans from dense air −1024 units (black) to bone >+400 units or greater to dense metallic objects, etc. +3071(white). Initially deployed as a tool for imaging the head, it enabled radiologists to examine the brain accurately for the first time without the overlying features of the bony skull obscuring vital soft-tissue information.

CT scanning, as it is now known, has benefited enormously from advances in technology and computer processing power. The entire body can now be scanned in a matter of seconds, and images can be reconstructed in any plane: axial, coronal, saggital, or oblique. While CT scanning is a routine tool in clinical medicine, it is a relatively expensive technique and has only fairly recently been used for postmortem and forensic examination and is not a widely available resource for the investigator. However, recent studies have shown that it can be a very effective tool at postmortem examination (Haglund and Fligner 1993; Hildebolt et al. 1990; Myers et al. 1999; Riepert et al. 1995; Rocha Sdos et al. 2003; Thali et al. 2003a, b, 2006; Uysal et al. 2005) and may offer the opportunity to gather data that may otherwise be impossible to collect. The ability of CT scanning to undertake 3D and multi-planar reconstructions offers the pathologist and anthropologist the opportunity to examine the underlying skeletal structure of fleshed remains, visualizing trauma, degenerative processes, and articular surfaces and taking accurate measurements (Thali 2000). There are at present a number of studies being undertaken worldwide to evaluate the possibilities of CT for forensic examination and identification, and it was recently announced that a mobile CT scanner has, for the first time, been used in the investigation of a multiple casualty incident (Rutty 2006).

Radiation Protection

Within three months of Roentgen's announcement, reports of the harmful effects of X-rays began to appear in the literature (Burrows 1986). Early experimenters and practitioners, however, took no steps to protect themselves against the effects of radiation. X-ray rooms and X-ray tubes were unshielded and emitted radiation in all directions. It was a common practice among early radiographers and radiologists to test the X-ray tube and determine the exposure required by taking an exposure of their own hand prior to each examination (Burrows 1986). In the UK, documentation of radiation injuries by Dr. John Hall-Edwards and Ernest Wilson led to the publication of a safe code of practice by Dr. Hall-Edwards in 1908 (Hall-Edwards 1908). Both men later died of their radiation-induced injuries.

Adequate protection and codes of practice did not become commonplace until the 1920s, and it was not until 1928 that the International Congress of Radiology in Stockholm adopted the third revised report of the British Radiological Protection Committee as the basis for international regulations (International X-ray Protection Committee 1928). It was not until the 1950s that it was understood that the low levels of radiation exposure used in diagnostic radiology represented a danger to patients. This resulted in the adoption of the radiation protection regulations that are now in use, based upon the risk to patients and operators from late effects of radiation upon patients and radiation workers following low-level exposure (Engel-Hills 2006).

There is no absolute evidence of a threshold below which no damage occurs. Even the lowest doses may cause damage to cells that might later lead to malignancy or hereditary effects if the cells irradiated are the germ cells in the gonads (Engel-Hills 2006). For this reason, radiation exposures should be limited and controlled by appropriate international, national, and state regulations, codes of practice, and schemes of work. X-ray and imaging equipment should be regulated, adequately maintained and inspected, and subject to regular quality control programs. Radiation workers should be appropriately trained in the use of such equipment for the purpose for which it is employed. This is particularly important for fluoroscopy, where the radiation exposure received by the operators can be significantly increased by the use of poor technique and by inexperienced operators using the equipment for longer periods than are necessary to gather the required information.

Provided that the appropriately qualified personnel are involved in planning, commissioning, and operating the equipment, most X-ray techniques can be performed safely in "field" conditions encountered in incident mortuaries following mass fatality incidents or during large-scale criminal investigations. The imaging equipment routinely required in such investigations (fluoroscopy, digital and digital dental radiography, and even CT scanning) is available in mobile or portable form and is routinely employed in military field hospitals or domicillary and veterinary radiological practices. There is therefore no logistical reason why incident mortuaries cannot benefit from the resources required to undertake a thorough investigation.

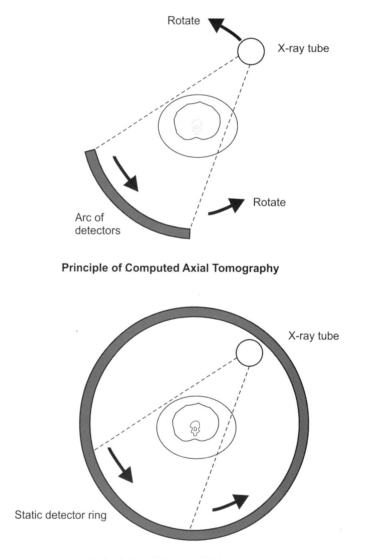

Principle of Computed Axial Tomography

Principle of Modern CT Scanner

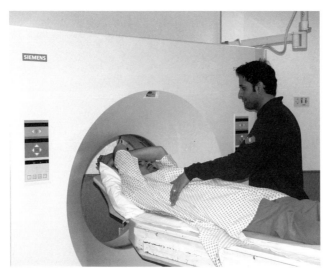

Fig. 8.9 The basic principles of computed axial tomography

Application of Radiographic Methods to Mass Fatalities

Whatever modalities are employed, the examination of commingled fragmented remains, particularly from large-scale incidents, will require systematic application of imaging so as to maximize the information gained while minimizing the time taken and preventing delays in the examination process. In planning the forensic protocol to include the use of radiological imaging, the following principles should be applied (Association of Forensic Radiographers 2004):

- Imaging will be useful as an initial screening tool at triage to determine the nature of the remains. This includes the presence of hazardous material, the remains of more than one individual, the presence of significant material and artifacts (e.g., personal effects and forensic evidence), and to locate and retrieve small, unassociated body fragments (e.g., teeth).
- Aside from dental radiography, the use of radiography for identification is likely to play a relatively small (but important) role in the identification process.
- Comparison views for identification will require accurate positioning and exposure. This is a time-consuming process and cannot be undertaken successfully until after the initial examination/search process is complete (Lichtenstein 1998). It is thus advisable to triage recovered remains so that detailed skeletal radiography for identification is undertaken only when indicated rather than as part of the routine forensic protocol.

Imaging techniques for mass fatalities are thus best deployed along the same lines as for the management of major trauma in the emergency room (Fig. 8.10):

- **Primary survey:** initial triage and assessment
- **Secondary survey:** standard examination of specific body parts (e.g., dentition)

PROCESS   OUTPUT

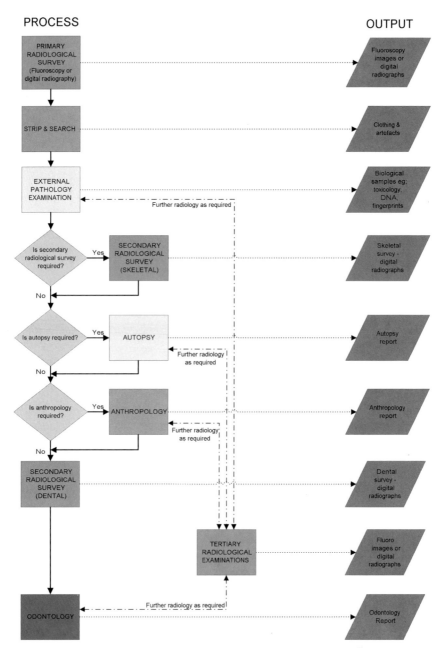

Fig. 8.10 Flowchart showing how radiology contributes to the examination of human remains in mass fatality investigations at each stage

- **Tertiary examinations:** specific examinations performed in response to findings during primary or secondary surveys or during pathology, odontology, or anthropology assessment

Primary Survey (Triage)

The purpose of the primary survey is to undertake an initial assessment of the remains. This should be considered essential in all cases but is particularly important for circumstances involving extensive fragmentation, decomposition, or intermixing with debris. In some cases the use of either computed radiography (CR) or direct digital radiography (DR) will deliver a high-quality image that can be subsequently evaluated by the pathologist, anthropologist, and odontologist without the need for further examination. The digital nature of these images will allow display of both hard and soft tissues, as well as metallic and nonmetallic artifacts and personal effects. In the absence of CR or DR, plain film radiography techniques will offer an alternative, but without the benefits of a digital image. DR has the advantage of being a far more rapid technique than film or CR, and it is particularly suited to use in the mass fatality situation when speed is of critical importance. Direct digital radiography should therefore be considered to be the modality of choice in such cases.

In the absence of DR, particularly in cases where large quantities of remains are recovered and commingled with one another and other evidential material, the advantages of fluoroscopy for mass fatality situations will become apparent at triage. The "real-time" nature of the fluoroscope image will enable rapid location and retrieval of items of interest, and the ability to rotate the C-Arm of the fluoroscope will enable superimposed structures to be more easily identified.

In all cases, the primary radiographic survey should be considered to be the first phase of the investigative process, particularly when examining remains from a crime scene. Imaging examination of the sealed body bag will yield all or some of the following information about the contents of the body bag:

- Recognition of body parts with discernable anatomical landmarks that can be used for body part identification, which is especially useful with cases of fragmentation and decomposition
- An indication of whether the remains of more than one individual are present
- The location and nature (if possible) of any hazardous material—unexploded ordnance, metallic sharps, glass, etc.
- The location and degree of skeletal trauma. This may include the location of any projectile fragments with possible associated bony injury
- The location of unassociated teeth and other small body parts useful for identification
- The location of personal effects, e.g., jewelry, cigarette lighters, keys, wallets, etc. (This may be particularly useful in cases of burned or exhumed remains, where these artifacts may be difficult to locate.)

- The presence of any unique identifying features (e.g., prosthetic hip replacement) that may require further radiographic investigation following autopsy
- The presence of previous healed fractures and other preexisting pathological or anatomical features that may be useful for identification purposes
- The presence of dental work (bridges, crowns, root canal treatments, etc.)

The information obtained from the primary survey should be recorded on a report form to aid subsequent pathology, anthropology, and odontology examinations. Examples of recording forms are shown in Fig. 8.11. If fluoroscopy is used, it is recommended that the entire examination is recorded using video or similar technology. Although hard- or soft-copy images should be taken of significant findings, fluoroscopy is a dynamic real-time examination, and it is advisable that the process is undertaken by a radiographer along with a forensic pathologist or anthropologist and appropriate law enforcement personnel to ensure continuity. The use of DR as a primary survey tool will result in a series of hard- or soft-copy images as a permanent record.

In cases with a large amount of fragmented commingled remains, a primary survey of body bags using digital radiography can be used to construct an image database to aid the identification process. Images can be categorized and filed according to observed anatomical parts, facilitating rapid retrieval for later comparison with antemortem radiographs should this prove necessary. It should be remembered that radiographs produced at the primary survey stage will not be of sufficient quality to permit accurate evaluation by a radiologist, due to the random nature of the anatomical positioning of the body parts within the body bag. Further radiography examinations may be required as part of the investigative process, as detailed below. These examinations, performed subsequent to the primary survey, should in all cases be correctly anatomically positioned so that the resultant radiographs replicate as far as possible the standard views that would be undertaken on a live subject.

Secondary Survey (Standard Radiographic Examination)

The secondary survey should be undertaken after the initial strip and search and external examination so that standard positions can be replicated without overlying clothing and other artifacts. In most cases, examinations can be undertaken following autopsy, but this will be dependent upon the precise nature of the examinations to be performed. Examinations of the skull, for example, are in most cases best undertaken prior to the cranial vault being opened.

The use of imaging to obtain standard projection radiographs as a routine part of the examination protocol should be restricted to those cases that are likely to yield the greatest benefit from the deployment of resources required. In the case of a mass fatality investigation, advances in other identification methods (e.g., DNA) have largely negated the need for the full skeletal survey examination deployed in previous incidents (Mulligan et al. 1988; Nye et al. 1996). In such cases, secondary surveys are now usually restricted to routine dental surveys as a means of collecting postmortem data for later comparison with antemortem films. As the incidence of dental X-ray examinations and the availability of dental records in Western populations are high, the likelihood of such antemortem data availability available makes the routine dental survey worthwhile. In other populations, where dental treatment is either rare or poorly documented, it may be decided that a routine dental radiography survey is not indicated. However, there may be value in routinely taking radiographs of the mandible in the region of the third molar in order to provide data for age estimation.

The precise requirements for dental radiography surveys will be determined by the working practices of the forensic odontologist. In the absence of a presumptive identification with antemortem data for comparison, a full sequence of intra-oral peri-apical films showing the entire dentition, together with bilateral bite-wing examinations, represents a thorough survey from which comparison can be made with antemortem data. In the case of large-scale examinations involving multiple fatalities, the secondary dental survey represents a significant and time-consuming part of the postmortem data collection process. A team approach, involving odontologists and experienced dental radiographers and nurses working together in the incident mortuary, can greatly increase the speed of the identification process and negate the requirement for body parts to be examined elsewhere (Viner et al. 2006).

Similar to the dental images, there may be other indications for including a series of cranial and postcranial projections in the routine postmortem examination protocol. For example, in the case of examining the remains from suspected atrocity crimes, the possibility of systematic antemortem torture and/or beatings may indicate routine examination of body parts, such as skull, limbs, and ribs for evidence of healed or healing fractures at the time of death (Tonello 1998; Viner 2001c).

In all events, the precise protocol deployed will be dependent upon a number of factors unique to the circumstances surrounding the death of the individual(s). The protocol will thus need to be agreed upon in consultation with the coroner, medical examiner, odontologist, anthropologist, radiologist, and radiographer in order to achieve the maximum benefit while limiting examination time and resources.

Tertiary Examinations (Special Circumstances)

As described earlier, a range of medical imaging techniques and examinations may be useful in determining the identity of an individual, his anthropological profile, or in determining the cause and manner of his death. The techniques employed will vary from case to case and will be determined by the nature, or suspected nature, of the incident under investigation. In most instances the requirement for further specific imaging will be determined as a result of data obtained at primary radiological survey or from the pathology, odontological, anthropological, or crime scene examinations. It should again be remembered that radiographs produced at the primary survey stage will not be of sufficient quality to permit accurate evaluation by a radiologist due to the random nature of the anatomical positioning of the body parts within the body bag. Examples of possible indications are

(a) RADIOGRAPHIC SURVEY FORM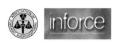

Artefact/Pathology location diagram

RIGHT   LEFT

KEY: (#1, #2 etc for multiple examples. Location: →)				
A: Intact Bullet	D: Cartridge Case	G: Needle	J: Jewellery	M: Metal (Unknown)
B: Bullet Fragment	E: Whole Round	H: Knife or Blade	K: Key	N: Radio / Remote
C: Shrapnel	F: Razor Blade	I: Glasses	L: Watch	O: Other (describe)

Date		Site Code & Body #	
Recorded by			
Signature		Page 4	MR22F (v8.1)

Fig. 8.11 (a) Examples of primary survey recording forms designed by the Inforce Foundation and the Association of Forensic Radiographers for use in the investigation of human remains exhumed from mass graves (continued)

(b)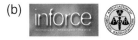

Artefact location diagram
For disarticulated remains. For articulated, please use next page.

Top of Bag

Right Side
of Bag

Left Side
of Bag

KEY: (#1, #2 etc for multiple examples. Location: →)				
A: Intact Bullet	D: Cartridge Case	G: Needle	J: Jewellery	M: Metal (Unknown)
B: Bullet Fragment	E: Whole Round	H: Knife or Blade	K: Key	N: Radio / Remote
C: Shrapnel	F: Razor Blade	I: Glasses	L: Watch	O: Other (describe)

Site Code & Body #		Date	
		Recorded by	
MR22F (v8.1)	Page 3	Signature	

Fig. 8.11 (b) allow the location of artifacts and pathology to be indicated on a grid system and anatomically as appropriate

- Any unique skeletal features or pathological conditions seen during the primary survey or identified during examination by the pathologist, anthropologist, or odontologist that may be useful for identification.
- To replicate poor-quality antemortem dental radiographs by undertaking subsequent examinations using substandard angulations to facilitate accurate comparison.
- In cases where evidence of trauma identified by the pathologist, anthropologist, or odontologist may indicate further imaging investigations to determine the nature of the injury or weapon used.
- To detect, locate, and retrieve items of forensic evidence seen during the primary survey but not located during examination by the pathologist.
- For those cases that are proving difficult to identify via other means, a full skeletal survey may be useful in determining age, sex, stature, etc., or for detecting unique skeletal features that have been previously documented in antemortem records.
- To document injuries and injury patterns for the purposes of the criminal investigation or as a means of negating the requirement for full autopsy where the cause of death is known.

In the last two cases, imaging examinations may be particularly useful in cases of fleshed remains where anthropological examination is difficult.

Case Studies

United Nations International Criminal Tribunal Investigations of Mass Graves in Croatia, Bosnia, and Kosovo 1996–2002

During the period from 1996 to 2002, the forensic teams of the Office of the Prosecutor for the United Nations International Criminal Tribunal for the Former Yugoslavia (ICTY) exhumed and examined several mass graves in Croatia, Bosnia and Herzegovina, and Kosovo as part of their investigation into alleged war crimes and crimes against humanity. Several mass graves, with wide variations in size and content, were exhumed, and the human remains were examined in mortuaries employing a modified mass fatality protocol. While the exhumation process was generally painstakingly carried out to the highest standards of forensic archaeology, some of the exhumed remains were inevitably commingled, particularly in "secondary" graves containing the remains of previous graves that had been "robbed" and reburied in an attempt to conceal them. Radiography played an important role in the examination of the remains from these graves. Fluoroscopy, radiography, and dental radiography were used, sometimes in "field" conditions, and were employed according to the following protocol.

Primary Survey

The primary survey (triage) was performed using fluoroscopy in all cases. All body bags were examined using a mobile C-Arm fluoroscope by a radiographer and pathologist or anthropologist working together. Fluoroscopy proved invaluable in the location of hazardous material including a number of live hand grenades (Fig. 8.12) and ammunition, razorblades, and other sharp objects. Its primary value was the location of projectile fragments (e.g., bullets and shrapnel), allowing the pathologists to locate and retrieve these at autopsy as well as locating personal effects, many of which carried identifiable markings. The examination of commingled remains using fluoroscopy enabled rapid evaluation of the contents of body bags and facilitated fast separation of human bone from soil, stones, and other artifacts.

Secondary Survey

Secondary surveys were only performed in specific circumstances. The incidence of any dental work among the population was generally very low and did not usually warrant a full dental radiography survey. In most cases, the secondary survey was limited to an oblique projection of both mandibular rami for age determination. In some specific investigations, however (where dental records were known to be available), a full-mouth dental radiography series was undertaken. In other investigations where systematic antemortem assault was alleged, a radiographic examination of the

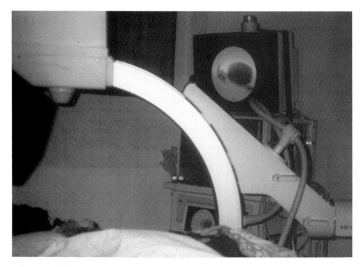

Fig. 8.12 The use of fluoroscopy for primary survey enables hazards to be identified and located. Fluoroscopy reveals the presence of a live grenade within the body bag (note image on screen in the background)

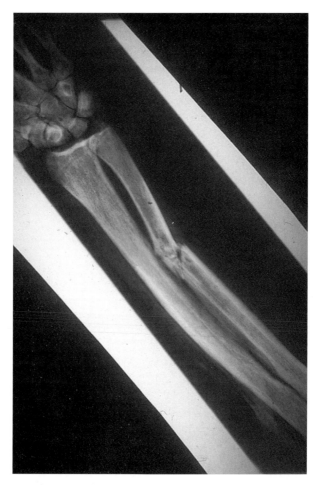

Fig. 8.13 Secondary surveys may sometimes be used to document perimortem injuries as in this case showing a defensive fracture of the radius and ulna

rib cage and extremities was undertaken to look for evidence of trauma and healing fractures (Fig. 8.13).

Tertiary Examinations

Fluoroscopy

The nature of the exhumed remains often rendered the physical location of items seen at primary survey difficult to locate during autopsy, particularly when these lay in clothing or decomposing tissue. Fluoroscopy was frequently employed during autopsy to locate and retrieve these items under X-ray control.

Radiography

Radiography was undertaken in a number of cases to document identifying features seen during the primary survey or at autopsy or anthropological examination. It was regularly employed to examine epiphyseal plates in young adults to assist with age determination, and, in some cases, it proved possible to establish identity by comparison of postmortem radiographs with ante-mortem films (Fig. 8.14). Generally, however, the incidence of antemortem films being available for comparison proved to be very low. Plain film radiography using high-definition techniques was also employed in some cases to determine whether bony trauma was associated with projectile fragments, particularly in cases where the exact nature of the injury could not be determined simply by physical examination.

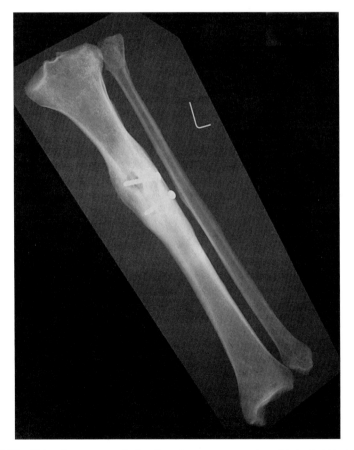

Fig. 8.14 Identifying features seen during the primary survey such as this healed fracture of the tibia with two orthopedic screws *in situ* were radiographed in true AP and lateral projections for the purpose of identification as a tertiary examination

July 7, 2005, London Bombings

On July 7, 2005, three terrorist bombs exploded on underground trains and a further bomb on a bus in London. Fifty-six people were killed in these explosions, and several hundred people were injured. Fifty-six cadavers were recovered from the scenes of the explosion together with a large number of fragmented remains.

In accordance with the London Resilience Mass Fatality Plan, the Association of Forensic Radiographers (AFR) mobilized its forensic radiography response team and equipment, some of which was provided on loan by the medical supply industry. A total of 27 radiographers worked in teams of between 6 and 8 for 12 hours per day during the subsequent 11 days (Viner et al. 2006). Two mobile C-Arm fluoroscopy units, a direct digital (DR) unit, a computed radiography (CR) unit, together with plain film radiography and dental radiography, were deployed according to the following protocol.

Primary Survey

Fluoroscopy was employed for the primary survey (triage) of the cadavers. Two radiographers, working together with a pathologist, examined each case documenting any identifying features, injuries, personal effects, and hazardous objects and printing hard-copy images via a thermal printer. The average examination time was 10 minutes.

Both digital radiography (DR) and computed radiography (CR) were employed for the primary survey of the body parts. The use of CR was abandoned after the first day as DR proved to be almost 10 times faster than CR in this application. Two radiographers examined each case using correct anatomical positioning where possible, which was facilitated by the use of transparent body part bags in many cases. Images were stored on a workstation accessible to pathologists and anthropologists for evaluation and written to CD-ROM as a permanent record.

The use of digital technology allowed images to be displayed to evaluate both soft-tissue and bony elements and facilitated rapid triage of commingled body parts for anthropological analysis and DNA testing. In many cases, subsequent radiography for analysis of bony elements was not required due to the high-definition nature of the images and the use of correct anatomical positioning. In this case, due to the rapid identification of victims by other means, it did not prove necessary to utilize the digital image database for comparison with antemortem skeletal radiographs. However, a number of dental fragments were recovered as part of the primary survey, and, in most cases, further radiography of these parts was not required, as the information obtained at primary survey was sufficient for odontological analysis and identification to be made.

Secondary Surveys

Dental radiography was undertaken as a routine part of the identification process using conventional intra-oral film radiography. Teams of experienced dental radiographers worked in conjunction with the forensic odontologists to undertake dental surveys *in situ*, shortening the odontological examination time.

Tertiary Examinations

Tertiary examinations of identifiable skeletal pathology were undertaken as part of the identification process, none of which contributed to a positive identification. A number of further examinations of fragmented remains were undertaken using both CR and DR. These enabled the anthropologists to examine bony elements for purposes of identification and documentation of injuries.

Conclusion

The science of medical imaging has developed rapidly over the last century since Roentgen's announcement of the discovery of X-rays and is continuing to develop at a rapid pace with each leap forward in computer technology. Medical imaging has an important and increasing role in forensic investigation, both in determining the cause of death or injury and in identifying the deceased. There is no one technique that will deliver all the answers, and its contribution to the analysis and identification of commingled human remains will be dependent upon the timely application of the most appropriate techniques. Close collaboration among investigators, pathologists, odontologists, anthropologists, and the radiology professionals (radiologists, radiographers, and physicists) is essential if the maximum benefit is to be obtained.

Acknowledgments Line drawings in Figures 8.1, 8.4b, and 8.9b from Ian Hanson, University of Bournemouth, UK. Photographs in Figures 8.4a, and 8.9a by kind permission of the Department of Radiology, St Bartholomew's and the Royal London Hospitals, London. Radiological Images in Figure 8.8 by kind permission of Sarah Bourne, The Royal London Hospital School of Dentistry, Queen Mary & Westfield College, University of London, London. Figure 8.10 by kind permission of The Inforce Foundation & The Association of Forensic Radiographers. Photographs in Figures 8.5, 8.6a, and 8.6b by kind permission of the Metropolitan Police, Scotland Yard, London. Photograph in Figure 8.7a and radiological image in Figure 8.7b by kind permission of the Department of Forensic Medicine University of Cape Town, South Africa and Lodox Ltd., Johannesburg, South Africa. Photograph in Figure 8.12 by kind permission of Patrick Reynolds. Radiological Images in Figures 8.13 and 8.14 by kind permission of the United Nations International Criminal Tribunal for the Former Yugoslavia, The Hague, Netherlands.

References Cited

Aitken, A. G., O. Flodmark, D. E. Newman, R. F. Kilcoyne, W. P. Shuman, and L. A. Mack 1985 Leg length determination by CT digital radiography. *AJR Am. J. Roentgenol.* 144(3):613–615.
Alexander, C. J. and G. A. Foote 1998 Radiology in forensic identification: The Mt. Erebus disaster. *Australas. Radiol.* 42(4):321–326.

Association of Forensic Radiographers 2004 Radiography facilities for temporary emergency mortuaries in the event of a mass fatality incident (unpublished paper). London.

Bass, W. M. 1990 Forensic anthropology. In *CAP Handbook for Postmortem Examination of Unidentified Remain; Developing Identification of Well Preserved, Decomposed, Burned, and Skeletonised Remains*, M. F. Fierro, ed. College of American Pathologists, Skokie, IL.

Beningfield, S., H. Potgieter, A. Nicol, S. van As, G. Bowie, E. Hering, and E. Latti 2003 Report on a new type of trauma full-body digital X-ray machine. *Emerg. Radiol.* 10(1):23–29.

Binda, M., C. Cattaneo, A. Bogoni, P. Fattorini, and M. Grandi 1999 Identification of human skeletal remains: Forensic radiology vs. DNA. *Radiol. Med. (Torino)* 97(5):409–411.

Bisset, R. A., N. B. Thomas, I. W. Turnbull, and S. Lee 2002 Postmortem examinations using magnetic resonance imaging: Four-year review of a working service. *BMJ* 324(7351): 1423–1424.

Brogdon, B. G. 1998a Radiological identification of individual remains. In *Forensic Radiology*, B. G.Brogdon, ed., pp. 149–187. CRC Press, Boca Raton, FL.

1998b Radiological identification: Anthropological parameters. In *Forensic Radiology*, B. G. Brogdon, ed., pp. 63–96. CRC Press, Boca Raton, FL.

Brogdon, B. G. and J. E. Lichtenstein 1998 Forensic radiology in historical perspective. In *Forensic Radiology*, B. G. Brogdon, ed., pp. 13–34. CRC Press, Boca Raton, FL.

Brogdon, B. G., H. Vogel, and J. McDowell 2003 *A Radiologic Atlas of Abuse, Torture and Inflicted Trauma*. CRC Press, Boca Raton, FL.

Brookes, J. A., M. A. Hall-Craggs, V. R. Sams, and W. R. Lees 1996 Non-invasive perinatal necropsy by magnetic resonance imaging. *Lancet* 348(9035):1139–1141.

Bryan, G. J. 1979 *Diagnostic Radiography*, 3rd ed. Churchill Livingstone, Edinburgh.

Buchner, A. 1985 The identification of human remains. *Int. Dent. J.* 35(4):307–311.

Burrows, E. H. 1986 *Pioneers and Early Years: A History of British Radiology*. Colophon Ltd., Alderney, Chanel Islands.

Chilvarquer, I., J. O. Katz, D. M. Glassman, T. J. Prihoda, and J. A. Cottone 1987 Comparative radiographic study of human and animal long bone patterns. *J. Forensic Sci.* 32(6):1645–1654.

Craig, E. A. 1995 Intercondylar shelf angle: A new method to determine race from the distal femur. *J. Forensic Sci.* 40(5):777–782.

Culbert, W. L. and F. M. Law 1927 Identification by comparison of roentgenograms of nasal accessory sinuses and mastoid processes. *JAMA* (88):1632–1636.

Dimond, B. 2002 *Legal Aspects of Radiography and Radiology*. Blackwell Science, Oxford.

Eckert, W. G. and N. Garland 1984 The history of the forensic applications in radiology. *Am. J. Forensic Med. Pathol.* 5(1):53–56.

Emerton, D., I. Honey, A. McKenzie, P. Blake, D. Annett, C. Lawinski, and H. Cole 2005 *Computed Radiography Systems for General Radiography (CR) Comparative Report, Edition 2, Report 05081*. NHS Purchasing and Supply Agency, Her Majesty's Stationery Office.

Engel-Hills, P. 2006 Radiation protection in medical imaging. *Radiography* 12(2):153–160.

Evans, K. T., B. Knight, and D. K. Whittaker 1981 *Forensic Radiology*. Blackwell Scientific, Oxford.

Fischman, S. L. 1985 The use of medical and dental radiographs in identification. *Int. Dent. J.* 35(4):301–306.

Glasser, O. 1931 First Roentgen evidence. *Radiology* (17):789.

Goodman, N. R. and L. B. Edelson 2002 The efficiency of an X-ray screening system at a mass disaster. *J. Forensic Sci.* 47(1):127–130.

Goodman, P. C. 1995 The new light: Discovery and introduction of the X-ray. *AJR Am. J. Roentgenol.* 165(5):1041–1045.

Gould, P. 2003 X-ray detectives turn images into evidence. *Diagn. Imaging* (Special edition).

Greulich, W. W. and S. I. Pyle 1959 *Radiographic Atlas of Skeletal Development of the Hand and Wrist*. Stanford University Press, Stanford, CA.

Haglund, W. D. and C. L. Fligner 1993 Confirmation of human identification using computerized tomography (CT). *J. Forensic Sci.* 38(3):708–712.

Hall-Edwards, J. 1908 On X-ray dermatitis and its prevention. *Arch. Roentgen Ray* (13):243–248.

Halperin, E. C. 1988 X-rays at the bar, 1896–1910. *Invest. Radiol.* 23(8):639–646.

Hansman, C. F. 1962 Appearance and fusion of ossification centers in the human skeleton. *Am. J. Roentgenol. Radium Ther. Nucl. Med.* 88:476–482.

Harcke, H. T., J. A. Bifano, and K. K. Koeller 2002 Forensic radiology: Response to the Pentagon Attack on September 11, 2001. *Radiology* 223(1):7–8.

Hart, D. and B. F. Wall 2002 *Radiation exposure of the UK population from medical and dental X-ray examinations.* National Radiological Protection Board-W4, Chilton.

Hildebolt, C. F., M. W. Vannier, and R. H. Knapp 1990 Validation study of skull three-dimensional computerized tomography measurements. *Am. J. Phys. Anthropol.* 82(3):283–294.

Hoerr, N. L., S. I. Pyle, and C. C. Francis 1962 *Radiological Atlas of the Foot and Ankle.* Charles C. Thomas, Springfield, IL.

International X-ray Protection Committee 1928 International recommendations for X-ray and radium protection. *Br. J. Radiol.* (1):358–363.

Jackowski, C., E. Aghayev, M. Sonnenschein, R. Dirnhofer, and M. J. Thali 2006 Maximum intensity projection of cranial computed tomography data for dental identification. *Int. J. Legal Med.* 120(3):165–167.

Jenkins, D. 1980 *Radiographic Photography and Imaging Processes.* MTP Press Ltd., Lancaster, UK.

Jensen, S. 1991 Identification of human remains lacking skull and teeth. A case report with some methodological considerations. *Am. J. Forensic Med. Pathol.* 12(2):93–97.

Kahana, T. and J. Hiss 1997 Identification of human remains: Forensic radiology. *J. Clin. Forensic Med.* 4(1):7–15.

Kahana, T., J. A. Ravioli, C. L. Urroz, and J. Hiss 1997 Radiographic identification of fragmentary human remains from a mass disaster. *Am. J. Forensic Med. Pathol.* 18(1):40–44.

Kirk, N. J., R. E. Wood, and M. Goldstein 2002 Skeletal identification using the frontal sinus region: A retrospective study of 39 cases. *J. Forensic Sci.* 47(2):318–323.

Krogman, W. M. and M. Y. Iscan 1986 *The Human Skeleton in Forensic Medicine,* 2nd ed. Charles C. Thomas, Springfield, IL.

Kurihara, Y., Y. Kurihara, K. Ohashi, A. Kitagawa, M. Miyasaka, E. Okamoto, and T. Ishikawa 1996 Radiologic evidence of sex differences: Is the patient a woman or a man? *AJR Am. J. Roentgenol.* 167(4):1037–1040.

Lawinski, C., A. McKenzie, H. Cole, P. Blake, and I. Honey 2005 *Digital Detectors for General Radiography: A Comparative Technical Report 05078.* NHS Purchasing and Supply Agency, Her Majesty's Stationery Office.

Levinsohn 1899 Beitraz zur feststellung der identitat. *Arch. Krim. Anthrop.* (2):221.

Lichtenstein, J. E. 1998 Radiology in mass casualty situations. In *Forensic Radiology,* B. G. Brogdon, ed., pp. 189–208. CRC Press, Boca Raton, FL.

Maresh, M. M. 1943 Growth of major long bones in healthy children. *Am. J. Dis. Child.* 66: 227–257.

Marlin, D. C., M. A. Clark, and S. M. Standish 1991 Identification of human remains by comparison of frontal sinus radiographs: A series of four cases. *J. Forensic Sci.* 36(6): 1765–1772.

Mason, R. and S. Bourne 1998 *A Guide to Dental Radiography,* 4th ed. Oxford University Press, Oxford.

McCormick, W. F. 1980 Mineralization of the costal cartilages as an indicator of age: Preliminary observations. *J. Forensic Sci.* 25(4):736–741.

Mora, S. et al. 2001 Applicability of the Greulich and Pyle standards. *Pediatr. Res.* (50):624–812.

Mulligan, M. E., M. J. McCarthy, F. J. Wippold, J. E. Lichtenstein, and G. N. Wagner 1988 Radiologic evaluation of mass casualty victims: Lessons from the Gander, Newfoundland, accident. *Radiology* 168(1):229–233.

Murphy, W. A., F. G. Spruill, and G. E. Gantner 1980 Radiologic identification of unknown human remains. *J. Forensic Sci.* 25(4):727–735.

Myers, J. C., M. I. Okoye, D. Kiple, E. H. Kimmerle, and K. J. Reinhard 1999 Three-dimensional (3-D) imaging in post-mortem examinations: Elucidation and identification of cranial and facial fractures in victims of homicide utilizing 3-D computerized imaging reconstruction techniques. *Int. J. Legal Med.* 113(1):33–37.

Nambiar, P., M. D. Naidu, and K. Subramaniam 1999 Anatomical variability of the frontal sinuses and their application in forensic identification. *Clin. Anat.* 12(1):16–19.

Navani, S., J. R. Shah, and P. S. Levy 1970 Determination of sex by costal cartilage calcification. *Am, J, Roentgenol. Radium Ther. Nucl. Med.* 108(4):771–774.

Nye, P. J., T. L. Tytle, R. N. Jarman, and B. G. Eaton 1996 The role of radiology in the Oklahoma City bombing. *Radiology* 200(2):541–543.

Pyle, S. I. and N. L. Hoerr 1955 *Atlas of Skeletal Development of the Knee.* Charles C. Thomas, Springfield, IL.

Reichs, K. and R. B. J. Dorion 1992 The use of computed tomography (CT) scans in the analysis of frontal sinus configuration. *Can. Soc. Forensic Sci. J.* (25):1.

Riepert, T., C. Rittner, D. Ulmcke, S. Ogbuihi, and F. Schweden 1995 Identification of an unknown corpse by means of computed tomography (CT) of the lumbar spine. *J. Forensic Sci.* 40(1): 126–127.

Rocha Sdos, S., D. L. Ramos, and G. Cavalcanti Mde 2003 Applicability of 3D-CT facial reconstruction for forensic individual identification. *Pesqui. Odontol. Bras.* 17(1):24–28.

Roentgen, W. C. 1895 A new kind of ray. *Phys.-Med. Ges.* (137):132–141.

Rogers, T. and S. Saunders 1994 Accuracy of sex determination using morphological traits of the human pelvis. *J. Forensic Sci.* 39(4):1047–1056.

Rutty, G. N. 2006 University of Leicester Announces World First Forensic Technique: A New Horizon for Mass Fatality Radiology, University of Leicester Press Release, Leicester.

Sanders, I., M. E. Woesner, R. A. Ferguson, and T. T. Noguchi 1972 A new application of forensic radiology: Identification of deceased from a single clavicle. *Am. J. Roentgenol. Radium Ther. Nucl. Med.* 115(3):619–622.

Scheuer, L. and S. Black 2004 *The Juvenile Skeleton.* Academic Press, London.

Schwartz, S. and E. D. Woolridge 1977 The use of panoramic radiographs for comparisons in cases of identification. *J. Forensic Sci.* 22(1):145–146.

Society of Radiographers 2005 Radiographers help identify London Bombing victims. *Synergy* September:1.

Sutherland, L. D. and J. M. Suchey 1991 Use of the ventral arc in pubic sex determination. *J. Forensic Sci.* 36(2):501–511.

Tanner, R. J., B. F. Wall, P. C. Shrimpton, et al. 2001 *Frequency of Medical and Dental X-ray Examinations in the UK, 1997–98.* National Radiological Protection Board.

Thali, M. J. et al. 2000 Improved vision in forensic documentation: Forensic 3D/CAD-supported photogrammetry of bodily injury internal structures to provide more leads and stronger practical forensic evidence. Paper presented at the International Society of Optical Engineers: 3D Visualisation for Data Exploration and Decision Making.

Thali, M. J., T. Markwalder, C. Jackowski, M. Sonnenschein, and R. Dirnhofer 2006 Dental CT imaging as a screening tool for dental profiling: Advantages and limitations. *J. Forensic Sci.* 51(1):113–119.

Thali, M. J., K. Yen, W. Schweitzer, P. Vock, C. Boesch, C. Ozdoba, G. Schroth, M. Ith, M. Sonnenschein, T. Doernhoefer, E. Scheurer, T. Plattner, and R. Dirnhofer 2003a Virtopsy, a new imaging horizon in forensic pathology: Virtual autopsy by postmortem multislice computed tomography (MSCT) and magnetic resonance imaging (MRI)—A feasibility study. *J. Forensic Sci.* 48(2):386–403.

Thali, M. J., K. Yen, W. Schweitzer, P. Vock, C. Ozdoba, and R. Dirnhofer 2003b Into the decomposed body-forensic digital autopsy using multislice-computed tomography. *Forensic Sci. Int.* 134(2–3):109–114.

Tonello, B. 1998 Mass Grave Investigations. Paper presented at the Imaging Science Oncologists, British Institute of Radiology.

Trotter, M. and G. C. Gleser 1952 Estimation of stature from long bones of American whites and Negroes. *Am. J. Phys. Anthropol.* 10:463–514.

1958 A re-evaluation of estimation of stature based on measurements of stature taken during life and of long bones after death. *Am. J. Phys. Anthropol.* 16:79–123.

Uysal, S., D. Gokharman, M. Kacar, I. Tuncbilek, and U. Kosa 2005 Estimation of sex by 3D CT measurements of the foramen magnum. *J. Forensic Sci.* 50(6):1310–1314.

Viner, M. D. 2001a Forensic investigation: The role of radiography. *Eur. Radiol.* Supplement to Volume 11(2):95.

2001b Forensic investigation: The role of radiography in forensic medicine. *ISRRT Newsletter* 37(2):4–7.

2001c The radiographers role in forensic investigation. *Hold Pusten: J. Norwegian Soc. Radiog.* (9/2001).

Viner, M. D., M. Cassidy, and V. Treu 1998 The Role of Radiography in a Disaster Investigation. Paper presented at the Imaging Science Oncolologists, British Institute of Radiology.

Viner, M. D., W. Hoban, C. Rock, and M. T. Cassidy 2003 The Role of Radiography in the Investigation of Mass Incidents. Paper presented at the American Academy of Forensic Science 55th Scientific Meeting, Chicago, IL.

Viner, M. D., C. Rock, N. Hunt, G. Mackinnon, and A. W. Martin 2006 Forensic Radiography: Response to the London Suicide Bombings on 7th July 2005. Paper presented at the American Academy of Forensic Science 58th Scientific Meeting, Seattle, WA.

Chapter 9
Detection of Commingling in Cremated Human Remains

Michael Warren

Introduction

Commercial cremation of human remains, as it is currently practiced in North America and most of Western Europe, results in commingling of the cremated remains (cremains) of more than one dead body. Locard's Principle of Exchange, also known as the theory of transfer, tells us that—in light of how cremations are performed—commingling is inevitable and will occur to some degree in every cremation. The extent of commingling is contingent upon several factors, including the specific protocol used by the cremationist and the design of the retort and processor. If commingling is expected, why has the issue of commingled cremains become an important legal issue? This chapter will discuss (1) the inevitability of commingling in cremation, (2) factors that lead to commingling, (3) how commingling becomes a legal issue, and (4) how commingling is detected and how it might be described to a jury or arbitrator, who ultimately must decide if the degree of commingling is incidental to the normal cremation process or the result of negligent cremation practice. The methodology is qualitative, focusing on a discussion of the probative value of evidence in determining if demonstrable commingling exists and to what extent. As the reader will see, experience plays a role in interpreting each piece of evidence. What might the investigator expect to find from previous cremations in the same retort? What biological and artifactual evidence might we expect to survive postprocessing of remains? What types of biological and artifactual evidence should we expect to find? Equally important, what types of evidence would we not expect to find, and what does that tell the investigator?

As cremation has become more popular, the cremation industry has inevitably become the target of civil litigation. Issues such as the commingling of the remains of more than one decedent, improper cremation practice, disputed identity of remains, and improper disposal are becoming increasingly popular courtroom subjects. Several class-action suits of note have involved literally hundreds of plaintiffs—each with potentially millions of dollars at stake (Bass and Jefferson 2003; Iverson 2001; Maples and Browning 1994). As a result, crematories and funeral homes have been placed under public scrutiny as industry standards and practices are developed and instituted. Specific legal issues, such

From: *Recovery, Analysis, and Identification of Commingled Human Remains*
Edited by: B. Adams and J. Byrd © Humana Press, Totowa, NJ

as establishing an "acceptable" amount of commingling, are presently being determined by the courts, and we can expect this process to continue over the next several years.

When plaintiffs have some reason to believe that the cremains in their possession are not those of their loved one, or that more than one person is represented, legal counsel will often consult with forensic experts to perform scientific analyses that might help resolve the dispute. Since cremains are principally composed of the fragmented remains of the skeleton, the expert usually takes the form of a forensic anthropologist, a specialist in skeletal anatomy, morphology, and taphonomy (literally, *burial laws*, but in a biological sense the processes that occur to a body after death). The anthropologist performs an examination of the cremated remains using microscopy, radiography, and other methods to find clues that might lead to identification. These clues generally come from two sources: the biological remains, consisting of osseous (bony) and dental fragments, and non-osseous artifacts. In almost every case, the evidence for identity is presumptive since positive lines of evidence such as DNA and fingerprints are lost during the cremation process (although in rare cases, an altered dental or medical appliance can be matched to antemortem radiographs, providing a positive line of identification).

Along with the anthropologist, the expertise of a forensic odontologist is warranted, especially for cases in which significant dental artifacts are found. The odontologist will recognize the types of dental artifacts within cremains and be able to better assess the antemortem dental records and radiographs than the anthropologist. In major cases, a multidisciplinary team has been retained, including an anthropologist, a pathologist, and an odontologist—each bringing a different area of expertise to bear.

The Inevitability of Commingling in Cremation

To understand the relevant findings in a forensic analysis of cremains, as well as the inevitable issue of commingling, one must have a thorough understanding of the cremation process (for a complete description of the cremation process, see Murad 1998). The process begins when the body is placed into an empty cremation retort. The body is usually within a cardboard or fiberboard container designed for cremation. The body is subjected to a direct flame and burns at temperatures ranging between 1400 °F to 1800 °F (760 °C to 982 °C) in the cremation chamber, for one to two hours. The specific protocol depends on the type of equipment, the size of the body, and whether or not the cremation is being performed in a preheated retort (i.e., whether the cremation is the first one of the day or is being performed immediately after a preceding cremation). The goal is *calcination*, the process of removing all water and organic matter using intense heat.

Once the body has been incinerated, the retort door is opened and the chamber is allowed to cool. Once the chamber temperature has cooled to a temperature that is bearable, the cremationist, using a long-handled wire-bristle brush or hoe, rakes the calcined bone fragments forward. Most retorts are built with an aperture near the door into which the fragments fall, eventually ending up in a receptacle beneath the door. At this point, the cremationist will usually remove larger foreign objects, including medical and dental hardware, casket hardware, and all magnetic debris. After the cremationist has removed these objects from the cremains, they are typically emptied into a machine that is variously known as a pulverizer, processor, or cremulator. This processor reduces the calcined bone fragments to small particles and ash suitable for inurnment or scattering (Warren and Schultz 2002).

After the cremains have been swept from the retort and removed from the collection bin, the retort is ready for another cremation. The next body is placed into the retort and the process is repeated. The above-mentioned Locard's Principle of Exchange—one of the central theories in the forensic sciences—tells us that it is impossible, even under ideal conditions, to introduce a body into an enclosed space and then remove it without leaving evidence of it having been there. Obviously, the cremation retort does not present ideal conditions. During cremation it becomes an extremely volatile environment in which fragments of calcined bone are blown about by large volumes of combustion air. When the cremated bone fragments and ash are removed from the retort by the cremationist, it is difficult for even the most well-trained and conscientious cremationist to perfectly clean out the deeper recesses of the retort floor. The retort is a relatively large space, and the areas in the back corners are difficult to reach with the standard issue long-handled broom and hoe. The cremation chamber is unlit, so the back areas are dark, making bone fragments and artifacts difficult to see and remove. Additionally, the retort is hot, especially if another body is to be cremated. These challenges lead to mistakes and lapses in procedure, which lead to, among other problems, significant commingling.

Factors That Lead to Excessive Commingling

Aside from the normal degree of commingling expected during a well-performed cremation, a number of other factors can lead to excessive amounts of commingling. Although commercial cremation has been practiced in North America since the 19th century (Prothero 2001), it has been within the last few decades that it has gained wide acceptance. The funeral industry, while closely regulated by various governmental agencies, began practicing cremation with relatively little oversight. Few, if any, industry standards were established. Most cremationists were, and continue to be, trained and certified by the manufacturers of the equipment. Therefore, there were no prohibitions against several practices, such as cremating more than one body simultaneously, that are uniformly considered unprofessional by current standards. In response, the funerary industry has been proactive in seeking remedies for earlier shortcomings, and many states have passed legislation that controls and permits action against crematories guilty of improper practices. For example, Arizona has passed laws that permit disciplinary action against crematories for "using a retort for any purpose other than the cremation of human remains," "cremating more than one dead human body at the same time in the same retort without the express written consent of the authorizing agents," and "introducing a second dead human body into a retort before reasonable efforts have been made to remove all fragments of the cremated remains from the preceding cremation without the express written consent of the authorizing agents." The inevitability of commingling is acknowledged in the legislation by specifically referencing "incidental and unavoidable residue remaining in a retort after a cremation" (Arizona State Legislation 32-1398; *Crematories; Disciplinary Action; Acts of Crematory*). This implies that "reasonable" efforts to remove all material from the retort will never be completely successful.

Another source of excessive commingling is simply the result of poor cremation practice and procedures. The process requires vigilance and good effort. Although some crematories are "direct cremation" businesses, most cremationists are associated with funeral homes and many are licensed funeral directors. The funeral industry is built on trust and compassion. A cremation performed by a well-meaning and thorough cremationist will generally keep the crematory out of legal trouble. In fact, most of the cremains examined by the author have been conducted in the proper manner and no evidence of wrongdoing can be found. On the other hand, some show evidence of haphazard procedure—insufficient temperature and/or duration, failure to remove magnetic debris, inadequate documentation and other signs that introduce doubt into the families of the decedents, as well as the jurors and arbiters hearing the case.

How Commingling Becomes a Legal Issue

A primary issue leading to litigation is that the family of the decedent is not informed about the cremation process and told about the inevitability of commingling. When told of the legal issues that arise in cremation cases, several colleagues—forensic pathologists—from Thailand failed to understand why commingling is an issue at all. Cremation is by far the preferred method of postmortem disposition of the body in Thailand, and the process is thoroughly understood by most Thai people because they participate in the cremation ceremony. Most Thai cremations are performed on a traditional pyre that is built for one cremation only, so the process results in very little commingling of remains. However, the families of the deceased see no problem with the prospect of their loved one's cremains containing some small quantity of another decedent's cremains. It seems that commingling of remains is not the primary issue, but it is instead the fact that the commingling can be readily detected and identified that creates a problem.

Many families receive an urn from the funeral home containing their loved one's cremains and never open the container. Most people do not have a clear understanding of what cremains should look like and, in fact, have little knowledge of the cremation process. When the urn is opened, some plaintiffs compare what they are seeing with a preconceived expectation that does not match. There are not enough cremains; there are too little; no "emotional attachment" is felt when viewing the cremains; the cremains do not look like ash but something else. This insecurity is compounded when a funeral home or crematory is publicly accused of misdeeds.

Legal action often follows when the cremains of a child are examined by the parents. The cremains of children are smaller in weight and volume and are often hand-processed, resulting in less reduction and larger bone fragments. Children have accrued less medical and dental artifacts than adults. When the parents examine their child's cremains and find remnants of denture material, surgical clips, or other artifacts, it is readily apparent that either they have the wrong set of cremains or the cremains of their child are commingled with those of an adult. It is this type of demonstrable commingling that proves problematic for the cremation industry and brings forensic experts to bear. In summary, two things are certain: (1) Commingling will occur with every cremation, and (2) legal issues will be resolved by the amount and quality of *demonstrable* commingling identified by forensic experts. The jury will be the arbiter of whether the cremationist was conscientious and thorough in the performance of the cremation, or whether the commingling is evidence of improper or negligent cremation practices.

How Commingling Is Detected

Cremains consist of both biological remains and cultural artifacts. Both biology and culture define one's identity. The analysis of cremated remains is focused on finding evidence for identity that corresponds to the known biological parameters of the decedent and any evidence that records the decedent's life history—most of which is found among various non-osseous artifacts.

A proper cremains investigation requires a well-equipped forensic laboratory containing a quality dissecting microscope, scales, testing sieves, photographic equipment, and access to radiologic and chemical testing equipment. The analysis involves careful examination of every fragment and artifact contained within the urn. Most examinations take from six to eight hours, exclusive of documentation and reporting, depending on the nature of the cremains and the amount and quality of the artifacts to be identified. Most examiners use testing sieves to segregate the particulates into like sizes so that emphasis can be placed on the larger, more diagnostic pieces. The fine ash that comprises variable portions of cremains is essentially pretreated for chemical analyses (e.g., induced-coupled plasma mass spectroscopy, or particle-induced X-ray emission spectroscopy). These chemical analyses can be employed should the examiner suspect that foreign material has been presented with—or in lieu of—human cremains.

The Biological Remains

The biological component of cremated remains consists of literally thousands of small, calcined bone and tooth fragments. These fragments, while distinguishable as bone and teeth, are almost uniformly unidentifiable in all other respects. With very few exceptions (most notably the ear ossicles), almost every fragment will be nondiagnostic in terms of whether the bone is human or nonhuman and which bone is represented. Therefore, information gleaned from the osseous remains usually results in only general statements about concordance of the remains with known information about the decedent. For example, if the decedent had teeth, one would typically find tooth enamel fragments among the cremains. An edentulous decedent should not contain numerous tooth enamel fragments; this is presumptive evidence of commingling. More specific information is rare, although evidence of specific pathology or skeletal anomalies is occasionally found (Warren et al. 1999). Obviously, the more completely the remains are processed, the less diagnostic the osseous fragments will be. The type and condition of the processor greatly affect the survivability of diagnostic bone and teeth fragments (Fig. 9.1).

A second consideration is the weight of the remains. The expected range of the weight of cremated remains is well documented and loosely correlated with such variables as cadaver stature and estimated skeletal weight (Warren and Maples 1997). If the weight of the cremated remains grossly exceeds the expected range, the investigator can only reach the conclusion that more than one decedent is represented. If the weight is considerably less than the expected range, several possibilities exist—either all of the remains are not present, or the remains are those of a smaller body (i.e., a child, or even a pet). Consideration of weights

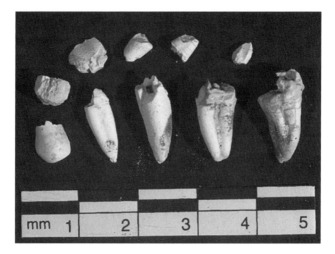

Fig. 9.1 Intact tooth roots that survived a rotary-bladed type of processor. The forensic odontologist will be able to identify which teeth are represented and compare the information with the clinical records of the decedent

must necessarily rely on the assumption that all of the remains are present. This problem is particularly vexing because it is not uncommon for cremated remains to be divided among family members. More research is needed to examine the full range of expected cremains weights from a number of different crematories, since it has been demonstrated that differences in mean weights exist from crematory to crematory—probably as a result of differing equipment and procedures (Bass and Jantz 2004; Birkby 1991).

The Non-osseous Artifacts

The material most informative about personal identity consists of medical, dental, mortuary, and other miscellaneous artifacts. These artifacts tell us something about the decedent's life history. As described above, larger orthopedic and dental prosthetics are usually found and discarded after cremation. However, many of these materials are manufactured of nonmagnetic and para-magnetic alloys and so are not picked up by the heavy magnet used by most cremationists (Fig. 9.2).

These artifacts represent presumptive evidence for identity and are key in building a case either against, or for, commingling. For example, it is common to find broken pieces of sternotomy wire sutures in the cremated remains of individuals who had undergone heart bypass surgery. Porcelain-like fragments are common and indicative of an individual cremated with their dentures in place. If the decedent was embalmed for visitation prior to cremation, at least one of the injector needles will inevitably find its way into the remains presented to the family. On the other hand, the artifacts found may be inconsistent with the known information about the

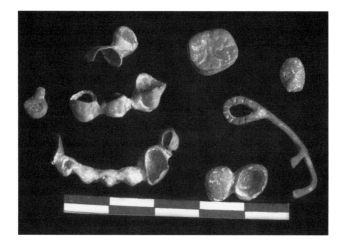

Fig. 9.2 Various dental artifacts presented with the cremains and found during examination. As in Figure 9.1, the forensic odontologist may be able to identify the types and locations of these dental appliances and compare that data with the antemortem dental records and radiographs of the putative decedent

decedent. A small section of pacemaker lead wire or porcelain fragments in the cremated remains of a child are telltale signs that at least some small portion of the cremains is that of an adult.

Personal Identification

The second phase of a cremains examination involves gathering antemortem data about the putative decedent. This can be accomplished by providing a questionnaire to the decedent's family or legal representative. Since this usually involves court orders and other forms of legal wrangling, this process should begin as soon as the expert is contacted and retained. Collection of antemortem data from the family members of the decedent is, of course, a familiar process to anthropologists working in human identification. Here, the context is different, resulting in a slightly different inquiry. Below is a reasonable list of questions that might bear fruit in establishing identity and/or determining whether commingling exists:

- Was the decedent male or female?
- What was the decedent's age at death?
- What was the decedent's height?
- What was the decedent's weight?
- What was the cause and manner of death?
- List surgical procedures and surgeon of record.
- List dental procedures and dentist of record.
- Did the decedent have any natural teeth remaining? Dentures or partial plates?
- Was the decedent embalmed prior to cremation (i.e., was there a "viewing or wake")?
- What clothing was on the body during cremation?
- Was the decedent cremated in a cardboard container, a wooden "cremation casket," a standard wooden casket, or without container or casket?
- Were any foreign objects cremated with the decedent (e.g., CDs, stuffed animals, flower arrangements)?
- Have the cremains been in an urn since cremation? What type? Was there a small memorial urn?
- Are all of the cremains present?

The crematory may be asked to answer some of the following questions:

- What is the brand of retort?
- Is the floor cast or brick?
- How old is the retort?
- Has the floor been replaced?
- What tools did the cremationist use to remove the cremains from the retort?
- Does the cremationist open the retort and stir the remains during the cremation cycle?
- What type of processor was used to pulverize the cremains?
- Was a magnet used to retrieve ferrous material from the cremains?

- Is the cremationist experienced? Did he receive training from the retort manufacturer?
- Was a cremation "tag" used and should it be with the cremains?
- If possible, enclose a copy or original of the temperature readout during the cremation cycle.
- When was the last EPA or OSHA inspection of the retort and/or facilities? Are there local inspectors?

With the above information in hand, the examiner can begin to compile a life history for the putative decedent. Once this biological profile and history are known, the examiner can generate a list of expected (and unexpected) findings. Here, experience in the analysis of cremains is important, because the examiner must know the aspects of the medical, dental, and mortuary history on which to focus. Some pathological conditions or treatments are more likely to produce evidence than others. Medical and dental records may be subpoenaed via the legal counsel (plaintiff or defense) for whom the examiner is consulting.

The fictitious list below might be relevant for a male decedent who died postoperatively following heart bypass surgery and who was embalmed prior to the cremation of his body in a cremation casket. If the decedent died while still in possession of his natural dentition, then enamel and root fragments would be placed in the "expected" list and artificial porcelain-like fragments would be included in the "unexpected" list.

Expected Biological and Artifactual Evidence	Present	Absent
Bone structure (e.g., trabecular bone, foramina, cortex)	X	
Diagnostic human bone	X	
Natural dental fragments (e.g., root apices, enamel fragments)	X	
Hospital bracelet clasp	X	
Hospital gown snaps		X
Ligation clips		X
Skin-closure staples	X	
Sternotomy sutures	X	
Mortuary injector needles	X	
Coffin hardware (e.g., screws, staples, brads)	X	
Jewelry (including slumped yellow metal and gemstones)		X

Unexpected Biological and Artifactual Evidence	Present	Absent
Porcelain or composite artificial dentition fragments (e.g., dentures, crowns, pontics)	X	
Dental posts, bridgework, or other metallic dental prostheses		X
Clothing snaps, hooks, clasps, zippers		X
Pacemaker or internal defibrillator lead wires		X
Embolism filters		X
Arterial stents		X
Artificial heart valves		X
Bra hooks and clasps		X

The list can be exhaustive provided the examiner gets good compliance with the request for antemortem information. The presence or absence of each finding can be considered presumptive evidence that either partially refutes or confirms the identity of the decedent. Mixed results (e.g., artifacts are present in both the expected and unexpected lists) suggest commingling of the remains of more than one individual.

How Is Commingling Described to a Jury?

The forensic consultant is an objective expert. Findings relevant to the case are disclosed to counsel whether the evidence supports or refutes the case for commingling, negligence, mistaken identity, or any other legal issue. However, attorneys for both the defense and plaintiff(s), armed with an impartial and fair assessment from their expert, can adopt a strategy for how evidence that supports their argument will be presented to the jury or arbitrator. Moreover, the expert may be able to initially provide the legal team with advice on which cremains within a "class" are most likely to demonstrate (or not) commingling.

The defendant's counsel may address the certainty of commingling based on Locard's principle. As mentioned above, legal issues will be resolved by the amount and quality of *demonstrable* commingling. Equipped with knowledge that, even following a well-performed and professional cremation, some degree of commingling has occurred, the defense attorney can argue that a small amount of *demonstrable* commingling does not imply poor cremation practice. This argument is best supported by a preponderance of presumptive evidence that supports the identity of the putative decedent. In the absence of supporting evidence, the expert must concede that the only evidence for identity is inconsistent with the known information for the decedent and that the most likely explanation is that the cremains are those of another individual. Attorneys for the defense tend to present evidence for commingling by reporting the weight of the artifacts and biological material as a (small) percentage of the overall weight of the cremains. For example, the inconsistent artifacts may "weigh about the same as a dime" or "weigh less than 1% of the total cremains weight."

Plaintiff's counsel will consider any demonstrable commingling as proof of improper practice or as introducing doubt as to the identity of the decedent. This doubt, they will point out, caused emotional or financial hardship and is what led the family to consider legal action as a remedy. The plaintiff's attorneys are inclined to focus on the quality and numerical quantity of the commingled evidence.

Case Study

The following case study is representative of a typical cremation investigation. The case, which involves the cremated remains of a fetus that was spontaneously aborted at $4^{1}/_{2}$ lunar months gestation, illustrates the amount of information that can be gleaned from a small amount of bone fragments (Fig. 9.3).

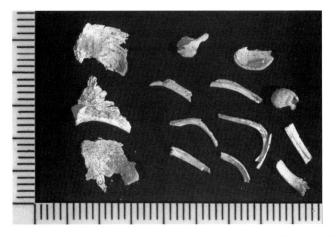

Fig. 9.3 Several bone fragments from a 4-lunar-month fetus. Among the fragments found intact were neural arches, cranial vault fragments, and intact long bone diaphyses

The author examined the remains at the C.A. Pound Human Identification Laboratory at the University of Florida. The cremains were mostly white in color, completely calcined and brittle, and produced a metallic sound when percussed with an instrument. The size of the cremains fragments was most consistent with a commercially available rotary-bladed processor.

The total weight of the bag of cremains was 225.0 grams. This weight is significantly less than the published mean of approximately 2430 grams for a mixed-sex sample of cremated adult remains, suggesting either that the remains were those of a subadult or that a portion of the cremains was not presented for examination. This weight is also significantly more than the cremains weight published for a fetus of roughly comparable gestational age as that reported for the putative decedent (Warren and Maples 1997).

Several intact bones were present that confirmed that the cremains were of human origin. An intact incus bone (one of the ear ossicles) was uniquely human in morphology. Among the cremains were several small but intact long bone diaphyses. An intact femoral diaphysis measured 23.5 millimeters, corresponding to a crown-to-heel length of approximately 19.644 centimeters using the established regression formulae of Fazekas and Kósa (1978); or alternatively, approximately 21.275 centimeters using published data from Warren (1999). This crown-to-heel length corresponded to a gestational age of between 4 and 5 lunar months, or 16 to 20 weeks. The degree of development of seven intact vertebral elements of the neural arch, two complete ribs, three additional long bone fragments, and a partial sphenoid bone all corresponded to a fetal developmental age of 4 to 5 lunar months gestation.

Two larger bone fragments were too large to be fetal material and represented commingled cremains from a previous cremation of an adult. No debris was found among the cremains, including staples or other casket hardware. Most importantly, no dental material was discovered, nor were any medical, dental, or mortuary artifacts noted at all.

A *Service of Answers to Interrogatories* (e.g., responses to a questionnaire similar to the one above) filled out by the putative decedent's family, and provided by plaintiff's counsel, provided the following information about the decedent. The decedent was a female who died of nonviable immaturity at 17 weeks gestation. No surgical, medical, or dental procedures had been performed, and the decedent had no natural teeth. It was unknown whether the decedent was embalmed prior to cremation. The family reported that no clothing or foreign objects were cremated with the remains and that all of the cremains were presented for examination.

In this case, several complete bones, as well as primary ossification centers representing elements of the vertebral column were noted and confirmed that the cremains were those of a human. The size and morphology of the bones and elements was consistent with a human fetus between 4 and 5 lunar months gestation, the developmental age of the putative decedent. In terms of commingling, two cortical bone fragments were too thick to represent fetal bones. The absence of dentition, as well as the absence of medical or dental artifacts, was consistent with expected findings for a fetus or infant.

One interesting note involved the cremains weight in this case. The cremains weight was more than the weights published for a decedent of similar age. However, the reference fetus documented in the published study (Warren and Maples 1997) was cremated in a stainless steel container placed within the retort. The presence of the two larger bone fragments in the case example presented here suggested that the fetus was most likely cremated on the floor of the retort and a small amount of unrelated ash and refractory material was added to the weight.

This case illustrates several points. First, doubt crept into the minds of the parents because they had no prior knowledge of the amount of cremains that should be expected after the cremation of a fetus. Second, it is easier to discover *demonstrable* commingling among the cremains of fetuses, infants, and children than it is among adults—both due to the lesser volume of material to be examined and the shorter time during which to accrue cultural artifacts related to life history. The presence of bone fragments diagnostic of gestational age, as well as the relatively small amount of commingling in this case, convinced the decedent's loved ones that the crematory had performed a conscientious and professional service and they returned home contented.

Conclusion

Contemporary commercial cremation represents an extreme taphonomic process that usually destroys all positive biological evidence of identity and leaves very little in the way of scientific evidence that might help resolve legal issues of commingling and improper cremation practice. However, several recent legal cases have drawn the attention of forensic scientists, who have responded by producing a growing body of literature outlining case histories and research projects that seek to improve our understanding of the cremation process and its effect on the human body. These efforts are not directed at resolving commingling during cremation but are instead aimed at increasing our ability to discover the extent and nature of commingling as a part of the cremation process.

References Cited

Arizona State Legislation 32-1398; *Crematories; Disciplinary Action; Acts of Crematory.*

Bass, B. and J. Jefferson 2003 *Death's Acre.* G.P. Putnam's Sons, New York.

Bass, W. M. and R. L. Jantz 2004 Cremation weights in east Tennessee. *J. Forensic Sci.* 49(5): 901–904.

Birkby, W. H. 1991 The Analysis of Cremains. Paper presented at the 43rd Annual Meeting of the American Academy of Forensic Science, Anaheim, CA.

Fazekas, I. and K. Kósa 1978 *Forensic Fetal Osteology.* Akademiai Kiado Publishers, Budapest, Hungary.

Iverson, K. V. 2001 *Death to Dust: What Happens to Dead Bodies?* 2nd ed. Galen Press, Ltd., Tucson, AZ.

Maples, W. R. and M. Browning 1994 *Dead Men Do Tell Tales: The Strange and Fascinating Cases of a Forensic Anthropologist.* Broadway Books, New York.

Murad, T. 1998 The growing popularity of cremation versus inhumation: Some forensic implications. In *Forensic Osteology: Advances in the Identification of Human Remains,* K. J. Reichs, ed. pp. 86–105. Springfield, Ill.: Charles C. Thomas.

Prothero, S. 2001 *Purified by Fire: A History of Cremation in America.* University of California Press, Berkeley.

Warren, M. W. 1999 Radiographic determination of developmental age in fetuses and stillborns. *J. Forensic Sci.* 44(4):708–712.

Warren, M. W., A. B. Falsetti, W. F. Hamilton, and L. J. Levine 1999 Evidence of arteriosclerosis in cremated remains. *Am. J. Forensic Med. Pathol.* 20(3):277–280.

Warren, M. W. and W. R. Maples 1997 The anthropometry of contemporary commercial cremation. *J. Forensic Sci.* 42(3):417–423.

Warren, M. W. and J. J. Schultz 2002 Post-cremation taphonomy and artifact preservation. *J. Forensic Sci.* 47(3):656–659.

Chapter 10
Models and Methods for Osteometric Sorting

John E. Byrd

Assemblages of commingled human remains present special problems in the identification process. Complete biological profiles of individuals cannot be developed until the remains have been segregated into individuals. Cause and manner of death cannot be properly evaluated without access to segregated, complete skeletons. Segregation is also a goal for reasons extending beyond the need for comprehensive analysis, as in forensic applications when remains must be returned to next of kin for disposition. Though the presence of soft tissue can, in some cases, usefully inform the process (i.e., hair color and texture, skin tone, etc.), most of the information used to resolve commingling is obtained from the skeleton. Charles Snow (1948) provided an early comprehensive overview of methods for sorting commingled skeletons that is still relevant today, though it predates some important new technologies such as DNA analysis. The primary categories of information used to sort commingled remains are age, articulation, visual pair-matching, size (osteometric sorting), robusticity ("build"), taphonomy, and DNA profile data. Osteometric sorting is but one of the many tools available to the anthropologist for sorting commingled remains. Descriptions of these methods are given in several publications (Adams and Byrd 2006; Byrd and Adams 2003; Snow 1948; Ubelaker 2002) and will not be repeated here.

An additional tool that can be invaluable in sorting commingled remains is the process of elimination (Adams and Byrd 2006). Most authors neglect this important aspect of segregating remains despite its fundamental relevance. However, before bones can be assigned to an individual on the basis of a process of elimination, one must be certain that the case includes only a specific, known number of individuals. We might say that such cases exhibit *epistemic closure* (De Cornulier 1988), meaning that the circumstances of the case permit one to make strong inferences on negative evidence. An example of the use of process of elimination is where we have two commingled individuals and seek to associate a left femur. One of the individuals has a right femur, but it is found to be of a size too large to match the left femur. We conclude that it must associate with the other individual because that is the only rational choice remaining post-analysis: The second individual is the only one *with no evidence against the association*. Following Snow, we advocate the systematic use of all of the aforementioned methods to sort commingled remains. Each step in the sorting process is documented and can (in

From: *Recovery, Analysis, and Identification of Commingled Human Remains*
Edited by: B. Adams and J. Byrd © Humana Press, Totowa, NJ

principle) be replicated by other anthropologists (Adams and Byrd 2006; Byrd and Adams 2003).

The segregation of commingled remains is inductive and should be viewed as a series of tests of possible associations between bones. The tests are performed using the methods listed above, with some methods being inherently more powerful than others. But the ability of a test to correctly segregate bones depends upon more than the power of a statistical model; it will also be determined by the condition of the case specimens themselves. For example, some articulations are more reliable than others for testing the association of adjoining bones (Adams and Byrd 2006). Unreliable articulations are those for which bones from different individuals can appear to fit at an uncomfortably high frequency. (The reverse—adjoining bones from a single individual not articulating—can be considered rare-to-nonexistent.) A test involving an "unreliable" articulation can nonetheless yield a convincing result when the fit is extremely poor (e.g., the bones cannot articulate). What we seek when conducting analyses are *severe tests* (Mayo 1996, 2003, 2004); that is, tests that follow the *severity principle*. Mayo states, "The intuition underlying the severity principle is a familiar one: we have a good indication that we are correct about a claim or hypothesis . . . just to the extent that we have ruled out the ways we can be wrong in taking the claim or hypothesis to be true" (Mayo 2003: 101). Thus, confidence in the negative test result with an unreliable articulation is based upon the fact that an extremely poor fit between two adjoining bones (from the same individual) will be a rare-to-nonexistent event. The rarity of a negative test result when the bones originate in one person grants the severity. Tests based on statistical hypotheses are capable of providing a measure of how strong the evidence against the null hypothesis (of an association) is. Statistical tests also permit one to measure the *severity* of the test, as defined by Mayo (Mayo 1996, 2003, 2004; Mayo and Spanos 2006). Osteometric sorting utilizes statistical tests.

Osteometric sorting depends upon the significant correlations among the sizes of the bones of the skeleton. A large humerus is associated with a large femur, a large metatarsal, etc. This isometric reality is exploited in the sorting process by formally comparing the sizes of two bones. Byrd and Adams (2003) have proposed that we test the statistical null hypothesis that the two specimens are of a size to have originated in the same individual. The original proposal relied upon the use of prediction intervals, following the Neyman–Pearson approach to hypothesis testing (cf. Neyman and Pearson 1967). This chapter will expand beyond the use of prediction intervals and present a means of assessing the strength of evidence obtained in a particular test as well as a means of comparing the strength of evidence for competing sorting options in a given analysis. These approaches require the calculation of statistical models from a large reference data set appropriate to the population of interest. This chapter presents three basic approaches to osteometric sorting: (1) comparison of left and right bones using models that key on shape; (2) comparison of adjoining bone with models responding to the correlation of corresponding regions at joints (see Buikstra et al. 1984);

and (3) comparison of the sizes of bones with the use of regression models. Each approach is described below following a brief description of the reference data.

Data Sources and Analytical Methods

Statistical models employed for hypothesis testing are only as good as the reference data they are built upon. Reference data should be appropriate to the problem at hand, meaning that they are representative of the same population as the case specimens in question, can be considered a random sample with regard to the attributes measured, and were collected according to a standard protocol. Since the ancestry and sex of commingled individuals are often unknown prior to sorting, reference data for osteometric sorting should be representative of multiple populations and both sexes. The reference data used in this study were developed at the Central Identification Laboratory, Joint POW/MIA Accounting Command (JPAC/CIL) for broad applications in research and casework. The data are comprised primarily of postcranial measurements. Included are the standard measurements found in the Forensic Databank at the University of Tennessee, Knoxville (Moore-Jansen et al. 1994), as well as new measurements designed to be taken on fragmented bones. The numbering scheme for new measurements was designed to integrate with the forensic databank. A considerable portion of the reference data consists of Forensic Databank data generously provided by Dr. Richard Jantz. The individuals in the reference data set are as listed in Table 10.1.

Table 10.1 Reference Sample Organized by Collection, Race, and Sex

COLLECTION	SEX	BLACK	WHITE	ASIAN	MEX	TOTAL
CIL	F	0	1	0	0	1
	M	5	55	5	0	65
CMNH-HT	F	2	2	0	0	4
	M	7	7	0	0	14
SI-TERRY	F	14	10	0	0	24
	M	14	2	0	0	16
UT-BASS	F	3	9	0	0	12
	M	4	7	0	0	11
FDB	F	12	46	0	0	58
	M	17	108	0	0	125
ICMP	F	0	0	0	0	0
	M	0	41	0	0	41
HARV-PEA	M	0	0	0	2	2
	F	0	0	0	3	3
TOTAL		78	288	5	5	376

CIL, JPAC Central Identification Laboratory. *CMNH-HT*, Cleveland Museum of Natural History Hamann-Todd collection. *SI-TERRY*, Smithsonian Institution Terry collection. *UT-BASS*, University of Tennessee Bass collection. *FDB*, University of Tennessee Forensic Databank. *ICMP*, International Commission on Missing Persons. HARV-PEA, Harvard University Peabody Museum.

Statistical calculations (described below) were performed using SPSS (2000), Microsoft Excel (2001), and the Resampling Stats Add-in for Excel (2006) as follows. Regression models were calculated in SPSS. Comparisons to the t-distribution and normal distribution were made in Microsoft Excel. Bootstrap analyses were conducted in Microsoft Excel using the add-in produced by Resampling Stats. Details of these statistical analyses will be presented in the appropriate sections ahead.

Models for Osteometric Sorting

The basic principle underlying osteometric sorting is that two bones that are of sizes more disparate than observed in most humans are likely to be commingled. In this, as in most forensic applications, we are working from the general patterns known to exist in the relevant population(s) to the specific patterns seen in case specimens. This approach can be contrasted with the more common goal of statistical analysis in science: to infer general population characteristics from the specific characteristics of samples. Thus, osteometric sorting depends upon our ability to formally characterize normal size and shape relationships among skeletal elements. This is accomplished by utilizing estimates of population parameters such as the mean and standard deviation calculated from the reference data. These parameters are then used to formulate the null hypothesis of a "typical" size (and/or shape) relationship that is subjected to significance testing as described by Fisher (1958). Conclusions are primarily supported by having rejected a null hypothesis, since accepting the null in-and-of-itself does not prove an association. The models are built from the reference data to address the problems encountered in the case (utilizing measurements that can be taken from the case specimens). An effort has been made to keep the statistical models as simple as possible. Simplicity serves two goals: The first is to avoid common problems with complex models, such as overfitting; the second is to make the method accessible to case analysts using only an osteometric board, calipers, and a spreadsheet.

Paired Elements

Models for comparison of right and left paired bones were developed that emphasize shape. These models respond to many of the same attributes that make visual pair-matching (Adams and Byrd 2006) possible and in most cases perform equally well. Measurements of length and of girth at numerous positions along each bone are utilized. Where length measurements are not available (due to fragmentation), models utilizing only girth measurements are calculated. These models take the general form

$$D = \Sigma(a_i - b_i), \tag{10.1}$$

where a is the right side bone measurement i, and b is the left side bone measurement i for each of the measurements included in the comparison. The null hypothesis of no difference is tested by comparing the value of D against "0" (no difference) and using the reference data standard deviation of D. The deviation from "0" divided by the reference data standard deviation is evaluated against the t-distribution with two tails to obtain a p-value. A low p-value provides a measure of the strength of evidence against the null, which can also be taken as evidence for how atypical the case specimens are assuming they originate in the same individual. The 0.10 significance level is recommended for most applications of this test, but recognize that the cut-off must be determined according to the needs of the investigation. (It is also worth emphasizing the need to use the test result in conjunction with independent lines of evidence.) This method has performed well in all test applications but would benefit from a larger reference sample.

Example 1. A left and right femur were randomly selected from the reference sample to serve as an example. Five measurements were chosen in this case (Fig. 10.1), as listed in Table 10.2.

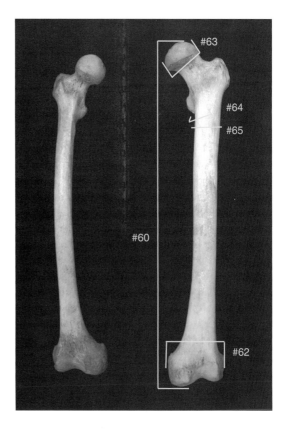

Fig. 10.1 Measurements used in Example 1 (see also Appendix). (Photograph by Charity Barrett.)

Table 10.2 Measurement Values and Statistics from Comparison of Randomly Chosen Left and Right Femurs in Example 1

Measurement[1]	Left	Right
60. Total length (mm)	505	448
62. Distal epiphysis breadth (mm)	82	86
63. Maximum diameter femur head (mm)	50	47
64. A-P subtrochlear diameter (mm)	29	27
65. M-L subtrochlear diameter (mm)	32	35
D	55.0	
Reference sample standard deviation ($N = 67$)	3.99	
t [calculated as $(D - 0)/3.99$]	13.8	
p (from t-distribution, d.f. = 66, 2 tails)	0.000	

[1] Measurement numbers correspond to Moore-Jansen et al. (1994).

We regard this result as relatively easy to interpret, since we can expect disparities between a left and right femur this large to be rare-to-nonexistent events when the bones are from the same individual. These bones would be segregated.

Articulating Bone Portions

Models for comparison of adjoining bones are calculated using the difference in sizes of adjoining portions as their basis (for an example of this approach, see Buikstra et al. 1984). For example, the innominate and femur are compared by subtracting the maximum diameter of the femur head (measurement #63 in Moore-Jansen et al. 1994) from the maximum diameter of the acetabulum (measurement described in Adams and Byrd 2002). The model takes the general form

$$D = c_i - d_j, \tag{10.2}$$

where measurement i of bone c is subtracted from measurement j of bone d. The null hypothesis that the two specimens are of an appropriate size to have originated in one individual is evaluated by comparing the D−value obtained from the case specimens to the mean D−value calculated from the reference data. The deviation of D from the reference data mean, divided by the reference data standard deviation, is evaluated against the t-distribution with two tails to obtain a p-value. A low p-value provides a measure of the strength of evidence against the null, which can also be taken as evidence for how atypical the case specimens are if we assume that they originate in the same individual. The 0.05 significance level is recommended, but larger or smaller significance levels can be assigned depending upon the circumstances of the investigation.

Example 2. A femur and tibia were randomly selected from the reference sample to serve as an example. Two measurements, one taken from the distal femur and the other the proximal tibia (Fig. 10.2), were used as the basis for the statistical test. Table 10.3 presents the data and results.

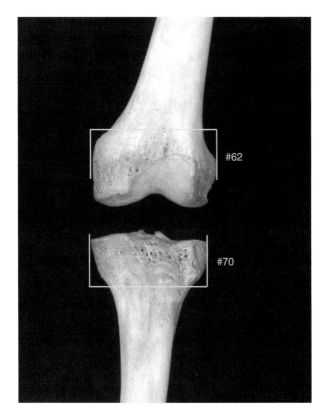

Fig. 10.2 Measurements used in Example 2 (see also Appendix). (Photograph by Charity Barrett.)

This result (*p*-value of 0.057) provides strong evidence that the two bones are not from the same individual. That said, strict adherence to the 0.05 cut-off could lead one to ignore this strong evidence for sorting. The decision to sort them apart depends upon the cut-off value chosen by the analyst along with other factors (such as independent lines of evidence, an evaluation of alternative associations, etc.).

Table 10.3 Measurement Values and Statistics from Comparison of Randomly Chosen Femur and Tibia in Example 2

Measurement[1]	Value
62. Femur distal epiphysis breadth (mm)	85.0
70. Tibia proximal epiphysis breadth (mm)	84.0
D	1.0
Reference sample mean ($N = 270$)	5.2
Reference sample standard deviation	2.2
t [calculated as $(D - 5.2)/2.2$]	1.91
p (from t-distribution with d.f. = 269, 2 tails)	0.057

[1] Measurement numbers correspond to Moore-Jansen et al. (1994).

Other Bone Portions

Models for comparison of different bone sizes are generally more complex in their derivation. After experimenting with numerous approaches, Byrd and Adams (2003) settled on the following linear combination as an acceptable index for bone size. The available measurements on a bone are simply summed and the natural logarithm of this sum is the value used in regression models. Since length measurements typically show the highest correlations with one another, models including length measurements perform best. The addition of breadths and girth measurements into the indices offers a slight, but noticeable, improvement in the statistical models. A surprising finding is that models utilizing several breadth and girth measurements, with no length measurements, perform nearly as well in some cases as those including lengths. This fact has great significance when working with highly fragmented assemblages.

Byrd and Adams (2003) originally advocated using the 90% prediction interval as the basis for the hypothesis tests. If the point representing the two bones fell within the prediction interval, then the null hypothesis of association was accepted; otherwise, it was rejected. There was no measure of how good or poor the "fit" of the case specimens was relative to the regression model. It is recommended here to derive the t-value from the case specimens using the following model, modified from the confidence interval model provided by Giles and Klepinger (1988):

$$t = |y^\wedge - y_i|/[(\text{S.E.}) \times \sqrt{[1 + (1/N) + (x_i - x)^2/(N \times S_x^2)]]}, \qquad (10.3)$$

where $y^\wedge$ is the predicted value from the regression model, y_i is the dependent variable value of the case specimen, S.E. is the regression model standard error, N is the sample size used in calculation of the regression model, x_i is the independent variable value of the case specimen, x is the reference sample mean for the independent variable, and S_x is the reference sample standard deviation of the independent variable. Note that the confidence interval model from which this formula was derived is shaped as a hyperbola, centered on the regression model line. The hyperbolic shape is sensitive to sample size and reflects the increasing uncertainty of regression model predictions as the independent variable value becomes more distant from the mean value (see Neter and Wasserman 1974). At large sample sizes, whence the lines of the hyperbola become flat, a simpler model can be derived by using the difference between the case specimen dependent variable value and the predicted value divided by the standard error of the estimate. The value resulting from this calculation can be compared to the t-distribution.

Example 3. A humerus and a femur were selected from two individuals in the reference sample. These individuals were designated "A" and "B." Comparisons were made (see Table 10.4) as though the true association of the bones was unknown and there were only two individuals commingled in the case. For ease of presentation, only one measurement for each bone (Fig. 10.3) was used rather than the combinations recommended in Byrd and Adams (2003).

Table 10.4 Model and Statistics for Comparison of Humeri and Femora in Example 3

Measurement[1]	Value	
40. Maximum length humerus (HUM) (mm)	A. 348 mm	B. 324 mm
60. Maximum length femur (FEM) (mm)	A. 505 mm	B. 468 mm
Regression model: HUM = 0.647(FEM) + 28.335		
N	274	
R	0.932	
F	1804.702	
P	0.000	
S.E. (standard error)	9.590	
X (mean FEM)	461.257	
S_{FEM} (standard deviation FEM)	43.541	
HUM A & FEM A	t: 0.735	p: 0.463
HUM B vs. FEM B	t: 0.742	p: 0.459
HUM A vs. FEM B	t: 1.756	p: 0.080
HUM B vs. FEM A	t: 3.228	p: 0.001

[1] Measurement numbers correspond to Moore-Jansen et al. (1994).

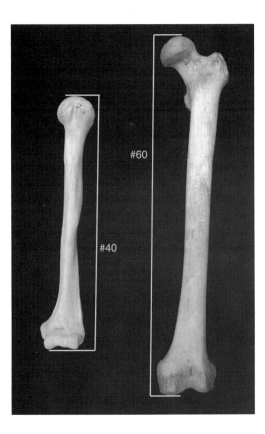

Fig. 10.3 Measurements used in Example 3 (see also Appendix). (Photograph by Charity Barrett.)

Assuming that epistemic closure holds for this case, we are faced with two courses of action: (1) Segregate humerus A from femur A, which forces the segregation of humerus B from femur B; or (2) segregate humerus A from femur B along with humerus B from femur A. Since the association of humerus B with femur A is rejected with $p = 0.001$, we would recommend the second of the two courses of action. Further evaluation of decisions where multiple options must be considered simultaneously is discussed below.

Assessment of Results

Sorting commingled remains is an inductive process. From a table of bones with varying elements, sizes, shapes, and condition, one must proceed stepwise through the assemblage using a variety of "tests" to infer whether each pair of bone specimens could have originated in the same individual. One does not seek a numeric probability of correct association since each segregation decision is either correct or incorrect. Rather, confidence is built by having subjected the sorting options to severe tests (Mayo 1996, 2003, 2004). Some tests are more powerful (i.e., visual pair-matching, osteometric pair-matching, comparison of DNA profiles) than others (i.e., assessment of age, comparison of taphonomy). In the end, we are hopefully left with segregated skeletons for which there is a high degree of confidence that every bone attributed to each skeleton originated from the same individual. There will rarely be *absolute* certainty in the resulting segregations, as induction by its nature does not lead to absolutes. However, inductive processes in science do lead to conclusions that are highly reliable (e.g., able to withstand scrutiny, exhibit low error rates, etc.). How reliable are the results of osteometric sorting?

Osteometric sorting proceeds by testing the null hypothesis that two bones under consideration are of a size (and, to some extent, shape) that could have originated in the same individual. Such tests are repeated as often as necessary to segregate the assemblage of bones. Byrd and Adams (2003) originally proposed the use of the prediction interval of a regression model as a basis for the test, where all case values falling outside the prediction interval were rejected. This Neyman–Pearson-type approach to hypothesis testing requires one to choose the prediction interval value (90% or 95%) in advance and then react only to whether the case values fell within or outside the interval. This approach has some notable limitations. First, it ignores important information, such as how far outside the interval a set of case specimens fall. If their test value was within the prediction interval, was it close to the boundary or near the value expected under the statistical model? Second, the original approach provides no objective method of assessing the family of results that are obtained when more than two bones are included in a test or when results of multiple tests must be evaluated. The method of hypothesis testing is redirected here to a form more in line with Fisher's (1958, 1959) significance testing.

Assessment of the results of a single test is straightforward: One relies upon the p-value, which indicates how often we should expect to see bone measurement values as disparate as observed in the case specimens when the bones originate in a single individual. A low p-value (e.g., $p < 0.10$) is interpreted to mean we do not expect to find bones of the sizes seen in this case unless (1) the bones are commingled from two individuals, or (2) an unlikely event has occurred. Since unlikely events are infrequent, it is rational to opt for the first interpretation. More complex is the issue of what to do with the multiple p-values resulting from multiple comparisons. The recommended method is a modification of Fisher's omnibus statistic, originally offered as a means of combining results of multiple chi-squared tests (Fisher 1958: 99–101). Fisher noted that

> When a number of quite independent tests of significance have been made, it sometimes happens that although few or none can be claimed individually as significant, yet the aggregate gives an impression that the probabilities are on the whole lower than would often have been obtained by chance. It is sometimes desired, taking account only of these probabilities, and not of the detailed composition of the data from which they are derived, which may be of very different kinds, to obtain a single test of the significance of the aggregate, based on the product of the probabilities observed. The circumstance that the sum of a number of values of X^2 is itself distributed in the X^2 distribution with the appropriate number of degrees of freedom, may be made the basis of such a test. (Fisher 1958: 99)

Fisher's method called for using twice the summation of the natural log of the respective p-values, with sign reversed, to obtain a new statistic. This statistic was itself compared to the chi-squared distribution to get a single p-value for the aggregate. Since we are not using chi-squared tests in osteometric sorting, Fisher's method is not directly applicable to the problem of assessing the multiple test results.

The tests performed in osteometric sorting utilize the t-distribution. We can devise an omnibus test applicable to our test results that is similar to Fisher's chi-squared version by first using the same basic statistic:

$$O = \sum - \ln(p_i), \qquad (10.4)$$

which is the summation of the natural log of each p-value, with sign reversed. Note that we do not double the value as Fisher did. We next calculate the mean and standard deviation of the omnibus statistic from the reference data. For application here, the add-in Resampling Stats for Excel was used to sample p-values from the reference data (where each individual's p-value was derived from application of a test to their measurement values), with replacement, for several thousand trial runs. P-values from combinations of two, three, four, and six of the trials were randomly associated with one another to create a simulation of the test, but where no bones are commingled (e.g., the null hypothesis is true). Thus, bootstrap estimates of the mean and standard deviation of the omnibus statistic were derived. The omnibus statistic calculated from the reference skeletal data is at least approximately normally distributed (see Fig. 10.4). It has been observed that the mean tends to be very close to (slightly less than) the number of tests in the aggregate, and the standard deviation tends to be very close to the square root of the number of tests. One can conservatively substitute these values for the sample statistics. Mean and standard deviation estimates for the omnibus statistic are then used to derive a z-score for each

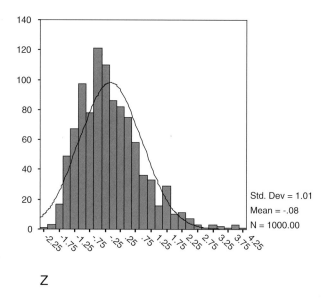

Z

Fig. 10.4 Z-scores calculated from the omnibus statistic. This example used data from comparison of the distal femur to the proximal tibia. *p*-values were calculated from the reference data and then sampled 1,000 times with replacement. This process was repeated 6 times to generate 1,000 randomly selected groupings of *p*-values. Z-scores were calculated using the value $O - 6$, divided by the square root of 6

aggregate of test results. The z-score is compared to the normal distribution to obtain the overall *p*-value. This should be viewed as a one-sided test since we are only interested in significantly high values of O. An alternative manner for obtaining the *p*-value is to use the bootstrap distribution; however, experimentation suggests that the normal distribution is simpler to use and gives approximately the same result.

The severity of tests used in osteometric sorting can be measured using the procedure given by Mayo (1996: 194) under her Rule of Rejection: Severity is 1 minus the probability of getting a statistical value as large as obtained, assuming that the bones are not commingled (the condition represented by the reference data). Thus, the smaller the *p*-value obtained, the greater the severity of the test. It is clear that the severity obtained in a test is determined by the power of the test *and* the scale of the difference observed in the case specimens. Severity can be achieved even with weak tests so long as the case specimens exhibit sufficient disparity in their values (relative to one another). Osteometric tests predictably lack severity when the sizes of the commingled individuals are approximately the same, but can be very severe indeed when the body sizes are disparate. For each test, there will be a degree of body size disparity at which osteometric tests will sort all measured bones with no error (severity = 1).

Example 4. Eleven airmen who were killed in 1944 when their B-24 bomber crashed into the jungle of Papua New Guinea were extensively commingled. Careful field recovery revealed that in some instances partially articulated skeletons could be recovered as a unit and that remains of the respective individuals were distributed in the site according to where they had been positioned in the aircraft. Two left innominates (AL and BL) and two right innominates (AR and BR) from one area within the site needed to be segregated in the laboratory. One of the left innominates (BL) was already associated with a partial skeleton. Fragmentation precluded the application of visual pair-matching. Due to the fragmentation, only one measurement (#59A; see Fig. 10.5) could be taken on all four bones. The standard deviation for the difference between left and right innominates for measurement #59A was calculated from the reference data. This value, along with the value for D [see Equation (10.1)], was used to test the null hypothesis (of no difference) for each of the possible pairings of the bones. Note that in this case we have two possible courses of action and a total of four pairings to evaluate: (1) AL and AR are paired along with BL and BR, or (2) AL and BR are paired along with BL and AR. We can objectively evaluate each course of action by testing the null hypothesis that the course of action combines two p-values expected by chance if the bones are correctly paired. Table 10.5 presents the results of the tests.

In this instance we have a clear interpretation of the results. Course of Action #1 is well within the limits of reasonable expectation for bones originating in a single individual. In contrast, Course of Action #2 is outside such limits, and it would be irrational to choose these associations. The severity of the test of Course of Action #2 is 0.9999.

Example 5. Remains of two Marines killed in action in 1943 on Tarawa Atoll were accidentally discovered during construction activities in 1999. The disturbance of the grave resulted in extensive commingling of the remains. After the legs had been sorted into two sets of limbs, there was a need to associate the lower limbs with hip and abdomen portions. This problem could be addressed by osteometric comparison

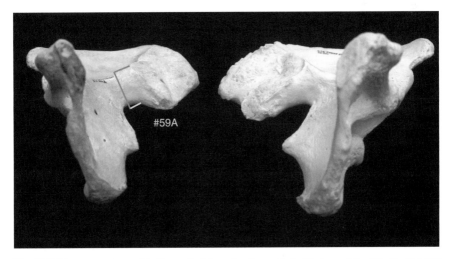

Fig. 10.5 Measurements used in Example 4 (see also Appendix). (Photograph by Charity Barrett.)

Table 10.5 Comparison of Right and Left Innominates from Example 4

Measurement[1]	Value	
59A. Max. thickness ilium at sciatic notch (mm)	AL: 21.6	AR: 23.2
	BL: 29.8	BR: 29.7
Course of Action #1		
AL & AR	t: 1.13	p: 0.265
BL & BR	t: 0.070	p: 0.944
Course of Action #2		
AL & BR	t: 5.70	p: 0.000
BL & AR	t: 4.64	p: 0.000
O (COA #1)	z: 1.39	p: 0.668
O (COA #2)	z: 25.98	p: 0.000

[1] Measurement described in Adams and Byrd (2002).

of the diameter of the acetabulum (measurement #59E) from one of the innominates with the maximum diameter of the femur head (measurement #63) from a femur representing each limb set (Fig. 10.6). Only one of the hip sets could be measured due to fragmentation. The data and statistics are presented in Table 10.6.

We have strong support for the segregation of the innominate from the second femur, which is notably smaller than the first. Since there are only two individuals involved in the case (i.e., we have epistemic closure), then by process of elimination

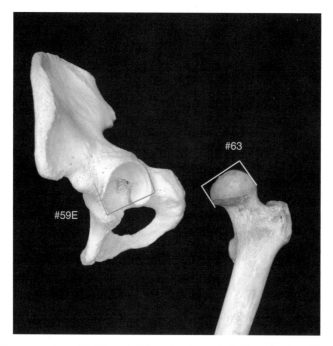

Fig. 10.6 Measurements used in Example 5 (see also Appendix). (Photograph by Charity Barrett.)

Table 10.6 Statistics from Comparison of Innominate and Femur from Example 5

Measurement[1]	Values	
59E. Max diameter of the acetabulum (mm)	Innom#1: 66	
63. Max diameter of femur head (mm)	Fem#1: 53.7	Fem#2: 46.9
Innom#1 & femur #1	t: 1.578	p: 0.117
Innom#1 & femur #2	t: 5.640	p: 0.000

[1] Measurement numbers correspond to Moore-Jansen et al. (1994) or Adams and Byrd (2002).

we can associate the second set of limbs to the second set of hips. The simplicity of the problem negated the need for an omnibus test. The severity of the second test is 0.9999.

Example 6. This example is taken from the case involving a B-24 aircraft crash that was described above. Two pairs of unassociated radii (designated A and B) were known to belong to either of two individuals represented by partial skeletons (I-09 and I-11). Both partial skeletons (I-09 and I-11) contained distal humeri. Osteometric sorting was attempted in order to sort the unassociated radii. A simple linear regression model relating one measurement (Fig. 10.7) of the radius (#47C) to two measurements of the humerus (#41 and #41A) was calculated from the reference data. As prescribed in Byrd and Adams (2003), the measurements for each bone were summed and the natural log taken to create the variables RAD and HUM, with

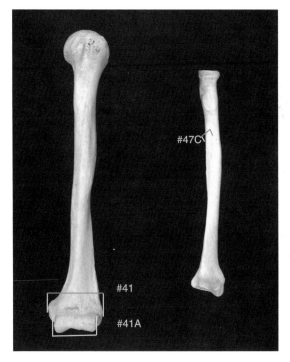

Fig. 10.7 Measurements used in Example 6 (see also Appendix). (Photograph by Charity Barrett.)

Table 10.7 Model and Statistics from Comparison of Humeri and Radii from Example 6

Measurement[1]	Value	
41. Epicondylar breadth humerus (mm)	I-09: 66	I-11: 61.5
41A. Capitulum-trochlear breadth humerus (mm)	I-09: 45.4	I-11: 41.6
47C. Minimum diameter diaphysis radius (mm)	A: 11.8	B: 11.0
HUM	I-09: 4.71	I-11: 4.64
RAD	A: 2.47	B: 2.4
Regression model: RAD = 1.099(HUM) – 2.737		
N	164	
R	0.801	
F	291.9	
P	0.000	
S.E. (standard error)	0.762	
x (mean HUM)	4.67	
S_{HUM} (standard deviation HUM)	0.091	
Course of Action #1		
HUM I-09 &. RAD A	t: 0.402	p: 0.688
HUM I-11 vs. RAD B	t: 0.493	p: 0.623
Course of Action #2		
HUM I-09 vs. RAD B	t: 0.514	p: 0.608
HUM I-11 vs. RAD A	t: 1.41	p: 0.161
O (COA#1)	z: –0.818	p: 0.793
O (COA#2)	z: 0.230	p: 0.410

[1] Measurement numbers correspond to Moore-Jansen et al. (1994) or Adams and Byrd (2002).

HUM being the independent variable. Next, four tests were conducted comparing the regression model predicted values for the two humeri to the measurement values for the two radii. In each instance we tested the null hypothesis that the radius was of the expected size, given the size of the humerus and the regression model statistics. Following the four tests of possible associations, the omnibus statistic was used to test each of the two possible courses of action in sorting. Results are presented in Table 10.7.

Upon viewing these results, one can be tempted to reject COA#2 on the basis that we are only interested in large positive z-scores, and the z-score for COA#2 is appreciably larger than that of COA#1. We cannot, however, interpret the results in this simplistic manner. Despite the larger z-score and corresponding smaller p-value, COA#2 is still well within the range of results we expect to obtain by chance when bones are legitimately associated. The severity of the test of Course of Action #1 is only 0.207 and is only 0.590 for Course of Action #2. No sorting is possible based on the osteometric results in this example.

Conclusion

Segregation of commingled remains is a process of induction whereby bones are systematically compared to one another in a series of tests. Confidence in results is greatest when the tests are severe. Less than severe test results must be combined with other lines of evidence before segregation is done. Osteometric sorting is an important sorting tool that permits objective assessments of the severity of its tests. The application of osteometric sorting in case work at the JPAC/CIL is currently done in an ad hoc manner, where the appropriate statistical models (utilizing measurements available in the case specimens) are calculated from the reference data as the need arises. Osteometric comparisons of paired bones and adjoining bones are most advantageous when sorting large assemblages where it is impractical to make visual comparisons of every possible match. Further, this method is superbly suited to computer automation. We hope to develop an approach whereby all available measurement values for the case specimens are entered in advance, and all relevant comparison results can be produced as the analysis proceeds, without having to generate the statistical models for each comparison as separate steps for the anthropologist. As specimens are sorted apart by the various methods described in this report, they can be eliminated from consideration within the software application.

References Cited

Adams, B. J. and J. E. Byrd 2002 Interobserver variation of selected postcranial measurements. *J. Forensic Sci.* 47(6):1193–1202.

Adams, B. J. and J. E. Byrd 2006 Resolution of small-scale commingling: A case report from the Vietnam War. *Forensic Sci. Int.* 156(1):63–69.

Buikstra, J. E., C. C. Gordon, and L. St. Hoyme 1984 The case of the severed skull: Individuation in forensic anthropology. In *Human Identification: Case Studies in Forensic Anthropology*, T. A. Rathbun and J. E. Buikstra, eds., pp. 121–135. Charles C. Thomas, Springfield, IL.

Byrd, J. E. and B. J. Adams 2003 Osteometric sorting of commingled human remains. *J. Forensic Sci.* 48(4):717–724.

De Cornulier, B. 1988 "Knowing whether," "knowing who," and epistemic closure. In *Questions and Questioning*, M. Meyer, ed. Walter de Gruyter Press, Berlin.

Fisher, R. A. 1958 *Statistical Methods for Research Workers,* 13th (Revised) ed. Hafner Publishing Company, New York.

Fisher, R. A. 1959 *Statistical Methods and Scientific Inference*. Hafner Publishing Company, New York.

Giles, E. and L. L. Klepinger 1988 Confidence intervals for estimates based on linear regression in forensic anthropology. *J. Forensic Sci.* 33(5):1218–1222.

Mayo, D. 1996 *Error and the Growth of Experimental Knowledge*. University of Chicago Press, Chicago.

Mayo, D. 2003 Severe testing as a guide for inductive learning. In *Probability Is the Very Guide of Life: The Philosophical Uses of Chance*, H. E. Kyburg, Jr. and M. Thalos, ed. Open Court, Chicago.

Mayo, D. 2004 An error-statistical philosophy of evidence. In *The Nature of Scientific Evidence: Statistical, Philosophical, and Empirical Considerations*, M. Taper and S. Lele, eds. University of Chicago Press, Chicago.

Mayo, D. and A. Spanos 2006 Severe testing as a basic concept in a Neyman-Pearson philosophy of induction. *Br. J. Philos. Sci.* 57(2):323–357.

Microsoft Corporation 2001 Microsoft Excel 2002.

Moore-Jansen, P. M., S. D. Ousley, and R. L. Jantz 1994 *Data Collection Procedures for Forensic Skeletal Material*. University of Tennessee, Department of Anthropology. Submitted to Report of Investigations no. 48.

Neter, J. and W. Wasserman 1974 *Applied Linear Statistical Models: Regression, Analysis of Variance, and Experimental Designs*. Richard D. Irwin, Inc., Homewood.

Neyman, J. and E. S. Pearson 1967 On the problem of the most efficient tests of statistical hypotheses. In *Joint Statistical Papers*. Cambridge University Press, Cambridge.

Resampling Stats Inc. 2006 Resampling Excel Add-in, Version 3.2.

Snow, C. 1948 The identification of the unknown war dead. *Am. J. Phys. Anthropol.* 6:323–328.

SPSS for Windows 2000 Version 10.1.0. SPSS, Inc.

Ubelaker, D. H. 2002 Approaches to the study of commingling in human skeletal biology. In *Advances in Forensic Taphonomy: Method, Theory, and Archaeological Perspectives*, W. D. Haglund and M. H. Sorg, eds. CRC Press, Boca Raton, FL.

Appendix

This appendix presents models and statistics that can be applied to whole and fragmented bones in case assemblages. The measurements used are described in Table 10.8. Measurements are numbered and defined as in Moore-Jansen et al. (1994), Adams and Byrd (2002), and Byrd and Adams (2003) unless otherwise noted.

Measurement Descriptions

Table 10.8 Measurements

Measurement	Definition
Scapula	
39B. Max. br. glenoid fossa	The maximum breadth of the glenoid fossa. Place one flat surface of the jaw of the calipers on the anterior side of the glenoid fossa and place the flat surface of the other jaw on the posterior side with both jaws oriented parallel to the long axis of the bone.
Humerus	
40. Max. length	The maximum length of the humerus taken on the osteometric board.
41. Epicondylar br.	The maximum breadth of the distal humerus taken on the osteometric board.
41A. Capitulum-trochlea br.	The breadth of the capitulum and trochlea at the distal humerus. One end of the sliding calipers is positioned parallel to the flat, spool-shaped surface of the trochlea, and the other end is moved until it comes into contact with the capitulum.
42. Max. vertical diam., head	Place the point of the fixed jaw of the sliding calipers on the most superior point of the head of the humerus on the perimeter of the articular surface. Place the movable jaw so as to find the maximum diameter without moving the fixed jaw from its position.
42A. A-P br., head	The maximum breadth of the humeral head taken in the anterior-posterior direction on the articular surface. This measurement is taken perpendicular to the vertical diameter of the humeral head.

(continued)

Table 10.8 (continued)

Measurement	Definition
Scapula	
44B. Min. diam. diaph.	The minimum diameter of the humeral diaphysis taken in any direction perpendicular to the shaft. This measurement should be taken on the oval part of the shaft, superior to the flattening observed around the olecranon fossa and the lateral supercondylar ridge. Often it is found near midshaft.
Radius	
45. Max. length	The maximum length of the radius taken on the osteometric board.
46. Sag. diam. midshaft	The sagittal diameter of the diaphysis taken at midshaft with sliding calipers.
47. Trans. diam. midshaft	The transverse diameter of the diaphysis taken at midshaft with sliding calipers.
47A. Max. diam. radial tub.	The maximum shaft diameter on the radial tuberosity. Position the calipers around the tuberosity and rotate the bone until the maximum distance is obtained.
47B. Max. diam. diaph. distal to radial tub.	The maximum shaft diameter distal to the radial tuberosity, *positioned along the interosseous crest.* The bone should be rotated to find the maximum distance.
47C. Min. diam. diaph. distal to radial tub.	The minimum shaft diameter anywhere distal to the radial tuberosity. The bone may be rotated to find the minimum distance.
47D. Max. diam. radial head	Position the calipers around the radial head and rotate the bone until the maximum distance is obtained.
Ulna	
48. Max. length	The maximum length of the ulna taken on the osteometric board.
49. Dorso-volar diam.	The diameter taken perpendicular to the transverse diameter at the same position along the diaphysis.
50. Transverse diam.	The diameter taken in the transverse dimension at the point of maximum expression of the interosseus crest.
51A. Min. diam. along interosseus crest	Locate the minimum diameter of the diaphysis along the portion of the bone that includes the interosseous crest. This measurement may not necessarily include the interosseous crest, but should be taken on that part of the shaft that exhibits the crest.
51C. Br. distal end of semi-lunar notch	This is a measure of only the distal surface of the semilunar notch (the base). In order to obtain the distance, one end of the calipers is positioned within the radial notch (approximate midpoint), roughly parallel to the shaft. The other end of the calipers is applied to the medial edge of the semilunar notch.

(continued)

Table 10.8 (continued)

Measurement	Definition
Innominate	
59A. Max thickness sciatic notch	The maximum thickness of the ilium at the sciatic notch. Place the fixed jaw of the sliding caliper on the anterior surface of the ilium adjacent to the apex of the auricular surface. Close the flat surface of the movable jaw onto the posterior surface.
59E. Max. diam. acetabulum	The maximum diameter of the acetabulum. Move the jaws of the sliding calipers around the perimeter of the acetabulum to find the maximum value.
Femur	
60. Max. length	The maximum length of the femur taken on the osteometric board.
62. Epicondylar br.	The breadth of the epicondylar region of the distal femur taken on the osteometric board.
63. Max. diam. head	The maximum diameter of the femur head taken with sliding calipers.
64. A-P subtrochlear diam.	The anterior-posterior diameter of the femur taken in the subtrochlear region.
65. Trans. subtrochlear diam.	The transverse diameter of the femur taken in the subtrochlear region.
68E. Max. diam. along linea aspera	The maximum shaft diameter at any point along the linea aspera. As the bone should be rotated to obtain the maximum distance, the measurement does not necessarily have to include the linea aspera.
69. Max. length	The condylar-malar length of the tibia.
Tibia	
70. Max br. prox. epiphysis	The maximum breadth of the proximal tibia taken on the osteometric board.
71. Max. br. distal epiphysis	The maximum breadth of the distal tibia taken on the osteometric board.
72. Max. diam. nut. foramen	The maximum diameter of the tibia at the nutrient foramen taken with sliding calipers.
73. Trans. diam. nut. foramen	The transverse diameter of the tibia taken at the nutrient foramen.
74B. Min. A-P diam. distal to popliteal line	Locate the smallest anterior-posterior distance at any point on the tibial shaft.
Fibula	
75. Max. length	The maximum length of the fibula taken on the osteometric board.
76. Max. diam. midshaft	The maximum diameter of the fibula at midshaft, taken with sliding calipers.
Talus	
79. Min. br. art. surface	The minimum diameter of the articular surface of the talus. Place the flat surfaces on the jaws of the sliding calipers on either side of the articular surface with the jaws (approximately) parallel to the long axis of the bone. Close the jaws to take the minimum value.

Paired Elements

Use Equation (10.1) to calculate D with the sets of measurements listed (Table 10.9) for each bone. Next, compare the value of "$|D - 0|$/standard deviation" to the t-distribution as a two-sided test with $N - 1$ degrees of freedom.

Articulating Bone Portions

Calculate the value for D as indicated as indicated in Table 10.10 [based on Equation (10.2)]. Next, compare the value of "$|D -$ mean$|$/standard deviation" to the t-distribution as a two-sided test with $N - 1$ degrees of freedom.

Other Bone Portions

Use the listed measurements to calculate the variable values given in Table 10.11. Next, enter the independent variable value from the first case specimen into the regression model equation in Table 10.12 to obtain the predicted value for the dependent variable. The predicted value of the dependent variable, the actual value of the dependent variable (from the second case specimen), the actual value of

Table 10.9 Statistics for Comparison of Paired Elements

Element	Measurements	N	Standard Deviation
Humerus	#40, #41, #42	113	5.28
Radius	#45, #46, #47	100	3.56
Ulna	#48, #49, #50	93	3.60
Femur	#60, #62, #63, #64, #65	67	3.99
Tibia	#69, #70, #71	87	3.68
Fibula	#75, #76	71	2.99
Fragmented Bones			
Humerus	#44B	73	0.72
Radius	#47A, #47B, #47C	52	1.34
Ulna	#49, #50, #51A	45	1.62
Femur	#64, #65	123	1.75
Tibia	#72, #73, #74B	44	2.62

Table 10.10 Models and Statistics for Comparing Bones from Selected Joints

Joint	D	N	Mean	Standard Deviation
Shoulder	(#42A - #39B)	159	6.61	2.35
Elbow 1	(#41A - #47D)	156	20.99	2.38
Elbow 2	(#41A - #51C)	166	20.49	2.39
Hip	(#59E - #63)	176	9.66	1.67
Knee	(#62 - #70)	270	5.20	2.20
Ankle	(#71 - #79)	147	17.91	2.85

Table 10.11 Variables

Variable	Measurements	N	Mean	Standard Deviation
HUM	LN(#40 + #41 + #42)	291	6.08	0.08
HUMFG	LN(#41A + #44B)	169	4.13	0.10
RAD	LN(#45 + #46 + #47)	282	5.61	0.11
RADFG	LN(#47A + #47B + #47C)	181	3.84	0.11
ULN	LN(#48 + #49 + #50)	277	5.68	0.10
ULNFG	LN(#49 + #50 + #51A)	177	3.73	0.12
FEM	LN(#60 + #62 + #63)	277	6.38	0.08
FEMFG	LN(#64 + #65 + #68E)	161	4.49	0.11
TIB	LN(#69 + #70 + #71)	277	6.23	0.10
TIBFG	LN((#72 + #73 + #74B)	180	4.44	0.12

Table 10.12 Models

Model	N	R	p	Std Err
RAD=1.01(HUM)–0.52	264	0.93	0.000	0.03
ULN=0.994(HUM)–0.35	259	0.93	0.000	0.03
HUM=0.95(FEM)+0.02	255	0.95	0.000	0.03
RAD=1.03(FEM)–0.93	248	0.92	0.000	0.03
ULN=0.99(FEM)–0.65	239	0.91	0.000	0.04
TIB=1.02(FEM)–0.29	255	0.96	0.000	0.02
HUM=0.88(TIB)+0.57	252	0.94	0.000	0.03
RAD=1.00(TIB)–0.61	249	0.96	0.000	0.03
ULN=0.97(TIB)–0.37	242	0.96	0.000	0.03
RAD=1.01(ULN)–0.13	261	0.99	0.000	0.02
Fragmented Bones				
RADFG=0.96(HUMFG)–0.14	161	0.89	0.000	0.05
ULNFG=1.07(HUMFG)–0.68	160	0.88	0.000	0.06
HUMFG=0.87(FEMFG)+0.22	139	0.85	0.000	0.06
RADFG=0.93(FEMFG)–0.37	141	0.85	0.000	0.06
ULNFG=0.96(FEMFG)–0.60	142	0.79	0.000	0.08
TIBFG=1.02(FEMFG)–0.15	144	0.90	0.000	0.05
HUMFG=0.77(TIBFG)+0.72	152	0.85	0.000	0.06
RADFG=0.83(TIBFG)+0.14	162	0.84	0.000	0.06
ULNFG=0.88(TIBFG)–0.18	165	0.82	0.000	0.07
RADFG=0.81(ULNFG)+0.83	172	0.87	0.000	0.06

the independent variable, the mean and standard deviation values of the independent variable (from Table 10.11), the standard error of the regression model (from Table 10.12), and the sample size(from Table 10.12) are entered into Equation (10.3) to obtain the value for t. This value is then compared to the t-distribution as a two-sided test with $N - 2$ degrees of freedom (where N is taken from Table 10.12).

Chapter 11
Patterns of Epiphyseal Union and Their Use in the Detection and Sorting of Commingled Remains

Maureen Schaefer

The utility of epiphyseal union as a means of estimating the age of juvenile remains is well known and documented. Less thoroughly investigated, however equally valuable, is the application of epiphyseal union in the recognition and sorting of commingled remains (Buikstra et al. 1984; L'Abbe 2005; Owsley et al. 1995; Schaefer and Black 2007). Detection of commingled remains is most easily accomplished through the recognition of duplicate elements within an assemblage, i.e., two left femora. In the absence of repeated elements, however, commingling episodes are more difficult to recognize and rely on the anthropologist to detect discrepancies between skeletal elements within the assemblage. Inconsistencies often include variations in size and shape of bilateral elements, disproportionate upper and lower body measurements, or discrepancies in the age, sex, or racial attributes of materials within the assemblage (Buikstra et al. 1984; Byrd and Adams 2003; L'Abbe 2005; Owsley et al. 1995; Snow 1948; Snow and Folk 1970). In much the same way, status of epiphyseal union can serve as a tool to recognize incongruities in the maturity level of different elements. This technique is useful for identifying commingling episodes between juvenile remains mixed with that of either additional juvenile or adult material. While discrepancies between juvenile and adult material may seem obvious, they are less conspicuous if the juvenile skeleton has approximated full maturity, and many epiphyseal elements would be expected to display complete union.

The ability to detect discrepancies in the developmental status of juvenile material nearing maturity requires an understanding of the association between union phases of different epiphyses. Three lines of evidence can be used to guide this understanding: (1) the sequence in which the epiphyses initiate union; (2) the sequence in which the epiphyses complete union; and (3) an understanding of the epiphyses that complete union before other epiphyses begin union. Sequences of "beginning" and "complete" union have been previously documented by Schaefer and Black (2007), while the relationship between beginning and complete union will be formally examined within this chapter. Once phase associations between epiphyses are understood, the documented patterns can serve as a reference from which to recognize potentially incompatible material. Epiphyseal elements that do

From: *Recovery, Analysis, and Identification of Commingled Human Remains*
Edited by: B. Adams and J. Byrd © Humana Press, Totowa, NJ

not conform to the documented patterns are likely to suggest the presence of more than one individual.

Once potentially incompatible material is identified, statistical analysis can be used to further support or reject suspicions of commingling. Statistical analysis is useful in that it simultaneously considers all epiphyseal relationships and mathematically considers the number of observations used to define each pattern. Although normally reserved for aging purposes and stature estimation within forensic anthropology (Lucy et al. 1996; Ross and Konigsberg 2002; Schmitt et al. 2002), Bayes' theorem was selected to perform the analysis, as it is an appropriate statistic to use with ordinal data such as epiphyseal scores (Lucy et al. 1996). Bayes' theorem supplies the probabilistic inference that a suspect element originates from the same individual as the other elements within an assemblage based on phases of epiphyseal union.

As a further component of this research, the utility at which epiphyseal phase associations can be applied to recognize the presence of developmentally incompatible material was tested on artificially commingled assemblages. In performing a validation study such as this, an understanding of the method's reliability was learned. This is an important consideration if the technique is to be potentially admissible in a court of law. Satisfaction of the *Daubert* criteria (U.S. Supreme Court 1993) for admissibility of evidence in a U.S. Federal Court is becoming a growing concern among forensic scientists (Koot et al. 2005; Ritz-Timme et al. 2000; Rogers 2005; Rogers and Allard 2004; Williams and Rogers 2006). This study attempts to improve the technique's acceptability through a validation of its reliability. Prior to discussion of the commingling test, an explanation of the three areas of epiphyseal documentation will be presented.

Reference Materials

Phase relationships among the epiphyses were defined using a Bosnian sample, including 256 identified male individuals between the ages of 14 to 30 who lost their lives during the fall of Srebrenica. For an age distribution of the sample, see Table 11.1. Data were collected on 21 epiphyses, including

- Proximal, medial, and distal humerus
- Proximal and distal radius
- Proximal and distal ulna
- Proximal and distal femur, greater and lesser trochanter
- Proximal and distal tibia
- Proximal and distal fibula
- Ischial tuberosity, iliac crest, and tri-radiate complex
- Medial clavicle
- Coraco-glenoid complex and acromion process

Table 11.1 Age Distribution of the Bosnian Sample

Age	n	% of Total
14	3	1
15	6	2
16	15	6
17	20	8
18	24	9
19	20	8
20	26	10
21	26	10
22	13	5
23	13	5
24	18	7
25	18	7
26	13	5
27	11	4
28	14	6
29	9	4
30	7	3
Total	256	100

The two complexes for which data were collected (tri-radiate and coraco-glenoid) are composed of multiple epiphyses, but they have been considered as one functional unit for the sake of simplicity. In this research, the tri-radiate complex consists of six epiphyses—the os acetabuli, superior and posterior epiphyses and the anterior, vertical, and posterior flange. Union considers both pelvic and acetabular surfaces. The coraco-glenoid complex comprises three components—fusion of the coracoid to the body of the scapula and the subcoracoid and glenoid epiphyses. The two complexes are abbreviated to cor and acet within the diagrams here in the effort to conserve space.

Each epiphysis for which information was recorded was scored according to a three-phased approach:

- Phase 0—open or no union
- Phase 1—active union (union had initiated, but parts of an epiphyseal line were retained)
- Phase 2—complete union (line of fusion was no longer present, although an epiphyseal scar could remain)

Sequence of Epiphyseal Union

Familiarity with epiphyseal union sequencing is one such means to recognize developmentally incompatible material. The sequence in which 21 epiphyses of the postcranial skeleton initiate and complete union has been previously documented utilizing the Bosnian sample (Schaefer and Black 2007). Documentation of both "beginning" and "complete" union was necessary as the two sequence patterns, although similar, were not identical. Sequence of beginning union reflects differential fusion times among the epiphyses, whereas sequence of complete union reflects differential timing as well as union duration. Thus, the epiphyses did not initiate union in exactly the same order that they completed. The inclusion of both sequences thereby provides a wider spectrum of evidence from which to recognize commingling in that maturational discrepancies can be identified not only between those that have completed union in relation to those that have not, but also in terms of those epiphyses that have begun union in relation to those that have not.

To define sequence patterns, the phase distributions of the 21 epiphyses were individually cross-referenced with those of the remaining 20 epiphyses to understand the fusing relationship between the 210 epiphyseal pairs. To determine which epiphysis of the pair initiated union first, comparisons were made between the number of individuals who displayed some form of union (i.e., active or complete) for one epiphysis while at the same time displaying no union for the second epiphysis. This was compared to the total number of individuals displaying some form of union (i.e., active or complete) for the second epiphysis while at the same time displaying no union of the first epiphysis. Ideally, only one of the two epiphyses would exhibit active union prior to the other epiphysis, indicating the consistency with which that epiphysis was observed to initiate first. Realistically, however, this was not always the case and variable sequence orders were frequently encountered between the two epiphyses. Table 11.2 displays the proximal fibula initiating union prior to the proximal humerus in the majority (five cases) of the sample but also illustrates observations of the reverse sequence order (two cases). Epiphyses that exhibit variation in their sequence order are important to be aware of to ensure that skeletons displaying less frequent but acceptable sequence patterns are not mistakenly considered as two individuals.

Establishing the sequence of complete union was accomplished using the same method; however, different variables were considered. To determine complete union sequencing, the number of individuals who displayed complete union of one epiphysis while at the same time displaying non-complete union (i.e., no or active union) of a second epiphysis were compared to the number of individuals displaying complete union of the second epiphysis while at the same time displaying non-complete union of the first. Table 11.2 provides an example in which no individuals were observed to display complete union of the proximal humerus prior to that of the proximal fibula. Thus, the relationship between "complete union" is

Table 11.2 Cross-Tabulation of Phase Frequencies Between the Proximal Fibula and Proximal Humerus; Displays Variation in the Sequence Order of Beginning Union and Consistent Sequencing in Terms of Complete Union

	Phase	Proximal Fibula		
		0	1	2
Proximal	0	28	4	1
Humerus	1	2	7	32
	2	0	0	134

more consistent than that of "beginning union" in that the proximal fibula always completed union first.

Sequence Trees

Sequence tree diagrams (Figs. 11.1 and 11.2) can be used to illustrate the overall sequence in which the epiphyses begin and complete union (Schaefer and Black 2007). Each figure displays a modal sequence pattern, as demonstrated by a majority of individuals in the sample, in addition to all observed variations to that pattern.

The modal sequence pattern is represented by the central "tree trunk" within the figure and demonstrates progressive maturity from top to bottom. Figure 11.1 reveals that the acetabulum (tri-radiate complex) was the first epiphysis observed to initiate union and the medial clavicle was last. Variations to the modal pattern are demonstrated through the use of "tree branches." Each "branch" signifies the extent of variation that occurs in relation to the reference "trunk" epiphysis. The "twig" projections extending from the branches identify those epiphyses that exhibit the minority pattern; those positioned to the left of the trunk were occasionally observed to commence (Fig. 11.1) or complete (Fig. 11.2) union **before** the referenced "trunk" epiphysis, while those located to the right were sometimes observed to commence or complete **after** the referenced "trunk" epiphysis. Also included with each "twig" epiphysis is the number of individuals that display the alternative pattern in relation to the total number of cases utilized for defining the sequence. Highly detailed information such as this is critical to demonstrate the confidence that an anthropologist can assign to the epiphyseal status.

Epiphyses that have no "branches" extending from their "trunk" were not seen to exhibit any variation in sequence order to that of the modal pattern in this sample. The relationship between a "trunk" epiphysis and an epiphysis not identified by a "twig" extending from the trunk's branch is also 100% in the reference sample. These "unvaried" relationships are most useful to the anthropologist, who must discriminate between commingled remains. An indication of the number of individuals utilized in defining the relationship is necessary, however, to avoid sample size problems. The numbers of individuals involved in determining the nonvaried epiphyseal relationship are provided in Tables 11.3 and 11.4.

Open Versus Complete Union

Understanding the sequence in which the epiphyses initiate and complete union provides a solid basis for the recognition of incongruous maturity relationships among epiphyses. Materials may still be present, however, that do not violate the sequence patterns but present incompatible maturity levels nonetheless. Incompatible relationships between "open" and "complete" epiphyses have not

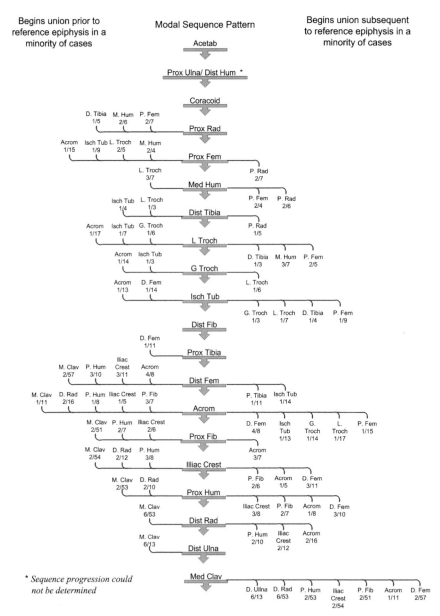

Fig. 11.1 Sequence of "beginning" union. Both a modal sequence pattern (represented by a majority of individuals within the sample) in addition to all observed variations to that modal pattern are provided

"Complete" Union

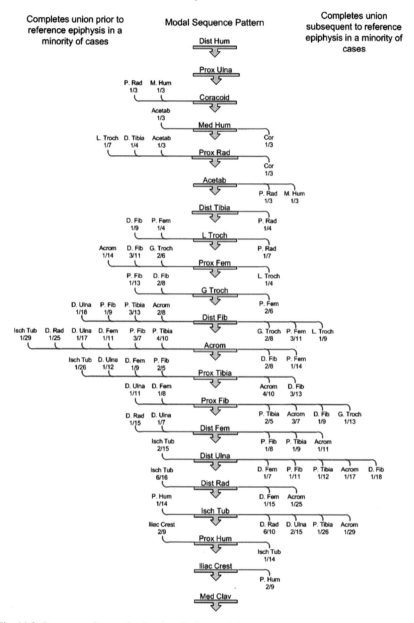

Fig. 11.2 Sequence of "complete" union. Both a modal sequence pattern (represented by a majority of individuals within the sample) in addition to all observed variations to that modal pattern are provided

Table 11.3 Number of Cases Utilized in Establishing Epiphyseal Relationships Associated with "Beginning" Union. Among the Relationships, the Epiphyses Listed Along the Vertical Axis Initiated Union Prior to Those Listed Along the Horizontal Axis

	Dist Hum	Prox Ulna	Cora-coid	Prox Rad	Prox Fem	Med Hum	Dist Tib	Lssr Troch	Gtr Troch	Isch Tub	Dist Fib	Prox Tib	Dist Fem	Acrom	Prox Fib	Iliac Crest	Prox Hum	Dist Rad	Dist Ulna	Med Clav
Acet	2	2	4	9	12	12	11	12	15	15	14	15	25	22	20	26	22	21	25	51
Dist Hum		No Info	2	10	14	14	13	15	19	22	15	21	31	29	28	33	34	36	44	46
Prox Ulna			2	10	13	13	13	15	18	20	16	20	29	28	26	31	32	37	45	83
Coracoid				5	7	8	6	7	10	11	9	11	20	18	15	18	18	18	21	46
Prox Rad					7	6	5	5	7	8	6	8	16	15	14	18	21	27	32	68
Prox Fem						4	1	5	5	9	5	10	19	15	18	24	22	24	31	71
Med Hum							1	7	5	18	4	7	16	15	14	12	21	25	32	70
Dist Tib								3	2	4	4	5	15	15	16	19	18	20	25	64
Lssr Troch									6	7	3	7	18	17	15	21	18	22	27	80
Gtr Troch										3	2	4	14	14	14	19	16	20	25	67
Isch Tub											2	2	14	13	13	18	15	18	24	63
Dist												1	12	10	12	14	3	17	22	60
Prox Tib													11	8	10	14	11	16	20	59
Dist Fem														8	5	11	10	11	15	57
Acrom															7	5	8	16	17	11
Prox Fib																6	7	7	11	51
Iliac Crest																	8	12	13	54
Prox Hum																		10	11	53
Dist Rad																			5	53
Dist Ulna																				13

Table 11.4 Number of Cases Utilized in Establishing Epiphyseal Relationships Associated with "Complete" Union. Among the Relationships, the Epiphyses Listed Along the Vertical Axis Completed Union Prior to Those Listed Along the Horizontal Axis

	Prox Ulna	Coracoid	Med Hum	Prox Rad	Acet	Dist Tibia	Lssr Troch	Prox Fem	Gtr Troch	Dist Fibula	Acrom	Prox Tibia	Prox Fibula	Dist Fem	Dist Ulna	Dist Rad	Isch Tub	Prox Hum	Iliac Crest	Med Clav
Dist Hum	8	7	14	14	9	18	24	28	30	27	38	37	35	48	51	56	66	80	84	165
Prox Ulna		2	5	7	4	8	13	17	18	19	29	27	25	37	43	48	53	70	70	153
Coracoid			3	3	3	5	11	10	13	11	18	14	12	21	17	20	26	35	37	78
Med Hum				3	3	5	8	12	13	16	24	22	22	32	39	45	50	67	68	148
Prox Rad					3	4	7	8	10	12	19	19	18	27	33	42	44	60	59	142
Acet						3	8	8	11	8	15	13	6	19	15	17	26	31	39	75
Dist Tibia							5	7	9	14	18	21	20	28	27	35	45	54	62	134
Lssr Troch								4	4	9	14	16	15	24	28	35	42	55	63	137
Prox Fem									6	11	14	14	13	22	26	32	39	51	60	134
Gtr Troch										8	10	12	13	20	24	31	38	51	59	133
Dist Fibula											8	13	9	15	18	25	32	42	48	121
Acrom												10	7	11	17	25	29	41	43	122
Prox Tibia													5	9	12	19	26	36	41	115
Prox Fibula														8	11	16	23	33	37	111
Dist Fem															7	15	17	31	37	112
Dist Ulna																8	15	27	28	111
Dist Rad																	16	18	19	101
Isch Tub																		14	19	95
Prox Hum																			9	83
Iliac Crest																				39

Table 11.5 Cross-Tabulation of Phase Frequencies Between the Medial Humerus and Distal Femur (In this example, the medial humerus always completes union prior to initiation of the distal femur.)

		Medial Humerus		
	Phase	0	1	2
Distal	0	17	4	12
Femur	1	0	0	20
	2	0	0	172

been previously explored and may provide further evidence of misplaced materials. This line of evidence requires the documentation of epiphyses that complete union prior to initiation of other epiphyses, and vice versa.

Documenting the relationship between "open" and "complete" epiphyses was accomplished utilizing the same Bosnian sample as employed in defining the sequence patterns. The 210 cross-tabulations displaying the phase distributions of each epiphyseal pair were again evaluated for analysis. From the data, three possible relationships were able to be defined and are illustrated by cross-tabulation in Tables 11.5, 11.6, and 11.7. The first type of relationship was characterized by one of the epiphyses in the pair always completing union prior to initiation of the second reference epiphysis (Table 11.5). The second relationship was defined by the dual possibility of observing one epiphysis in the pair completing union before initiation of the second reference epiphysis in addition to observations of the two epiphyses undergoing active union concurrently (Table 11.6). The third relationship was characterized by those epiphyses that never complete union prior to the second reference epiphysis (Table 11.7).

Table 11.6 Cross-Tabulation of Phase Frequencies Between the Proximal Femur and Distal Femur [In this example, the proximal femur sometimes completes union prior to initiation of the distal femur (4 cases) and sometimes undergoes union concurrently (6 cases).]

		Proximal Femur		
	Phase	0	1	2
Distal	0	18	15	4
Femur	1	0	6	18
	2	0	0	179

Table 11.7 Cross-Tabulation of Phase Frequencies Between the Proximal Fibula and Distal Femur (In this example, the proximal fibula never completes union prior to initiation of the distal femur.)

		Proximal Fibula		
	Phase	0	1	2
Distal	0	30	0	0
Femur	1	5	11	7
	2	0	1	168

Antenna Diagram

The interphase relationships as defined above can be illustrated by the use of an antenna diagram (Fig. 11.3). Located along the central body of the diagram is a list of epiphyses that serve as a reference for the attachment of antennae. The order of the central-bodied epiphyses follows according to the modal sequence of complete union, although this order is not overly important to the diagram; it simply places the early uniters toward the top of the page and those that fuse later toward the bottom. The antennae extending from the reference epiphyses connect to bubbles that further identify a list of epiphyses. Those listed in bubbles located on the left of the page are epiphyses that have been identified as **always** completing union prior to initiation of union of the reference epiphysis, while those listed in the bubbles toward the right of the page are those that **sometimes** complete union prior to initiation of the reference epiphysis. The epiphyses that **never** complete union prior to initiation of the reference epiphysis are understood through their exclusion as they are the epiphyses not listed within either the right or left bubble. The first few reference epiphyses included toward the top of the diagram do not have any antennae associated with them, thus indicating that no other epiphysis completes union before its initiation. This is not surprising, as the first few epiphyses represent those that fuse early.

Also included within each bubble is the number of observations from which the data were extracted. Thus, the bubbles on the left portray the number of individuals who display completion of the named epiphysis while at the same time displaying open union of the reference epiphysis. The bubbles on the right display a ratio; the first number represents the number of individuals displaying completion of the named epiphysis while at the same time displaying open union of the reference epiphysis, and the second number represents the frequency in which the two epiphyses were observed to be simultaneously in the process of uniting. The frequency at which various patterns are observed is important to understand in that an "always" relationship that is based on too few examples may in the future prove to be a "sometimes" relationship, and thus there are simply too few examples to assign great confidence to the relationship. In addition, less emphasis may be placed on a "sometimes" relationship that only exhibits one individual whose epiphyses are fusing concurrently while providing many examples in which the epiphysis completes before the other begins.

Testing for Commingled Remains

The utility of epiphyseal union as a means of detecting commingled remains was tested by artificially combining materials of known provenance. The two sequence trees, in addition to the antenna diagram, were used to identify potentially incongruent material, while Bayesian analysis was subsequently used to accept or reject suspicions. Bayesian analysis is not typically associated with accept/reject approaches, as it offers a real probability rather than a *p*-value. The posterior probability that

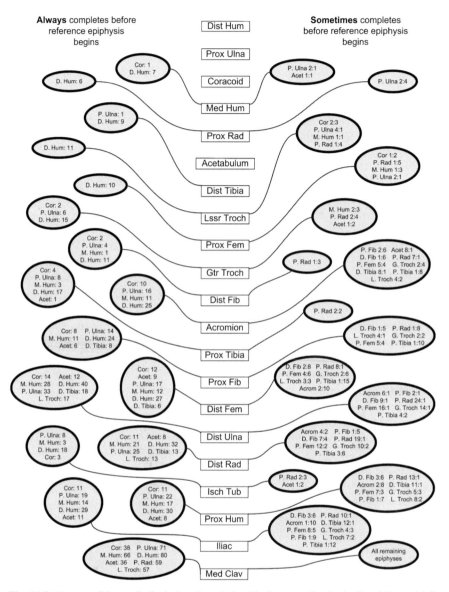

Fig. 11.3 "Antenna Diagram" displaying the relationship between "beginning" and "complete" union. Numbers on the left display the frequency at which the epiphysis was observed to complete prior to initiation of the reference epiphyses. Numbers on the right display a ratio of the frequency at which union completes prior to initiation of the reference epiphysis in relation to the frequency at which the two epiphyses were observed to be simultaneously in the process of uniting

is offered does, however, provide the anthropologist with a certain degree of confidence as to the likeliness of the observation. With this information, the anthropologist can then base his decision as to whether the element should be removed from the assemblage.

Testable Materials and Assemblage Composition

A subset of the Scheuer collection housed at the University of Dundee was utilized to test the ability with which epiphyseal phase relationships can be applied to recognize the presence of commingled remains. Six juvenile individuals from a modern Portuguese population were selected as their ages fell within the confines of the years of epiphyseal union and their integrity as single individual assemblages could be verified.

To initiate the test, skeletal elements from these six individuals were artificially commingled by an independent observer. Because of the potential of recognizing incongruent elements using more common commingling identification techniques, such as variations in size and shape, much care went into combining materials to ensure that only indicators of incompatible maturity were selected. The assemblages were therefore not randomly selected, but were instead well-thought-out combinations of materials. If the original individual was slight, for example, then only gracile material could be substituted as a replacement. Both right and left elements were also commonly replaced to avoid discrimination on the basis of bilateral shape differences. If only one side of the substitute material was available, then sides of other elements would also be removed to ensure that the absence of a bone did not provide indication of commingling. In addition to finding suitable material that emulates the overall impression of the skeleton, a further requirement was that the replacement element had to be of a different maturity level than the original element; otherwise, the test could not possibly discriminate between individuals.

Fifteen assemblages were combined and examined over a period of two months. As only six individuals were available for analysis, a greater number of assemblages were produced than the total number of represented individuals; thus, materials were reused in different combinations. Assemblages could include any number of elements from one individual as well as any number of misplaced elements. For example, one assemblage may combine the upper and lower limbs of two individuals, while the next may be mainly represented by a single individual with only one misplaced element. There was also the potential that everything in the assemblage belonged to only one individual and nothing was misplaced or that more than two individuals were represented.

A maximum of four assemblages were generated for analysis at any one time over a two-month period. The extended timescale was beneficial in that it allowed the researcher to forget elements that might belong together. This offered additional security that misplaced elements were detected solely on the basis of epiphyseal status and not memory recall.

Test Design

Phase of union was recorded for each epiphysis within the assemblage. Sequence trees for both "beginning" and "complete" union as well as the "antenna diagram" were used to cross-reference the union phases to determine whether any epiphyses were found to contradict the established pattern. Bayesian analysis was then run utilizing the Bosnian data to calculate the probability of the suspect element(s) exhibiting its phases of union based on the fusing status of the remaining epiphyses within the assemblage. Calculations were achieved utilizing the commercial software package Bayesware Discoverer. To make the method accessible for general use, the raw data set will be provided in future publications; however, it is available from the author until that time.

Before running the analysis, it was first necessary to define individual Bayesian networks for each assemblage. Bayesian networks provide a graphical representation of dependency relationships among variables, depicted through a system of nodes and arcs that ultimately inform the program how to calculate the final posterior probability. For an in-depth discussion of Bayesian networks in relation to forensic science, see Taroni and colleagues (2006). The presence of varying epiphyses and suspect elements within each assemblage required that a new network be defined for each case. Figure 11.4 provides an example of a network in which the greater trochanter, proximal femur, and proximal humerus will be used to predict the probability of the proximal tibia displaying its phase of union. Dependencies between the indicator epiphyses and the proximal tibia were artificially designed to allow the prediction, while the dependency between the greater trochanter and the proximal humerus and femur were mathematically derived. The mathematically learned dependencies act to influence the likelihood ratio, which ultimately affects the calculation of the final posterior probability. Thus, these dependencies are important to learn.

Bayesian analysis also requires knowledge of prior probabilities [for an in-depth discussion of the three components of Bayes' theorem, including that of a prior probability, see Lucy (2005) and Lucy et al. (1996)]. Despite the criticism that

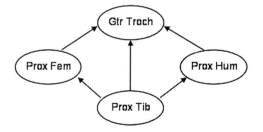

Fig. 11.4 Bayesian network displaying artificially derived dependencies between the proximal tibia and the three indicator variables (prox fem, gtr troch, and prox hum) to use in predicting the probability of observing the phase of union displayed by the proximal tibia. A mathematically derived dependency is also displayed between the greater trochanter and the proximal femur and humerus

reference priors have received in the past (Chamberlain 2000; Gowland and Chamberlain 1999), the Bosnian sample was used as a source to obtain priors within this study. Reference priors have been previously criticized as a result of their undue influence over the distribution of the final predictions, which ultimately reflect that of the reference sample rather than that of the population to which the remains belong (Bocquet-Appel 1986; Bocquet-Appel and Masset 1982; Chamberlain 2000; Gowland and Chamberlain 1999). To avoid this pitfall, researchers have suggested the use of an appropriate model that more realistically represents the population profile of the remains in question (Chamberlain 2000; Gowland and Chamberlain 1999). The fundamental challenge, however, is the selection of an *appropriate* model. When applying Bayesian analysis to detect improbable maturity relationships among epiphyseal elements, the selection of an appropriate prior is difficult at best. Evaluation of maturity relationships between the epiphyses requires a model that offers frequencies associated with the three phases of union for a particular population. This type of information is neither straightforward nor easy to obtain. Although the analysis is not age-dependent, phase frequencies are understandably heavily dependent on the ages of individuals within the model. A model that only includes individuals between the ages of 0 to 16 years, for example, will be heavily biased toward phase 0 (open union), whereas if the entire life cycle of a population is included, then frequencies will be heavily biased toward phase 2 (complete union). Therefore, it is likely that the best model is one that reflects the possible ages of the set of remains for which possible commingled elements are being tested. As the Bosnian sample represents a fairly good distribution of individuals within the years of epiphyseal union, it was selected as a source to learn prior probabilities within this analysis. The Bosnian sample may not, however, be suitable under other circumstances, and it is therefore the responsibility of the anthropologist to select what constitutes an appropriate prior for her own cases.

Results

Details regarding the composition of each assemblage, including the epiphyses that were present, the maturity level of the present epiphyses via epiphyseal scores, elements predicted as not belonging, and the final answers, are provided in Table 11.8. To gain a better appreciation of the way in which an element was predicted as not belonging, case 11 will be highlighted and discussed. The significant epiphyseal elements within case 11 included an open proximal humerus, an actively uniting proximal femur, greater trochanter and lesser trochanter, and a closed proximal tibia. When relating this material to the sequence in which the epiphyses complete union, a major contradiction is encountered. The documented sequence provides no examples of the proximal tibias ever completing union prior to the proximal femur or the greater or lesser trochanter. In addition to the sequence violation, this assemblage also defies established patterns between epiphyses that complete union before initiation of others. Documented relationships in the antenna diagram provide

Table 11.8 Contents of Each Assemblage Labeled as Cases (1–15), Including Which Epiphyses Were Present and the Scores Assigned to Each Epiphysis [Elements that were identified as "suspicious" are listed (prediction) as well as those that were in fact misplaced (answers).]

Epiphysis	Case 1	Case 2	Case 3	Case 4	Case 5	Case 6	Case 7	Case 8	Case 9	Case 10	Case 11	Case 12	Case 13	Case 14	Case 15
Prox Hum	2	2	2	2	0	2	2		2	0	0	2		0	2
Med Hum	2	2	2	2	2	2	2		2	2	2	2		2	2
Dist Hum	2	2	2	2	2	2	2		2	2	2	2		2	2
Prox Rad	2	1	2	2	2		2								1
Dist Rad	2	0	2	2	2		2								0
Prox Ulna	2	2	2	2	2		2				2	2			
Dist Ulna	2	0	2	2	0		2				0	0			
Prox Fem	2	1	1		1	1	2	2	2	1	2	2	2	2	2
Gtr Troch	2	0	1		1	1	2	2	2	1	2	2	2	2	2
Lsr Troch	2	0	1		0	0	2	2	2	1	2	2	2	2	2
Dist Fem	2	0	0		0	0	2	2	2	1	2	2	2	2	2
Prox Tibia	1	0			0		1	1		2			2	2	
Dist Tibia	2	0			0		2	2		2			2	2	
Prox Fibula	1				0	0	2	2		1	1	1		2	
Dist Fibula	1					0	2	2		2	1	1		2	
Cor-glen	2	2	1			1			1		2	2	1		2
Acromion	2	2	0			1			0		2	2	0		2
Med Clav											1	1			1
Acetabulum	2	2	2		2	2	2	2	2		2	2	2	2	
Iliac Crest	1	1	1		1	1	0	0	1		1	1	1	0	
Ischial Tub	2	2	2		2	2	1	1	2		2	2	2	1	
Prediction:	Tibia & Fibula	Scapula Femur	Femur Scapula	Scapula Tibia	Tibia	Tibia	Humerus	Tibia & Pelvis	Scapula Tibia	Scapula Tibia	Scapula Tibia	Ulna & Fibula	Scapula	Humerus & Pelvis	Radius
Answers:	Same	Same	Same	Same	Tibia & Femur	Same	Same	Same	Same	Same	Same	Same	Same	Same	Radius & Clavicle

no examples of the proximal tibias ever completing union prior to the proximal humerus beginning union. As such, the documented patterns provide evidence that the tibia is unlikely to belong to the other materials within the assemblage.

Utilizing the sequence trees and antenna diagram, 19 of 21 total misplaced elements were able to be identified. Two elements were unable to be identified as misplaced, including the femur in case 5 and the clavicle in case 15. No elements were inaccurately segregated. Thus, this method was successful in fully recognizing the presence of commingled elements in 13 out of 15 cases.

Probabilities associated with the epiphyses of known misplaced elements exhibiting each of the three phases of union were calculated and are provided in Table 11.9. A probability of less than 0.05 assigned to at least one epiphysis of a bone was accepted as the point at which that element could be rejected as not belonging to the assemblage. It is important to note that posterior probabilities are not p-values; however, the standard 0.05 was selected as a cut-off point as it represents a critically low probability, thereby guarding against false negatives. Interestingly, of the two cases that were not identified as misplaced, Bayes' theorem was able to successfully identify one of them as not belonging, based on the probabilities assigned to their observed phases. In a real case scenario, however, it may be impractical to calculate the probability of every element without justifiable cause. Thus, if no pattern violation occurred, then the statistical test may never have been performed in the first place.

Implications of the Test

While Bayes' theorem can be used to quantify the probability that an element belongs to an assemblage, the critical component in its application is the ability to identify suspicious elements from which to run the analysis. As such, the diagrams documenting the three lines of evidence are still required to permit recognition of suspect epiphyses.

As is common with other commingling identification techniques, the tested method is designed only to determine elements that do not belong, but it cannot be used to identify elements that do belong (Byrd and Adams 2003). The technique may also be able to permit skeletal reassociations, but only through the process of eliminating remains to which the element cannot belong. Within this study, a posterior probability of 0.05, calculated for at least one epiphysis on an element, was accepted as the point at which that element was identified as not belonging. Despite the low cut-off probability, this method was able to successfully identify 20 out of 21 misplaced elements, while no elements were falsely judged as not belonging.

The decision as to what constitutes an acceptable cut-off probability is a subjective area that must be judged independently by each anthropologist, depending on the circumstances of the case. More conservative probabilities will work to lower the possibility of false negatives; however, false negatives may at times be deemed as preferential to false positives. For example, in the case of large-scale identification

Table 11.9 Probabilities Assigned to the Three Possible Phases of Each Epiphysis of a Misplaced Element (The phase that was actually observed on the epiphysis is listed in the Obs column.)

Case 1	Obs	0	1	2
Prox Tibia	1	0.00	0.00	1.00
Dist Tibia	2	0.00	0.00	1.00
Prox Fibula	1	0.00	0.00	1.00
Dist Fibula	1	0.00	0.00	1.00

Case 2	Obs	0	1	2
Coracoid	2	0.06	0.940	0.00
Acromion	2	1.00	0.00	0.00

Case 3	Obs	0	1	2
Prox Fem	1	0.00	0.00	1.00
Gtr Troch	1	0.00	0.00	1.00
Lsr Troch	1	0.00	0.00	1.00
Dist Fem	0	0.00	0.001	0.999

Case 4	Obs	0	1	2
Coracoid	1	0.00	0.00	1.00
Acromion	0	0.00	0.001	0.999

Case 5	Obs	0	1	2
Prox Fem	1	0.013	0.620	0.367
Gtr Troch	1	0.042	0.686	0.272
Lsr Troch	0	0.022	0.484	0.494
Dist Fem	0	0.694	0.306	0.00
Prox Tibia	0	0.105	0.887	0.008
Dist Tibia	0	0.001	0.320	0.679

Case 6	Obs	0	1	2
Prox Tibia	1	0.00	0.00	1.00
Dist Tibia	2	0.00	0.00	1.00

Case 7	Obs	0	1	2
Prox Hum	2	0.985	0.015	0.00
Med Hum	2	0.080	0.777	0.143
Dist Hum	2	0.068	0.072	0.860

Case 8	Obs	0	1	2
Prox Tibia	1	0.00	0.00	1.00
Dist Tibia	2	0.00	0.00	1.00
Acet	1	NA	0.00	1.00
Iliac	0	0.00	0.202	1.00
Ischial	1	0.00	0.093	0.798

Case 9	Obs	0	1	2
Prox Tibia	0	0.00	0.00	1.00
Dist Tibia	0	0.00	0.00	1.00

Case 10	Obs	0	1	2
Coracoid	0	0.00	0.00	1.00
Acromion	0	0.00	0.00	1.00

Case 11	Obs	0	1	2
Prox Tibia	2	0.00	1.00	0.00
Dist Tibia	2	0.00	0.456	0.543

Case 12	Obs	0	1	2
Prox Ulna	2	0.00	0.00	1.00
Dist Ulna	0	0.00	0.00	1.00
Prox Fib	1	0.00	0.00	1.00
Dist Fib	1	0.00	0.00	1.00

Case 13	Obs	0	1	2
Coracoid	1	0.00	0.00	1.00
Acromion	0	0.00	0.003	0.997

Case 14	Obs	0	1	2
Prox Hum	0	0.00—	0.165	0.835
Med Hum	2	0.00	0.00	1.00
Dist Hum	2	0.00	0.00	1.00
Acet	1	NA	0.00	1.00
Iliac	0	0.00	0.171	0.829
Ischial	1	0.00	0.093	0.907

Case 15	Obs	0	1	2
Prox Ulna	2	0.00	0.00	1.00
Dist Ulna	2	0.00	0.00	1.00
Med Clav	0	0.055	0.507	0.437

procedures, further confirmatory tests (e.g., DNA analysis) may be performed on elements that are suspected of not belonging to further resolve the issue. If DNA analysis counteracts suspicions of an element not belonging, then the element can once again be returned to its appropriate remains without having harmed identification proceedings. Given this situation, relaxing the cut-off probability to identify more potentially incompatible material may serve to better ensure that all episodes of commingling are detected and that each assemblage constitutes one individual.

One overriding limitation of the method is that the commingled assemblage must include osseous material of differing levels of maturity. Failing this requirement, the technique cannot detect incompatible material, as it is likely that the developmental status of any bone would be nearly identical to that of the second individual. Even if the two individuals display differential maturation, the technique may still prove inadequate based on the elements present and the union that they display. The fewer the number of bones that are available within the assemblage, the less evidence that is provided and the less likely that commingling episodes will be recognized. This difficulty is illustrated by cases 5 and 14 in which a femur and clavicle were unable to be identified as misplaced due to the limited number of elements available within the assemblages.

This study offers validation and support to the technique's reliability in attempts of satisfying the *Daubert* criteria for admissibility in a U.S. Federal court of law. While no indication as to the method's future performance can be provided, the test within this study achieved an accuracy of 90.5%, clearly demonstrating the potential of the method. All errors were the result of false negatives, meaning that some misplaced elements were not identified. No errors were the result of false positives, meaning that no elements were wrongfully identified as not belonging. This is most likely the result of the cautious measures taken in this research, which accepts all elements as belonging unless proven as otherwise to below a 0.05 probability.

In conclusion, documentation of acceptable phase relationships between 21 epiphyses of the postcranial skeleton can be used as a successful tool to help with the detection of commingled remains, given that the individuals involved display differential maturity.

Acknowledgments I would like to thank ICMP for allowing me to conduct this research. Thanks also to Prof. Sue Black for her participation in designing the assemblages used within the commingling test, in addition to her input and advice on my Ph.D. thesis, from which this chapter is based.

References

Bocquet-Appel, J. 1986 Once upon a time: Palaeodemography. *Mitteil. Berlin Gessell. Anthropol. Ethnol. Urges* 7:127–133.
Bocquet-Appel, J. and C. Masset 1982 Farewell to paleodemography. *J. Hum. Evol.* 11:321–333.
Buikstra, J. E., C. C. Gordon, and L. St. Hoyme 1984 The case of the severed skull: Individuation in forensic anthropology. In *Human Identification: Case Studies in Forensic Anthropology*, T. A. Rathbun and J. E. Buikstra, eds., pp. 121–135. Charles C. Thomas, Springfield, IL.

Byrd, J. E. and B. J. Adams 2003 Osteometric sorting of commingled human remains. *J. Forensic Sci.* 48(4):717–724.

Chamberlain, A. 2000 Problems and prospects in palaeodemography. In *Human Osteology: Archaeology and Forensic Science*, M. Cox and S. Mays, eds. Greenwich Medical Media Ltd., London.

Gowland, R. and A. Chamberlain 1999 The use of prior probabilities in aging perinatal skeletal remains: Implications for the evidence of infanticide in Roman Britain. *Am. J. Phys. Anthropol. Suppl.* 28:138–139.

Koot, M. G., N. J. Sauer, and T. W. Fenton 2005 Radiographic human identification using bones of the hand: A validation study. *J. Forensic Sci.* 50(2):263–268.

L'Abbe, E. N. 2005 A case of commingled remains from rural South Africa. *Forensic Sci. Int.* 151(2–3):201–206.

Lucy, D. 2005 *Introduction to Statistics for Forensic Scientists*. John Wiley and Sons, Ltd., West Sussex.

Lucy, D., R. G. Aykroyd, A. M. Pollard, and T. Solheim 1996 A Bayesian approach to adult human age estimation from dental observations by Johanson's age changes. *J. Forensic Sci.* 41(2): 189–194.

Owsley, D. W., D. H. Ubelaker, M. M. Houck, K. L. Sandness, W. E. Grant, E. A. Craig, T. J. Woltanski, and N. Peerwani 1995 The role of forensic anthropology in the recovery and analysis of Branch Davidian Compound victims: Techniques of analysis. *J. Forensic Sci.* 40(3):341–348.

Ritz-Timme, S., C. Cattaneo, M. J. Collins, E. R. Waite, H. W. Schutz, H. J. Kaatsch, and H. I. Borrman 2000 Age estimation: The state of the art in relation to the specific demands of forensic practise. *Int. J. Legal Med.* 113(3):129–136.

Rogers, T. L. 2005 Determining the sex of human remains through cranial morphology. *J. Forensic Sci.* 50(3):493–500.

Rogers, T. L. and T. T. Allard 2004 Expert testimony and positive identification of human remains through cranial suture patterns. *J. Forensic Sci.* 49(2):203–207.

Ross, A. H. and L. W. Konigsberg 2002 New formulae for estimating stature in the Balkans. *J. Forensic Sci.* 47(1):165–167.

Schaefer, M. C. and S. M. Black 2007 Epiphyseal union sequencing: Aiding in the recognition and sorting of commingled remains. *J. Forensic Sci.* 52(2):277–285.

Schmitt, A., P. Murail, E. Cunha, and D. Rouge 2002 Variability of the pattern of aging on the human skeleton: Evidence from bone indicators and implications on age at death estimation. *J. Forensic Sci.* 47(6):1203–1209.

Snow, C. 1948 The identification of the unknown war dead. *Am. J. Phys. Anthropol.* 6:323–328.

Snow, C. C. and E. D. Folk 1970 Statistical assessment of commingled skeletal remains. *Am. J. Phys. Anthropol.* 32:423–427.

Taroni, F., C. Aitken, P. Garbolino, and A. Biedermann 2006 *Bayesian Networks and Probabilistic Inference in Forensic Science*. John Wiley and Sons, Ltd., West Sussex.

U.S. Supreme Court 1993 *Daubert v. Merrell Dow Pharmaceuticals*, 509 US 579.

Williams, B. A. and T. Rogers 2006 Evaluating the accuracy and precision of cranial morphological traits for sex determination. *J. Forensic Sci.* 51(4):729–735.

Chapter 12
How Many People? Determining the Number of Individuals Represented by Commingled Human Remains

Bradley J. Adams and Lyle W. Konigsberg

Introduction

Much of the literature that deals with various quantification techniques comes from faunal analysis. Generally, these techniques have two goals when working with animal remains. The first is to quantify the deposited/recovered faunal assemblage and from this data extrapolate information about past hominid behavior. The results of such studies attempt to draw conclusions concerning human diet, animal procurement strategies, and predator–prey relationships (Lyman 1987). The second goal is directed toward quantifying the recovered faunal assemblage in order to reconstruct the living community of animals. The results of these types of studies attempt to draw conclusions concerning faunal turnover and succession, reconstruction of paleoenvironmental conditions, and geographic faunal patterns (Lyman 1987). When working with commingled human remains, the goal of quantification is obviously to estimate the total number of dead, and many of the techniques developed for faunal analysis are not appropriate. Two exceptions are the Minimum Number of Individuals (MNI) and the Lincoln Index (LI). In paleodemographic studies, estimation of the number of individuals is critical for the interpretation of past cultures, while in the forensic context it is vital for the identification process and for possible criminal trials.

With few exceptions, the extent of discussions concerning commingled human remains revolves almost exclusively around the MNI. Certainly, one of the reasons for the popularity of the MNI is due to the ease of its calculation. Another reason is that most physical anthropologists are not familiar with other options. Recent research has shown that the Lincoln Index (LI) is a viable option for dealing with human remains and is not significantly more complicated than the MNI in its calculation (Adams 1996). A more statistically accurate modification of the LI has been presented called the Most Likely Number of Individuals, or MLNI (Adams and Konigsberg 2004). These alternatives to the MNI provide physical anthropologists with more analytical power when dealing with commingled remains. The key difference between the MNI and the LI or MLNI is that both the LI and MLNI estimate the *original* number of individuals represented by the osteological assemblage, while the MNI only estimates the *recovered* assemblage. In cases of taphonomic loss, this distinction can be quite important since the values presented by the MNI may provide misleading number estimates. The LI and MLNI, on the other hand, will present a more accurate estimate of the original population size that can be used for paleodemographic or forensic purposes. Furthermore, it is possible to provide confidence intervals with the LI and MLNI, but not with the MNI.

Factors Affecting Quantification: Bone Preservation and Scale of the Incident

There are two critical components to consider when determining the appropriate quantification technique: (1) bone preservation and (2) scale of the incident. Probably the more important of the two is preservation. Extremely fragmentary or poorly preserved remains are not amenable to any meaningful quantification techniques. In these situations, the MNI is the best quantification technique to utilize, but the results may not provide an accurate estimate of the true population of dead. Regarding the scope of the incident, most commingled sites can be considered to be either small-scale or large-scale. Everything else being equal, it will generally be easier to determine the number of individuals with small-scale incidents. Large-scale scenarios become more complicated from both an analytical and logistical perspective (Byrd et al. 2003). Obviously, it will be much easier to deal with a small-scale incident involving 5 people as opposed to a large-scale incident involving 500.

Taphonomy is defined as the "science of the laws of embedding or burial" (Lyman 1994: 1). The field of taphonomic study involves *any* organism and its geological context, but human remains are of particular interest to physical anthropologists. An accurate understanding and recognition of the potential taphonomic changes that can occur to skeletal remains prior to recovery is essential for a meaningful interpretation of the assemblage, especially for quantification studies. It would be an unusual occurrence for 100% of the skeletal elements deposited at a site to be recovered during excavation. Whether data loss occurs from chemical breakdown of the bone, transport away from the site, or recovery bias, some degree of data loss is nearly impossible to avoid. Lyman (1987, 1994) outlines four general taphonomic effects that occur after death: disarticulation, scattering/dispersal, fossilization, and mechanical alteration. At each of these stages, there is the potential for data loss. In addition, bone assemblages can still undergo detrimental changes after recovery unless adequate measures are implemented for their curation.

With human remains, disarticulation generally occurs as the result of animal scavenging or the natural putrification process. It is also possible as a result of traumatic events, such as a plane crash or explosion. Scattering/dispersal may occur simultaneously with disarticulation but is expressed in varying degrees depending on the distance between previously articulated elements. This could range from only a few millimeters to many miles. With remains deposited on the surface, dispersal may result from animal scavenging. It is also possible that intentional site tampering may occur, resulting in further commingling and data loss. Several such examples of clandestine body removal and mass grave relocation have been documented in the former Yugoslavia (Skinner et al. 2002).

Fossilization refers to the changes that occur as the result of the associated soil matrix and also includes surface weathering. Gordon and Buikstra (1981), for example, have shown how the pH level of the soil is directly related to the state of preservation encountered at mortuary sites. Mechanical alteration results in fragmentation and/or abrasion due to mechanical or physical processes (e.g., fluvial transport and compression). Fragmentation occurs by the loading of force on a bone and its failure to withstand the pressure, while abrasion is the result of frictional forces on the bone surface. Mechanical alteration can occur at any time between death (possibly associated with death) and recovery. Bone porosity and density are important factors for preservation during both fossilization and mechanical alteration. Several studies have shown that larger and denser bones have a better chance of survival than the delicate elements (Brain 1976; Lyman 1993; Waldron 1987; Willey et al. 1997).

Quantification Techniques

Minimum Number of Individuals (MNI)

The MNI is arguably the most popular method of quantification in any type of commingled osteological analysis. Many researchers credit T. E. White (1953) with its initial use for abundance studies in archaeology. For interpreting population size from a skeletal assemblage, the MNI (as the name suggests) presents the minimum estimate for the number of individuals that contributed to the sample. In order to deal with fragmentary remains, specific segments of an element (e.g., distal femur) can be used for the calculation of the MNI. Every fragment must share a unique landmark to ensure that fragments do not originate from the same skeletal element. The basic principle of an MNI estimate is to avoid counting the same individual twice.

Unless all of at least one type of skeletal element is recovered, the MNI will not provide an accurate estimate of the original (i.e., true) number of individuals represented by the remains. In their discussion of faunal remains, Fieller and Turner (1982: 56) wrote, "... the very presence of unmatched bones indicates that the MNI estimate is necessarily an underestimate of the number comprising the death assemblage." The MNI simply states how many individuals would have been necessary to provide the recovered skeletal elements but says nothing about the original death population. Since the MNI varies depending on the recovery rate, it may be of limited interpretive value in some instances.

Figure 12.1 shows the results of 1,000 computer-simulated tests at each of 9 different recovery rates that track the behavior of the MNI. At each of the recovery rates, a random draw on the binomial for the left and right sides produces two bone counts, for which the larger of the two represents the MNI. As is clear from the histogram, the value of the MNI is a direct indication of the representation of skeletal elements. In this example, a true population of 40 individuals is presented. When

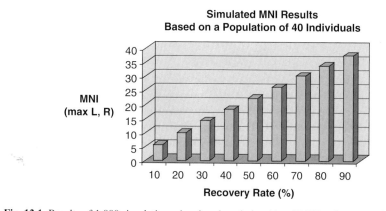

Fig. 12.1 Results of 1,000 simulations showing the relationship of MNI estimates to the recovery of skeletal elements when the true population is 40 individuals. Chart shows that the MNI estimate increases in proportion to the percentage of bones recovered

only 50% of the major elements are recovered, the MNI will be close to 20. If 90% are recovered, the MNI will be around 36, and it is only when almost 100% are recovered that the MNI will be a true reflection of the actual number, in this case 40. Granted that the original population estimate determined through the recovery of ancient remains can almost never be verified, but the general trend of the MNI's behavior proves the need for caution with its use as a quantifier of abundance. Even in circumstances of near-complete recovery, it will still be an underestimate of the original population.

Calculation of the MNI

The most common derivation of the MNI used for the analysis of human remains is simply calculated by sorting the bones by side and element and then taking the greatest number as the estimate. In other words, it is the most repeated element after sorting by element and side, Max (L, R), where L signifies left, R signifies right. It is equivalent to assuming that all of the less frequently observed bones are paired with the more frequently observed bones and subsequently provides a rather unlikely estimate in situations where the recovery is less than 100%. There is another variant of the MNI, sometimes referred to as the Grand Minimum Total, that will usually provide higher estimates than the standard MNI estimate. It is calculated as L + R − P, where L signifies left, R signifies right, and P signifies pairs. With this quantification technique, unpaired bones from different sides are assumed to come from different individuals. Take, for example, a scenario where femora were the most numerous elements recovered from a site. There were 145 lefts, 130 rights, and 95 pairs within this group. The MNI derived as Max (L, R) would be 145, while the Grand Minimum Total would be 180.

Lincoln Index and the Most Likely Number of Individuals

The Lincoln Index (LI) has been almost exclusively utilized and discussed concerning zooarchaeological remains and population studies of living animals (Allen and Guy 1984; Chapman 1951; Chase and Hagaman 1987; Fieller and Turner 1982; Horton 1984; Klein and Cruz-Uribe 1984; Plug 1984; Ringrose 1993; Seber 1973; Turner 1980, 1983, 1984; Turner and Fieller 1985; Wolter 1990; and many others). The LI was first developed for population studies of living animals based on capture-recapture techniques and was later adapted for application to zooarchaeological faunal assemblages. The Most Likely Number of Individuals (MLNI) is a slight variation of the LI that improves the accuracy of the estimates (Adams and Konigsberg 2004). With both the LI and MLNI, it is critical that elements can be accurately pair-matched.

The key feature for the use of the either the LI or MLNI with skeletal remains that separates them from the MNI is that accurate estimates of the original population can be derived from samples in which taphonomic data loss has occurred. The theoretical basis of the formula is that it is used on populations in which all of the animals (living or dead) need not be observed. This has particular utility with archaeological samples or in forensic situations when the recovery of major skeletal elements is less than 100%. When working with the LI or MLNI, it is important that the data loss occurs randomly (Ringrose 1993).

Calculation of the LI

In capture-recapture studies of living animals, a group of n_1 animals is initially trapped. These animals are then tagged and returned to the wild. Some time later, a second group of n_2 animals is captured. The number of tagged animals recaptured from the initial catch is then counted as m. With the assumption that the proportion of initially tagged animals present in the second sample is roughly the same for the entire population, the estimated population size ($\hat{N}$) can be derived by the simple equation

$$\hat{N} = n_1 n_2 / m.$$

The formula from the capture-recapture studies has been adapted for the same purpose of determining population size with zooarchaeological faunal remains. By using the bones of dead animals, the technique can achieve results similar to those obtained from the living animals. As previously stated, the goal of the implementation of the LI is to estimate the actual population that is represented by the skeletal assemblage, that is, the size of the community at death instead of at recovery.

When working with skeletal elements, the LI is calculated based on pair-matching. Pair-matching involves the comparison of right and left elements to determine if they are from a single individual. The bones from one side of the skeleton, e.g., left (L), are analogous to the initial stage of the capture-recapture procedure (n_1). The bones from the other side of the skeleton, e.g., right (R), are analogous to the second stage of the capture-recapture procedure (n_2). The number of elements that can be matched from the right and left sides as coming from the same individual (P) is analogous to the recapture of initially tagged animals (m). An estimate of the original death assemblage (LI) represented by the skeletal elements is

$$LI = LR/P.$$

Calculation of the MLNI and Confidence Intervals

A simple modification to this formula is recommended by Seber (1973) to account for possible sample bias. Recently, Adams and Konigsberg (2004) have shown that this formula represents the maximum likelihood estimate; referred to as the Most Likely Number of Individuals, or MLNI. It is simply calculated as

$$\text{MLNI} = \frac{(L+1)(R+1)}{(P+1)} - 1.$$

The resulting MLNI value should be presented as an integer value without rounding (i.e., any decimal value should be truncated), such that a value of 58.7 would be presented as 58. While both the LI and the MLNI will provide very similar results in most situations, it is recommended that the MLNI should be used in all circumstances since it was derived specifically in order to remove bias from the estimate. Using our example from above with 145 left, 130 right, and 95 pairs of femora, the resulting MLNI estimate would be 198 individuals. This value is considerably higher than both the Max(L, R) MNI value of 145 and the Grand Minimum Total of 180. The MLNI equation, using the hypergeometric probability function, is currently available in an Excel^{TM} spreadsheet for instances involving single elements or multiple elements at http://konig.la.utk.edu/MLNI.html.

With the LI and MLNI, it is possible to calculate confidence intervals, a feature not possible with MNI estimates. An approximate confidence interval can be calculated using the following variance equation:

$$v^* = \frac{(L+1)(R+1)(L-P)(R-P)}{(P+1)^2(P+2)}.$$

For example, an approximate 95% CI can then be calculated as MLNI $\pm 1.96\sqrt{v^*}$. Remember that the lower limit of the CI should never be reported as less than the MNI value of $L + R - P$.

Because the number of individuals, N, follows a discrete distribution, it is not statistically accurate to give customary confidence intervals, such as the 95% intervals discussed above. Adams and Konigsberg (2004) discuss a more appropriate technique called the "highest density region" (HDR) (see Lee 1997: 49), which is preferable to classical confidence intervals. For more information on the HDR and its calculation, see Adams and Konigsberg (2004) and the Website http://konig.la.utk.edu/MLNI.html. The Website gives Excel™ spreadsheets for instances involving single elements or multiple elements.

Comparison of the MNI and MLNI

In situations where accurate pair-matching is possible, the MLNI will provide much more accurate results than the MNI. Table 12.1 shows the behavior of the MNI and MLNI with differing population sizes and recovery rates. Each value is based on 1,000 computer simulations. Note how the MLNI value estimates the true population at low recovery rates, while the MNI does not reflect the true population. Also note that the MLNI estimates are very accurate when recovery rates reach 50%, while the MNI estimates are still quite low. Robson and Regier (1964) suggest that bias in the MLNI will be negligible if there are more than seven pairs.

Test for the Accuracy of Pair-Matching

The primary danger involved with the use of the LI or MLNI for quantification from skeletal elements is the misidentification of pairs. Because of the multiplicative nature of these techniques, it is more vulnerable than other methods to fragmentation and misidentification of pairs. In extremely fragmentary situations, thorough pair-matching may be impossible and the LI or MLNI should not be used. With good preservation, the step of pair-matching will be substantially facilitated by accurate field excavation notes, consideration of general morphology, and taphonomic similarities. Of course, extensive osteological experience will be one of the most important factors for an accurate analysis.

As accurate pair-matching is critical to the use of the LI and MLNI, it was necessary to examine this facet of the technique more in depth. In theory, any paired element in the body could be used for the calculation of the LI and MLNI. In practice, though, particular parts of the skeleton will be more useful than others. Important criteria to consider for choosing appropriate skeletal elements are their size, presence of distinct morphological traits, potential for age and sex determination, and likelihood of survival. In order to examine the reliability of pair-matching bones of the same element type (e.g., right and left femora), an experimental test was performed using an archaeologically recovered assemblage of well-preserved human skeletal remains. The accuracy of pair-matching was tested using only gross morphological characteristics.

In order to perform a verifiable test of gross pair-matching abilities, a random sample was drawn from an archaeological skeletal collection housed at the University of Tennessee, Knoxville. Larson Cemetery (39WW2) is an Arikara site associated with the Post-contact Variant of the Coalescent Tradition (Owsley 1994;

Table 12.1 Average Abundance Estimates Derived from Differing Population Sizes and Recovery Rates

		Recovery Rate										
		10%		20%		30%		50%		70%		90%	
		MLNI	MNI	MLNI	MNI	MLNI	MNI	MLNI	MNI	MLNI	MNI	MLNI	MNI
Original Population	10	2.6 (2.2)	1.5 (0.9)	5.8 (3.6)	2.7 (1.1)	8.3 (4.1)	3.8 (1.3)	10.0 (3.3)	5.9 (1.3)	10.0 (1.6)	7.8 (1.1)	10.0 (0.4)	9.5 (0.7)
	20	6.5 (4.4)	2.7 (1.3)	14.7 (7.9)	4.9 (1.6)	19.8 (9.4)	7.1 (1.7)	20.0 (5.7)	11.2 (1.9)	20.1 (2.2)	15.27 (1.6)	20.0 (0.5)	18.7 (1.0)
	50	25.6 (13.7)	6.1 (1.9)	51.3 (25.5)	11.6 (2.4)	55.8 (23.8)	16.8 (2.8)	51.1 (8.0)	27.0 (2.9)	50.0 (3.0)	36.9 (2.6)	50.0 (0.8)	46.2 (1.7)
	100	73.6 (33.2)	11.7 (2.6)	114.1 (53.5)	22.3 (3.4)	107.7 (32.1)	32.6 (3.8)	101.0 (10.4)	52.8 (4.1)	100.0 (4.4)	72.6 (3.6)	100.0 (1.1)	91.8 (2.4)
	150	134.4 (60.5)	17.0 (3.2)	170.0 (70.9)	32.8 (4.3)	156.7 (36.2)	48.2 (4.6)	150.9 (12.6)	78.3 (4.9)	150.0 (5.1)	108.1 (4.5)	150.0 (1.4)	137.0 (3.0)

Number in parentheses is the standard deviation. MNI is derived by the Max(L, R) method. MLNI is derived as $\frac{(L+1)(R+1)}{(P+1)} - 1$.

Owsley et al. 1977). Initial occupancy at Larson is suspected to have begun about A.D. 1680 and to have ended by A.D. 1700 (Johnson 1994). Larson Cemetery was excavated during the 1966–1968 field seasons under the direction of William M. Bass through the University of Kansas. A total of 621 individuals was recovered (Owsley et al. 1977). Based on the demographic analysis of the remains, the cemetery appears to have been the sole repository for the village dead (Bass and Rucker 1976).

Two computer-generated lists simulated a 60% recovery sample of tibia, femora, and humeri from both adult and subadult primary burials from Larson Cemetery, one derived from an original population of 15 individuals and one from 30 individuals. The samples drawn for the test consisted of both complete and fragmentary elements. The randomly selected elements were commingled on a table without any assistance by the observer (BJA), and any identifying labels (e.g., catalog numbers) were covered. These procedures removed any chance of bias to the observer during the test. Furthermore, the simulated recovery rate of 60% was also unknown to the observer.

Conjoining of fragmentary remains should be attempted prior to pair-matching. After all potential matches between fragments are exhausted, pair-matching should be performed. Morphological indicators to use in the matching process include length, robusticity, muscle markings, epiphyseal shape, and general symmetry between elements. Taphonomic variables include the state of preservation (e.g., degree of weathering and color), presence of burning, presence of cut marks, and presence of animal damage. Because of the potential variation that is possible from differential preservation, taphonomic indicators should not be weighted as heavily as gross morphological features during pair-matching.

Although limited, results of the Larson Cemetery pair-matching test suggest that pair-matching can be accurately performed by experienced osteologists (Tables 12.2 and 12.3). It was found that it is more likely for errors in pair-matching to occur from overlooking true pairs, as opposed to the pairing of unrelated elements. It is suspected that this tendency may change if the sample size is substantially increased since variation between individuals may not be as obvious. The main reason for any difficulty in pair-matching is that fragmentation, even minimal, can obliterate key areas used for identifying a match. Overall, the Larson Cemetery pair-matching test provided encouraging results.

Table 12.2 Results of the 15 Individual Tests for Pair-Matching

Element	Pairs	Unpaired Lefts	Unpaired Rights
Femur	6	3	3
Tibia	4	3	3
Humerus	3* (4)	4* (3)	6* (5)

*Indicates that an error was made and the number in parentheses is the correct answer.

Table 12.3 Results of the 30 Individual Tests for Pair-Matching

Element	Pairs	Unpaired Lefts	Unpaired Rights
Femur	11	4	10
Tibia	10* (11)	9* (8)	8* (7)
Humerus	11* (12)	9* (8)	7* (6)

* Indicates that an error was made and the number in parentheses is the correct answer.

Test Application of the MNI and MLNI: Larson Village

Commingled skeletal remains from Larson Village (39WW2) were utilized as a test for quantification using the MNI and MLNI. Larson Village an Arikara site that is associated with Larson Cemetery (described above in the pair-matching section). Larson Village was excavated during the summers of 1963 and 1964 as a salvage program of the Smithsonian Institution River Basin Surveys. Although 29 circular lodge depressions were visible on the ground surface at the village site, only 3 were completely excavated (Lodges 1, 21, and 23).

Initial discovery of scattered burials on the lodge floors led to suspicion of an epidemic disease (smallpox) as a cause (see Bass and Rucker 1976), but subsequent analysis revealed extensive perimortem trauma suggesting warfare (Owsley et al. 1977). The state of the skeletons encountered within the lodges was a clear indication that intentional burial did not occur. It appeared as though the individuals were massacred and placed within the lodges or were left to decompose where they were killed. The majority of the remains were discovered on the floor of Lodge 21 (Fig. 12.2). Owsley et al. (1977: 121) state in their analysis of the warfare evident at the site, "Due to disturbance and mixture of the skeletons ... it was necessary to treat the bones as if they came from an ossuary."

The bones from Larson Village are generally in an excellent state of preservation and exhibit minimal fragmentation, weathering, or abrasion. There was extensive commingling that appears to have been largely the result of carnivore scavenging. This was demonstrated by numerous examples of tooth puncture marks on the bones. A study by Hudson (1993) showed that limb bones tend to dominate animal-scavenged assemblages. This is an important pattern to acknowledge, especially for quantification techniques such as the LI that rely on paired elements. Similarly, Marean and Spencer (1991) showed through an actualistic study of carnivore ravaging that the ends of limb bones are often destroyed while the shafts are preserved. When carnivore activity is apparent, they stress the need to include long bone shafts into quantification procedures and not to rely solely on the more easily identifiable epiphyses.

A second agent responsible for disarticulation was the human factor. Many elements show evidence of cut marks, suggesting that parts of the victim's bodies were removed as trophies. Scalping and dismemberment of victims during warfare is not an uncommon event on the Great Plains, as is evident by the literature documenting this type of trauma from the ethnographic and osteological record (Catlin 1989; Denig 1961; Grinnell 1910; Hollimon and Owsley 1994; Olsen and Shipman 1994;

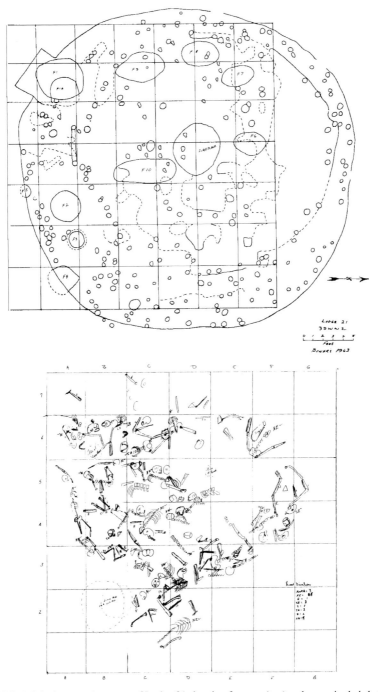

Fig. 12.2 Original excavation maps of Lodge 21 showing features (top) and commingled skeletons (bottom)

Owsley 1994; Owsley et al. 1977; Willey 1990). Scalping may be the most widely
recognized type of mutilation associated with Native American warfare, but hands,
feet, heads, noses, and limbs were also removed from the recently deceased as
trophies. Sometimes the violence and dismemberment were quite extensive, as is
exemplified by the Crow Creek massacre, where one-fourth of the victims were
decapitated (Willey 1990). At Larson Village, there is evidence that heads, hands,
and possibly feet were removed from several individuals. These disarticulated parts
would most likely have been transported away from the massacre site, creating a
systematic bias (nonrandom) and providing a viable rationale for excluding these
elements from any type of quantification study.

In order to observe the estimates generated by the MNI and the MLNI regarding
Lodge 21, four paired elements were selected for study. Sorting and pair-matching
procedures were performed on all of the humeri, os coxae, femora, and tibia discovered in the lodge. The MNI results derived by Max(L, R) from these elements
revealed an estimate of 43 individuals based on the counts of the femur (Table 12.4).

Calculation of the MLNI provided a higher population estimate. All of the MLNI
point estimates derived for each of the four elements inventoried from Lodge 21 are
between 49 and 51 individuals (Table 12.4). By assuming independence and combining the estimates from each of the four elements, an approximate 95% HDR (confidence interval) of 48 to 52 individuals was derived, with a point estimate of 50 individuals. A formatted spreadsheet is available at http://konig.la.utk.edu/MLNI.html
that calculates MLNI and HDR values from single elements or multiple elements.
The slightly higher MLNI estimate (approximately 7 more than the MNI) provides
evidence for the high recovery rate achieved at Larson Village, but it also shows that
data loss did occur and that the MNI is an underestimate of the true population.

Results from the Larson Village analysis are reasonably supportive of Badgley's (1986) view toward the MNI, which suggests that in situations of good preservation, near-complete recovery, and deposition resulting from a single event, the
MNI estimates will be close to the original population. Similarly, in this type of
situation, the LI results should be extremely accurate, and agreement between the
two techniques can be used to prove that a high degree of recovery was achieved. It
is considered advisable to compute the MLNI whenever it is feasible since it will be
much more accurate than the MNI when recovery is not quite so complete.

Table 12.4 Pair-Matching Results and Population Estimates from Lodge 21 (Larson Village)

Element	Pairs	Total Lefts	Total Rights	MLNI	MNI(Max L, R)
Tibia	20	30	34	**50** (44–62)	34
Os coxa	29	37	39	**49** (47–55)	39
Humerus	22	31	37	**51** (46–62)	37
Femur	31	43	36	**49** (48–54)	43
Combined				**50** (48–52)	**43**

*Note: The number in parentheses represents the approximate 95% HDR (confidence interval).
The lower limit of the interval cannot be less than L + R − P.

Summary and Conclusions

Data loss from skeletal assemblages can occur as a result of many distinct processes, i.e., taphonomic forces. Some of these include disarticulation, dispersal, fossilization, and mechanical alteration (Lyman 1987, 1994). Haglund and Sorg have published two edited volumes dealing precisely with forensic taphonomy (1997, 2002) showing that data loss is possible in both ancient and recent contexts. Any study that attempts to draw conclusions based on commingled human remains needs to implement the most appropriate quantification technique available.

This chapter has discussed three different quantification techniques, the MNI, the LI, and the MLNI. For human skeletal remains, the most common option employed by physical anthropologists for the purpose of estimating the original population size has been the MNI. The results revealed through computer simulation and the analysis of an actual commingled assemblage show that the MLNI is the best estimator of the original death assemblage, not the MNI. The strength of this technique is that it can account for taphonomic biases, which are an inherent part of archaeological samples and forensic contexts, with negligible effects to the estimate. The MLNI provides a more realistic reconstruction of past population counts from commingled situations and supplies researchers with more accurate figures from which to present demographic results and/or to establish identifications. The MNI should still be reported, but alongside the MLNI instead of alone. Similar results between the MNI and MLNI only provide added support for the reliability of the estimates and a high recovery rate. Discrepancies between the two methods demonstrate the MNI's correlation with the recovery rate and its inability to estimate the original population when data loss has occurred.

Overall, positive results were found for the reliability of pair-matching selected skeletal elements. If fragmentation is extensive or preservation is extremely poor so that accurate pair matches are impossible to determine, the MLNI is prone to gross miscalculations due to the multiplicative nature of the procedure. In situations of recovery greater than 50%, good preservation, and at least seven pairs, the use of the MLNI provides an accurate assessment of the actual population that contributed to the recovered osteological assemblage. It is also possible to apply confidence intervals to these estimates, a feature not available with the MNI.

References Cited

Adams, B. J. 1996 *The Use of the Lincoln/Peterson Index for Quantification and Interpretation of Commingled Human Remains.* Unpublished Master's thesis, Department of Anthropology, University of Tennessee, Knoxville.

Adams, B. J. and L. W. Konigsberg 2004 Estimation of the most likely number of individuals from commingled human skeletal remains. *Am. J. Phys. Anthropol.* 125(2):138–151.

Allen, J. and J. B. M. Guy 1984 Optimal estimations of individuals in archaeological faunal assemblages: How minimal is the MNI? *Archaeol. Oceania* 19:41–47.

Badgley, C. 1986 Counting individuals in mammalian fossil assemblages from fluvial environments. *Palios* 1:328–338.

Bass, W. M. and M. D. Rucker 1976 *Preliminary investigation of artifact association in an Arikara Cemetery (Larson Site), Walworth County, South Dakota.* National Geographic Research Reports, 1968 Projects.

Brain, C. K. 1976 Some principles in the interpretation of bone accumulations associated with man. In *Human Origins*, G. L. Isaac and E. R. McCown, eds., pp. 97–116. W.A. Benjamin, Menlo Park, CA.

Byrd, J. E., B. J. Adams, L. M. Leppo, and R. J. Harrington 2003 Resolution of large-scale commingling issues: Lessons from CILHI and ICMP. Paper presented at the Paper presented at the 55th Annual Meeting of the American Academy of Forensic Sciences, Chicago, IL.

Catlin, G. 1989 *North American Indians.* Viking, New York.

Chapman, D. G. 1951 Some properties of the hypergeometric distribution with applications to zoological sample census. *University of California Publications in Statistics* 1:131–159.

Chase, P. G. and R. M. Hagaman 1987 Minimum number of individuals and its alternatives: A probability theory perspective. *OSSA* 13:75–86.

Denig, E. T. 1961 *Five Indian Tribes of the Upper Missouri.* University of Oklahoma Press, Norman.

Fieller, N. R. J. and A. Turner 1982 Number estimation in vertebrate samples. *J. Archaeol. Sci.* 9:49–62.

Gordon, C. C. and J. E. Buikstra 1981 Soil pH, bone preservation, and sampling bias at mortuary sites. *Am. Antiquity* 46(3):566–571.

Grinnell, G. B. 1910 Coup and scalp among the Plains Indians. *Am. Anthropol.* 12:296–310.

Haglund, W. D. and M. H. Sorg (editors) 1997 *Forensic Taphonomy: The Postmortem Fate of Human Remains.* CRC Press, Boca Raton, FL.

2002 *Advances in Forensic Taphonomy: Method, Theory, and Archaeological Perspectives.* CRC Press, Boca Raton, FL.

Hollimon, S. E. and D. W. Owsley 1994 Osteology of the Fay Tolton Site: Implications for warfare during the Initial Middle Missouri Variant. In *Skeletal Biology in the Great Plains: Migration, Warfare, Health, and Subsistence*, D. W. Owsley and R. L. Jantz, eds., pp. 345–353. Smithsonian Institution Press, Washington, DC.

Horton, D. R. 1984 Minimum numbers: A consideration. *J. Archaeol. Sci.* 11:255–271.

Hudson, J. 1993 The impacts of domestic dogs on bone in forager camps. In *From Bones to Behavior*, J. Hudson, ed. pp. 301–323. Occasional Paper No. 21. Southern Illinois University, Carbondale.

Johnson, C. M. 1994 *A Chronology of Middle Missouri Plains Village Sites.* National Museum of Natural History, Smithsonian Institution. Submitted to Draft Report Prepared for the Department of Anthropology.

Klein, R. G. and K. Cruz-Uribe 1984 *The Analysis of Animal Bones from Archeological Sites.* University of Chicago Press, Chicago.

Lee, P. M. 1997 *Bayesian Statistics: An Introduction,* 2nd ed. Oxford University Press, New York.

Lyman, R. L. 1987 Zooarchaeology and taphonomy: A general consideration. *J. Ethnobiol.* 7:93–117.

Lyman, R. L. 1993 Density-mediated attrition of bone assemblages: New insights. In *From Bones to Behavior*, J. Hudson, ed., pp. 324–341. Center for Archaeological Investigations, Carbondale, IL.

Lyman, R. L. 1994 *Vertebrate Taphonomy.* Cambridge University Press, Cambridge.

Marean, C. W. and L. M. Spencer 1991 Impact of carnivore ravaging on zooarchaeological measures of element abundance. *Am. Antiquity* 56(4):645–658.

Olsen, S. L. and P. Shipman 1994 Cutmarks and perimortem treatment of skeletal remains on the Northern Plains. In *Skeletal Biology in the Great Plains: Migration, Warfare, Health and Subsistence*, D. W. Owsley and R. L. Jantz, eds., pp. 377–387. Smithsonian Institution Press, Washington, DC.

Owsley, D. W. 1994 Warfare in Coalescent Tradition populations of the Northern Plains. In *Skeletal Biology in the Great Plains: Migration, Warfare, Health and Subsistence*, D. W. Owsley and R. L. Jantz, eds., pp. 333–344. Smithsonian Institution Press, Washington, DC.

Owsley, D. W., H. E. Berryman, and W. M. Bass 1977 Demographic and osteological evidence for warfare at the Larson Site, South Dakota. *Plains Anthropol.* 13:119–131.

Plug, I. 1984 MNI counts, pits and features. In *Frontiers: Southern African Archaeology Today*, M. Hall, G. Avery, D. M. Avery, M. L. Wilson, and A. J. B. Humphreys, eds., pp. 357–362. British Archaeological Reports International Series 207, Oxford.

Ringrose, T. J. 1993 Bone counts and statistics: A critique. *J. Archaeol. Sci.* 20:121–157.

Robson, D. S. and H. A. Regier 1964 Sample size in Petersen mark-recapture experiments. *T. Am. Fish Soc.* 93:215–226.

Seber, G. A. F. 1973 *The Estimation of Animal Abundance and Related Parameters.* Griffin, London.

Skinner, M. F., H. P. York, and M. A. Connor 2002 Postburial disturbance of graves in Bosnia-Herzegovina. In *Advances in Forensic Taphonomy: Method, Theory, and Archaeological Perspectives*, W. D. Haglund and M. H. Sorg, eds., pp. 293–308. CRC Press, Boca Raton, FL.

Turner, A. 1980 Minimum number estimation offers minimal insight in faunal analysis. *OSSA* 7:199–201.

1983 The quantification of relative abundances in fossil and subfossil bone assemblages. *Ann. Trans. Mus.* 33:311–321.

1984 Behavioural inferences based on frequencies in bone assemblages from archaeological sites. In *Frontiers: Southern African Archaeology Today*, M. Hall, G. Avery, D. M. Avery, M. L. Wilson, and A. J. B. Humphreys, eds., pp. 363–366. British Archaeological Reports International Series 207, Oxford.

Turner, A. and N. R. J. Fieller 1985 Considerations of minimum numbers: A response to Horton. *J. Archaeol. Sci.* 12:477–483.

Waldron, T. 1987 The relative survival of the human skeleton: Implications for palaeopathology. In *Death, Decay, and Reconstruction*, A. Boddington, A. N. Garland, and R. C. Janaway, eds., pp. 55–64. Manchester University Press, Manchester.

White, T. E. 1953 A method of calculating the dietary percentage of various food animals utilized by aboriginal peoples. *Am. Antiquity* 4:396–398.

Willey, P. 1990 *Prehistoric Warfare on the Great Plains: Skeletal Analysis of the Crow Creek Massacre Victims.* Garland, New York.

Willey, P., A. Galloway, and L. Snyder 1997 Bone mineral density and survival of elements and element portions in the bones of the Crow Creek Massacre victims. *Am. J. Phys. Anthropol.* 104:513–528.

Wolter, K. M. 1990 Capture-recapture estimation in the presence of a known sex ratio. *Biometrics* 46:157–162.

Chapter 13
Assessment of Commingled Human Remains Using a GIS-Based Approach

Nicholas P. Herrmann and Joanne Bennett Devlin

Introduction

The quantification of fragmentary human remains offers a challenge for physical and forensic anthropologists. Physical anthropologists frequently borrow methods and quantification techniques developed by zooarchaeologists to assess such collections. Traditionally, zooarchaeological examinations deal with highly fragmentary, commingled samples from numerous contexts. As such, the archaeofaunal literature is rich with analytical approaches to assess these complex assemblages. However, the appropriate application of zooarchaeological approaches to human bone assemblages is uncertain.

The present study examines the commingled burned human remains from the Walker-Noe site (15Gd56) in Garrard County, Kentucky. The site is a small, early Middle Woodland Adena crematory located on the southern periphery of the Bluegrass physiographic region of the state of Kentucky. Extreme fragmentation of the remains precludes the use of a simple elemental coding system to generate a skeletal inventory. This chapter details the application of a geographic information systems (GIS)-based approach developed by zooarchaeological researchers (Marean et al. 2001) to provide both a minimum number of elements (MNE) and minimum number of individuals (MNI) estimate. The methods presented in this study have applications for both bioarchaeology and forensic anthropology. The physical anthropologist needs tools to accurately quantify the number of elements and individuals recovered from a commingled context, whether prehistoric, historic, forensic, or part of a human rights investigation.

Issues of Fragmentary and Commingled Human Remains

Though several measures exist for quantifying individuals represented in an assemblage, most frequently, biological anthropologists seek to estimate the minimum number of individuals (MNI). Simply, the MNI is generated by sorting elements to side of the body and recognizing the highest value as an indicator of the number of individuals present (Grayson 1984). This generates an approximation of the minimal number of individuals represented in the assemblage but cannot be

From: *Recovery, Analysis, and Identification of Commingled Human Remains*
Edited by: B. Adams and J. Byrd © Humana Press, Totowa, NJ

considered as a reflection of the size of the population that produced the recovered assemblage. Estimations of the original population size are possible (see Adams and Konigsberg 2004); however, extreme bone fragmentation limits the accuracy of such approaches and renders pair-matching impossible. For most examinations of extremely fragmentary remains, the estimation of the MNI is an appropriate approach.

At the core of MNI assessments must lay an accurate determination of the minimum number of skeletal elements (MNE) present in a collection. Seemingly straightforward, the relationship between the MNE and MNI is, in practice, a complex one. The MNE is defined as a derived quantitative measure (Lyman 1994) and, as such, requires explicit definition as to its calculation. Lyman presents multiple examples of MNE definitions that would result in several different estimates. Similarly, MNI calculations based on elemental coding systems are susceptible to the same problems of over- or underestimation as the MNE. Given the basic practice of sorting and coding elements by context to side of body and recognizing the highest count as indicative of the MNI, it is apparent how such values can underrepresent or potentially inflate the MNI. Recently, Adams and Konigsberg (2004) proposed a technique for estimating the most likely number of individuals (MLNI) as a variation of the Lincoln Index (LI). However, these techniques, predominantly based upon pair-matching, are poorly suited to extremely fragmented and cremated assemblages, as noted by Adams and Konigsberg (2004). Further, in an overview of methods for interpreting cremated remains, Mayne Correia and Beattie (2002) illustrate the lack of a cohesive analytical approach to estimating the MNI from cremated remains.

Osteological data collection manuals are lacking in coding systems for highly fragmented and taphonomically modified deposits. Buikstra and Ubelaker's (1994) osteological standards manual does provide for analysis of commingled remains, but the system is primarily useful when dealing with large fragments. Elements are to be coded according to the presence of specific percentages for the diaphysis (in thirds) and articular ends for long bones. Whole cranial elements and specific axial elements or groups of midline bones are to be recorded as such. The database recording structure presented in the standards manual (Buikstra and Ubelaker 1994) does allow for bone identification, element completeness, MNI count (based on identifiable elements), and demographic parameters. While providing a good structure for complete or near-complete skeletal recording, the methods presented in the standards manual (Buikstra and Ubelaker 1994) do not provide enough detail for highly fragmentary remains, cremations, or large commingled samples.

Church and Burgett (1996) and Burgett (1990) adapted a zooarchaeological coding system in an attempt to capture the variation in extremely fragmentary human remains. Burgett (1990) initially developed this information recording and retrieval system to document *in situ* commingled and fragmentary faunal remains. Church and Burgett (1996) describe the coding system as an alphanumeric identification hierarchy within which element, portion, and segment of the bone are identified. In addition to the identification hierarchy, Church and Burgett (1996) incorporate basic bone properties and taphonomic attributes. The properties fields constitute size, age, sex, fusion/development, and pathological conditions. The taphonomic attributes include weathering, gnawing, modification, breakage, burning, and trauma. While this system deals with fragmentary remains far better than the *Standards* (Buikstra and Ubelaker 1994) approach for human remains, it still has several shortcomings. The element, portion, and segment identification hierarchy can often become cumbersome when dealing with small identifiable fragments. The analyst decides whether an element is included in the calculation of the MNE or MNI. Small fragments typically do not represent the entire coded specimen and are given a "partial" or "fragment" segment code within this system. Clearly, the inclusion of partial/fragment codes in the summary analysis would result in overestimations of both the MNE and MNI, while excluding these specimens could seriously underestimate the MNE and MNI for fragmentary samples. This is problematic, given that an accurate estimation of the number of individuals represented in an assemblage is often crucial to the interpretation of site formation processes. Often with cremated and extremely fragmentary commingled remains, it is possible to identify very small fragments to side and exact position. However, these identifications may not be such that can be incorporated into an existing database or calculation system. Absent in the literature to date is a detailed recording system in biological anthropology that allows an analyst to accurately assess and estimate the MNE and MNI for commingled human remains.

Many of the problems considered herein are confronted in the technique developed by Marean and colleagues (Abe et al. 2002; Marean et al. 2001). A customized ArcView extension, *BoneEntryGIS,* utilizes an element-specific GIS to calculate MNE estimates. In effect, this approach facilitates a systematic means to overlay all identifiable elements, thereby generating a count of the minimum number of each element present in an assemblage. For the Walker-Noe site, we use this approach as a means to overcome the inadequacies of traditional inventory systems in managing fragmentary and highly modified remains such as cremated samples. The GIS approach provides a visual inventory and an efficient method to quantify the MNE. In the present discussion, we focus on the cranial elements of an archaeologically derived assemblage from the Walker-Noe site, Kentucky. In an attempt to thoroughly document both the number of individuals represented in the collection and taphonomic attributes of heat exposure as an indicator of cremation practice, identifiable bone fragments were digitized and assessed using a modified version of the *BoneEntryGIS* software extension. The results highlight the utility of this system for documenting highly fragmentary and taphonomically modified human remains, while also identifying potential problems in the application of this technique to human bone assemblages from both archaeological and forensic contexts.

Walker-Noe (15Gd56)

The Walker-Noe site (15Gd56) represents a small, early Middle Woodland period mound situated in the south-central Bluegrass Region of Kentucky (Fig. 13.1), supported by radiocarbon dates spanning from 170 B.C. to A.D. 130 (Pollack

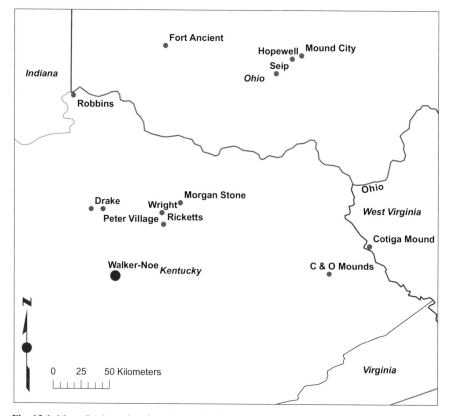

Fig. 13.1 Map of Adena sites found near the Kentucky Bluegrass region (modified from Pollack et al. 2005)

et al. 2005). Excavations at the site were conducted during the fall of 2000. Ceramics and lithic artifacts associate activity at the mound with the Adena culture. The radio-carbon dates firmly place the Walker-Noe site within the Middle Woodland period of the eastern United States. Adena is typically considered an early woodland cul-ture throughout much of the Ohio River Valley; however, Late Adena does extend into the Middle Woodland period (see Anderson and Mainfort 2002; Clay 1998, 2002; Railey 1990). Commonly, Adena mounds identified in Kentucky are charac-terized by extended interments with few cremations within large mounded burial facilities (Railey 1990). Walker-Noe can be considered as "event-centered" site a là Clay (1998, 2002), but it is not an accretional mound. Walker-Noe appears to have been a short-use facility where the local population cremated a small number of their dead (see Pollack et al. 2005).

The extensive presence of cremains at Walker-Noe suggests a fairly unique crematory pattern from that of other documented Woodland Period mounds both in design and in use in this region. In particular, Walker-Noe is rather distinct in the apparent existence of *in situ* cremations evidenced by substantial burned soils. The site is marked by a centrally located feature, a 1.25-square-meter deposit

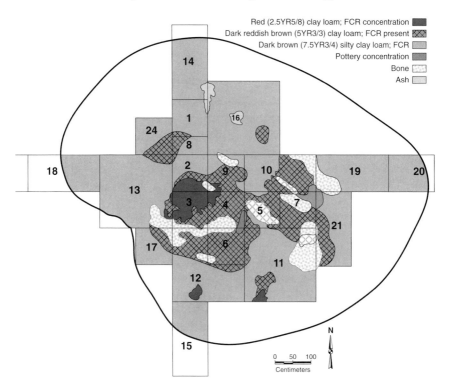

Red (2.5YR5/8) clay loam; FCR concentration
Dark reddish brown (5YR3/3) clay loam; FCR present
Dark brown (7.5YR3/4) silty clay loam; FCR
Pottery concentration
Bone
Ash

Fig. 13.2 Plan map of the Walker-Noe mound (modified from Pollack et al. 2005)

5 centimeters in depth, of burned clay loam (Fig. 13.2). The area of burned soil surrounding the central feature contained large amounts of fire-cracked dolomite (150 kilograms in total). Concentrations of cremated bone were identified directly above and around the central burned area. In addition, aggregations of burned bone were present in peripheral regions of the site. All skeletal material was located in association with wood charcoal, ash, and burned soils (Pollack et al. 2005). Several recovered projectile points/knives (PP/K) demonstrate attributes that suggest a contextual association with the cremation practices at the mound. Six PP/Ks do not exhibit any use-wear, interpreted to represent their preparation as ceremonial objects. However, two PP/Ks demonstrate heat alteration, indicating direct association with cremation practices. The Walker-Noe mound has been posited as a primary site for both cremation and interment, as supported by excavation and artifactual evidence (Pollack et al. 2005).

Walker-Noe Skeletal Analysis

A thorough examination and analysis of the human remains recovered at Walker-Noe is crucial in characterizing the mound as a crematory. Fieldwork yielded over 18 kilograms of charred and calcined human bone. The majority of fragments are less than 3 centimeters in diameter, with nearly all specimens exhibiting classic characteristics of extensive heat alteration, extreme fragmentation, and particular surface colors. All elements exhibit burning on both the internal and external surfaces. Little variation in color was noted across the cremation sample, with nearly all fragments displaying surface colors of gray and whitish gray, which is evidence of calcination. Surface colors associated with incomplete combustion of the organic components (i.e., browns and blacks) were not observed. In addition, fragments display extreme shrinkage and moderate degrees of warping, though the latter does vary throughout the assemblage. In addition, surface cracking and fracturing are apparent on the majority of specimens, on both endocranial and ectocranial surfaces. The condition of the skeletal material from the Walker-Noe site reflects a thorough incineration process. The consistency of these heat alteration attributes across the sample may be indicative of intentional processing and/or repeated exposure.

Preliminary assessments of the osseous material from Walker-Noe demonstrated that (1) identifiable cranial fragments far exceeded recognizable postcranial elements, and (2) the bone fragments examined in this study represent the commingled remains of numerous individuals (Bennett Devlin et al. 2006; Herrmann et al. 2005). We suspect that identification of cranial fragments over postcranial remains is common in most archaeologically derived cremains. The concentration of discrete and recognizable hard-tissue features of the skull compared to undifferentiated features of long bone shafts makes the use of cranial fragments more appropriate. Given this pattern, the present discussion incorporates data only from select cranial material.

GIS Analysis

The examination of the fragmentary human remains was conducted in several stages. Bone fragments were initially sorted into three categories of cranial, postcranial, and indeterminate elements. When possible, fragments were identified to particular element, though they were not sorted to side of the body. Due in part to this result, we focus upon several craniofacial elements: frontal, zygomatic, maxilla, and mandible. These elements were selected for several reasons: (1) They have a high likelihood of recovery; (2) these elements are readily identifiable (by osteologists) in fragmentary form; and (3) these four craniofacial elements possess multiple features that facilitate recognition of small, cremated fragments as a particular portion of the bone. The last of these criteria is the most important given the structure of the *BoneEntryGIS* system and approach.

Shapefile templates of the four cranial elements were created according to the methods described by Abe and Marean (n.d.). Within *Adobe Photoshop*, composite images of the four craniofacial elements were created that displayed both endocranial and ectocranial surfaces as well as other important elemental surfaces. For paired elements, these images were flipped horizontally to create the antimere image. The composite images were then georeferenced to four coordinate points within *Erdas Imagine*. The coordinate points are visible as the four symbols on the

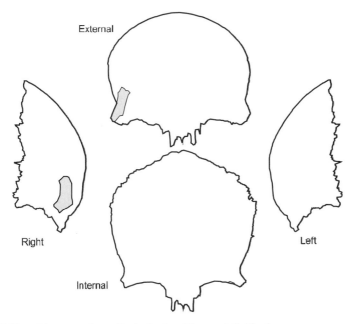

Fig. 13.3 Frontal bone template with single placed fragment digitized

images (see Figs. 13.3 and 13.4 for examples). The images were converted to a 1-bit grid and then changed to a shapefile to capture the perimeter of the bone surfaces. The element shapefile could then be edited, cut, and coded based on the observed fragments.

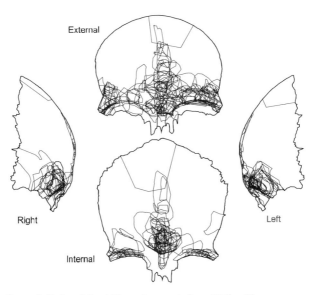

Fig. 13.4 Outlines of all placed frontal bone fragments from Walker-Noe

Fragmentary specimens were initially identified to one of four bones of the craniofacial skeleton. Fragments were separated based on field data. Subsequent examination sought to identify the particular area or region of the bone that the fragment represents. A substantial number of fragments were identifiable to a particular bone but did not contain specific features to facilitate identification to an exact location and were not digitized. A total of 396 specimens was subjected to further assessment (see Table 13.1). These specimens were identifiable to an exact location on the complete bone, herein referred to as "placeable." Researchers were able to "place" 112 frontal, 45 zygomatic, 59 left and 58 right maxillae, and 122 mandibular fragments to a particular location on the respective element. In addition, these fragments were macroscopically assessed in terms of surface colors, level of distortion, apparent degree of shrinkage, and overall fracture and cracking patterns. Each of these placeable fragments was assigned a specimen identification number as dictated by the *BoneEntryGIS* extension, which incorporated the field specimen number (fs) to enable consideration of fragment distribution across the site and site formation processes.

Surface colors were assessed on all identifiable specimens using an *X-rite CA22* spectrophotometer. This handheld device systematizes color evaluation by measuring areas on the sample greater than $1/4$ inch and relays color data to a host computer running *Matchrite ColorDesigner* software. As illustrated in Table 1, major and minor surface colors were noted and are represented as an average across the sample in the Mean Color column. Color data were recorded in the Lab color system, a numerical-based system that represents colors in terms of three dimensions. The extreme light and dark colors were also noted, as they are indicative of more unique heat exposure situations. Lab color values were then converted to Munsell colors (Munsell Soil Color Charts 2000) using the Munsell Color Conversion software (version 6.5.17; http://wallkillcolor.com/). Although time-intensive, the GIS system as used here provides the means to accurately quantify fragmentary and taphonomically modified skeletal material.

The nearly 400 placeable fragments were digitized using a modified version of the *BoneEntryGIS* software for ArcView 3.3 (Marean et al. 2001). Utilizing the software extension, skeletal fragments were recorded by location on two-dimensional images of the complete element. Multiple views of each element are included to ensure proper placement of each bone fragment. Figure 13.3 illustrates the process involved in "placing" a single fragment of the frontal bone. The overall shape,

Table 13.1 Lab and Munsell Color and MNE Estimate by Elements

Element	Placed Elements	Mean Color	Extreme Light Color	Extreme Dark Color	MNE
Frontal	112	8.9YR 6.4/2.8	9.7YR 8.8/1.0	8.6YR 3.4/2.1	26*
Malar	45	9.0YR 6.4/2.9	8.6YR 8.4/2.2	1.3Y 5.1/1.5	17
Maxillae R/L	59/58	8.9YR 6.2/3.0	9.3YR 8.1/2.4	9.5YR 4.5/2.1	20/21
Mandible	122	8.9YR 6.4/2.9	8.9YR 8.3/2.3	8.2B 4.5/0.48	21
Total	396				21

*Please see discussion of MNE determination in text.

location, and dimensions of the fragment are recorded as the specimen is positioned on the appropriate images that illustrate all views of the element. Each entry is saved as a shapefile, which can be merged (or layered) to demonstrate the density (i.e., numbers present) at a particular skeletal location. Figure 13.4 illustrates all of the data cells for identifiable fragments of frontal bone. Note the overlapping outlines of fragments. This information can then be interpreted and quantified as representing the number of elements present. Further, data such as fracture pattern, external and internal color, and other traditional human skeletal characteristics (pathology and discrete variants) can be recorded into a linked database. Data concerning recovery location may also be managed in this system. This technique generates a system that enables quantification of the MNI (and MNE) and allows collection and management of data illustrative of taphonomic processes, undoubtedly facilitating interpretation of numerous aspects of site use and formation.

Based on a weighted consideration of the number of identifiable fragments for each of the five cranial elements, an MNI of 21 individuals is indicated. Each craniofacial element was assessed individually, as illustrated in Fig. 13.5 and reported in Table 13.1. The highest density of "placeable" fragments per element, signified by an increasingly darker color, reflects specimen overlap, i.e., redundancy in fragments. The variation in MNE values noted for the individual elements examined reflects the fragmentation process due to thermal damage. For example, fragments from the orbital margin of the frontal are highly identifiable and placeable. However, delaminated endocranial surfaces of the frontal and fragments of the frontal plate are not locationally distinct and, as such, these fragments could rarely be specifically placed. The parietal bone was not selected for this study for these exact reasons.

Analysis of the frontal fragments indicates a maximum of 26 shared locations, or cells, within the GIS, indicating the minimum number of elements recovered from the site. Malar/zygomatic specimens support a minimum number of 17 elements. Fragments of the mandible and right maxilla indicate 21 elements, while the left maxilla suggests a minimum of 20 elements present. Although per-element MNE values range from 17 to 26, and the nature of MNI estimation suggests this should be the value presented for this collection, based upon the limited degree and the particular location of fragment redundancy, it is proposed that an MNI of 21 is most appropriate. No other skeletal element examined produced MNE values close to the lateral frontal determination of 26. All other elements fall near an MNE of 21. The marked difference in MNE values highlights a specific problem with template selection and digitizing of fragments. The lateral view of the frontal, specifically at the orbital margin, represents the entire depth of the frontal bone from nasion to the zygomatic process. The ability of the observer to accurately "place" or digitize a frontal bone fragment on either an anterior or posterior view is relatively simple. Determining accurate outlines of the same fragment in a lateral view is difficult, and we suspect that digitization errors have resulted in the high MNE estimate for the frontal bone based on the lateral view. The compression of three-dimensional distance across two-dimensional space will lead to digitizing problems for any analyst. We would argue that areas encompassing substantial depth should be identified and eliminated from the final MNE determination. Recent three-dimensional

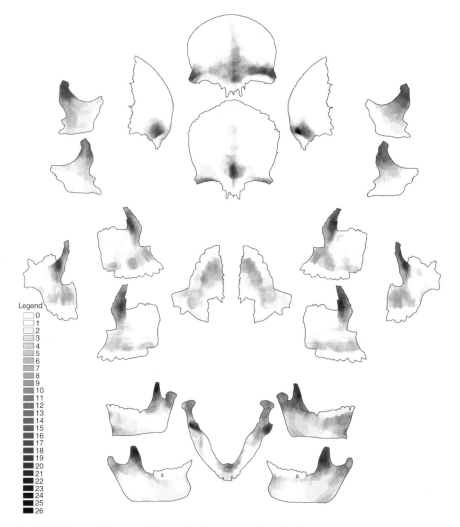

Fig. 13.5 Composite image of all cranial elements examined in this study

technologies would allow for the capture of all fragments either by computer tomography or by three-dimensional laser scanning. The scanned fragments could then be placed on a generalized three-dimensional element template. Such an approach would eliminate the problem associated with digitizing on a two-dimensional template.

Of interest is that the high representation of cranial fragments at Walker-Noe may also result from the common practice at Adena mortuary sites of including isolated crania, or trophy heads, in the burial context (Fenton 1991; Webb and Baby 1957). However, the *in situ* relationship of the skeletal material on the central platform is unknown due to a prior disturbance. No cutmarks were observed on any cranial elements, while several fragments did have surface fractures and cracking suggestive of a dry bone cremation. As such, it may be desirable to calculate an MNE from postcranial elements to compare with the cranial value. However, as previously stated, identification of highly fragmented postcranial elements is more difficult than cranial element recognition. We are currently evaluating the utility of a specific bony landmark inventory approach to deal with postcranial elements.

Conclusion

The initial cursory examination of the material from the Walker-Noe site indicated an MNI of less than 10 (Sharp et al. 2003). With application of the method described here, the value increased tremendously. Additional data concerning each fragment are collected during the laboratory analysis. Such information can be project-specific and allows the recorder to address specific research questions. In this case, we recorded surface modification and color changes related to heat. The implications for site use at Walker-Noe are directly impacted by findings from this study.

Although the GIS technique cannot be criticized for artificially inflating the values, it can, however, be faulted on several levels: (1) the extreme length of time involved in identifying and recording data for each fragment; (2) the reliance upon elements that include clearly identifiable and unique attributes; and (3) to be accurate and effective, the analysis *must* be completed exclusively by highly skilled osteologists. Although there may appear to be limitations to this image-based approach, in particular with regards to individual and population morphological variations, these concerns are manageable. Cranial and postcranial templates for infants and younger subadults should be developed separate from the adult templates. The database can be formulated to enable compilation of major skeletal parameters such as age distinctions (e.g., between adults and older subadults) or sexual dimorphism. Age and morphological variation does not impact the digitization of fragments. In effect, size and shape particulars are disregarded during the digitizing process, as all are reproduced onto the same generalized element created for the system. The element shapefiles produced in this approach reflect a standardized presence of the bone fragments, while the linked database provides fragment specific information for user queries. A key to this approach is template creation and selection. Specific element surfaces with significant depth should be reviewed and possibly eliminated from final templates to reduce the potential for MNE inflation due to fragment placement errors.

The accuracy of this method may result in higher counts for assemblages than those generated using more traditional quantification approaches. This system allows extremely precise estimation of the number of elements and individuals represented and further provides a systematic means for tracking patterns across an assemblage.

Acknowledgments We would like to thank David Pollack, the Kentucky Archaeological Survey, and the William S. Webb Museum of Anthropology at University of Kentucky for access to the Walker-Noe skeletal material. Curtis Marean of Arizona State University provided the *BoneGISEntry* extension and manual. Jonathan Bethard and Anne Kroman assisted in sorting the Walker-Noe material, and Sherri Turner performed data entry. The William M. Bass Endowment provided funding for the Xrite CA22 spectrophotometer.

References Cited

Abe, Y. and C. Marean n.d. Bone Entry GIS and Bone Sorter Manual: For recording, sorting, and analyzing bones using GIS. Unpublished manual distributed with the BoneEntryGIS software extension.

Abe, Y., C. Marean, P. Nilssen, Z. Assefa, and E. Stone 2002 The analysis of cutmarks on archaeofauna: A review and critique of quantification procedures, and a new image-analysis GIS approach. *Am. Antiquity* 67:643–663.

Adams, B. J. and L. W. Konigsberg 2004 Estimation of the most likely number of individuals from commingled human skeletal remains. *Am. J. Phys. Anthropol.* 125(2):138–151.

Anderson, D. and R. Mainfort (editors) 2002 *The Woodland Southeast*. The University of Alabama Press, Tuscaloosa.

Bennett Devlin, J., N. Herrmann, and D. Pollack 2006 GIS analysis of commingled and cremated bone. Poster presented at 71st Annual Meeting of the Society for American Archaeology, San Juan, Puerto Rico.

Buikstra, J. E. and D. H. Ubelaker (editors) 1994 *Standards for Data Collection from Human Skeletal Remains, Proceedings of a Seminar at The Field Museum of Natural History (Arkansas Archeological Survey Research Series No. 44)*. Spiral ed. Arkansas Archeological Survey, Fayetteville.

Burgett, G. 1990 The bones of the beast: Resolving questions of faunal assemblage formation processes through actualistic research. Unpublished dissertation, Department of Anthropology, The University of New Mexico, Albuquerque.

Church, M. and G. Burgett 1996 An information recording and retrieval system for use in taphonomic and forensic investigations of human mortalities (abstract). *Proc. Am. Acad. Forensic Sci. 48th Sci. Meeting* 2:167–168.

Clay, B. 1998 The essential features of Adena ritual and their implications. *SE Archaeol.* 17:1–21.

Clay, B. 2002 Deconstructing the Woodland Sequence from the Heartland: A review of recent research directions in the Upper Ohio Valley. In *The Woodland Southeast*, D. Anderson and R. Mainfort, Jr., eds. University of Alabama Press, Tuscaloosa.

Fenton, J. P. 1991 The Social Uses of Dead People: Problems and Solutions in the Analysis of Post Mortem Body Processing in the Archaeological Record (Mortuary Analysis). Unpublished dissertation, Columbia University, New York.

Grayson, D. K. 1984 *Quantitative Zooarchaeology*. Academic Press, New York.

Herrmann, N., J. Bennett Devlin, and D. Pollack 2005 GIS analysis of the cremated skeletal material from the Walker-Noe site, Kentucky. *Am. J. Phys. Anthropol. Suppl.* 40:11.

Lyman, R. L. 1994 *Vertebrate Taphonomy*. Cambridge University Press, Cambridge.

Marean, C., Y. Abe, P. Nilssen, and E. Stone 2001 Estimating the minimum number of skeletal elements (MNE) in Zooarchaeology: A review and a New Image-analysis GIS Approach. *Am. Antiquity* 66:333–348.

Mayne Corriera, P. and O. Beattie 2002 A critical look at methods for recovering, evaluating and interpreting cremated human remains. In *Advances in Forensic Taphonomy: Method, Theory and Archaeological Perspectives*, W. Haglund and M. Sorg, eds., pp. 435–450. CRC Press, Boca Raton, FL.

Munsell Soil Color Charts 2000 *Munsell Soil Color Charts*. Munsell Color GretagMacbeth, New York.

Pollack, D., E. Schlarb, W. Sharp, and T. Tune 2005 Walker-Noe: An early middle Woodland Adena mound in Central Kentucky. In *Woodland Period Systematics in the Middle Ohio Valley*, D. Applegate and R. Mainfort, Jr., eds., pp. 64–74. The University of Alabama Press, Tuscaloosa.

Railey, J. 1990 Woodland Period. In *Archaeology of Kentucky: Past Accomplishments and Future Directions*, D. Pollack, ed., pp. 247–374. Kentucky Heritage Council, Frankfort.

Sharp, W., D. Pollack, E. Schlarb, and T. Tune 2003 Walker-Noe: A middle Woodland mound in Central Kentucky. Paper presented at the 68th Annual Meeting of the Society for American Archaeology, Montreal, Canada.

Webb, W. S. and R. Baby 1957 *The Adena People*. No. 2. Papers in Archaeology. Ohio Historical Society, Columbus.

Chapter 14
The Application of Traditional Anthropological Methods in a DNA-Led Identification Process

Laura Yazedjian and Rifat Kešetović

About ICMP

The International Commission on Missing Persons (ICMP) was created in 1996, following the G-7 Summit in Lyon, France, to address the issue of persons missing as a result of the different conflicts relevant to Bosnia and Herzegovina, the Republic of Croatia, and Serbia and Montenegro between 1991 and 1995. In 1999 and 2001, ICMP expanded its operations to address missing persons cases from Kosovo and the Former Yugoslav Republic of Macedonia, respectively.

ICMP endeavors to secure the cooperation of governments and other authorities in locating and identifying missing persons and to assist them in doing so. ICMP also supports the work of other organizations in their efforts, encourages public involvement in its activities, and contributes to the development of appropriate expressions of commemoration and tribute to the missing.

Within ICMP, the Forensic Science Department (FSD) is responsible for developing, implementing, and managing the technical processes of assisting governments in exhumations, examinations, and identifications of the missing. The FSD established the use of a population-based, DNA-led system of identifications, which matches blood samples collected from family members of missing persons to bone samples from exhumed mortal remains.

It is estimated that as many as 40,000 people went missing as a result of the recent conflicts in the former Yugoslavia. As such a large number of individuals had never before been identified with a DNA-led approach, ICMP pioneered a high-throughput system, based in the affected regions. This strategy has made the DNA-led identification program feasible by reducing the cost. In addition, it has augmented the scientific capacity of the countries in the Balkans affected by the conflicts and created an interdependent system in the region that incorporates and trains local scientists under a multi-ethnic umbrella. The overall result has been to significantly increase the rate of positive identifications of exhumed remains.

From: *Recovery, Analysis, and Identification of Commingled Human Remains*
Edited by: B. Adams and J. Byrd © Humana Press, Totowa, NJ

The Podrinje Identification Project[1]

In July 1995, Bosnian Serb forces overran the UN Safe Haven of Srebrenica and almost 8,000 Bosnian Muslim men disappeared (Honig and Both 1997; Rohde 1998). It became clear early in the subsequent identification process that random and disorganized attempts with classical methods of identification, including the use of dental records, medical records, and anthropological analysis of remains for biological profiles, would not be effective for determining the identity of these individuals. Therefore, in 1999, ICMP established the Podrinje Identification Project (PIP) to address the question of their fate.

The PIP comprises a range of professionals: a project manager; a team leader, who coordinates the case work; four case managers, who contact families when a DNA matching report is issued for a set of mortal remains; a criminologist, who photographs all of the personal effects and clothing associated with the remains; a pathologist, who has the legal authority to issue death certificates; and, since 2003, a full-time anthropologist.

In 2000, a facility was built on land donated by the city to house the exhumed remains and provide examination and storage space. This mortuary, located in the northeastern city of Tuzla, has a refrigerated space with shelves for 867 complete (fleshed) bodies, but usually contains between 3,500 and 4,000 cases of skeletal remains exhumed from single and mass graves (Fig. 14.1).

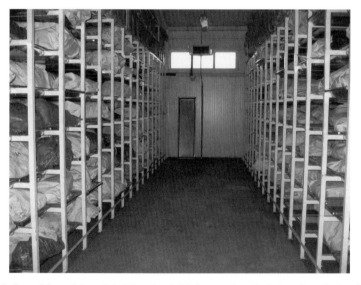

Fig. 14.1 One of four aisles of shelving that hold the remains of victims from Srebrenica. The paper bags above the body bags hold clothing

---

[1] Podrinje is the region of Eastern Bosnia where the town of Srebrenica and all of the graves relating to the fall of the UN Safe Haven are located.

A Challenging Task

There are several reasons that the identification of the victims from the fall of Srebrenica is particularly problematic: taphonomic processes, the demographic composition of individuals who were killed, and the lack of antemortem information available. With such a large number of missing, these factors practically ensured that the vast majority of individuals killed during the fall of Srebrenica would never be identified using traditional methods. Until the first "blind" DNA match on November 16, 2001, the project had managed only 222 identifications. Fifty-one were identifications based on excellent circumstantial evidence, such as documents found with the remains, combined with the recognition of clothing by family members and supporting information from examination of the remains. The remaining 171 cases were presumptive DNA identifications, that is, with weaker supporting material requiring samples to be sent to outside labs for confirmation by DNA. All of these identifications were virtually complete bodies recovered from primary graves.

Taphonomy

The majority of the remains from Srebrenica are disarticulated and/or commingled due to various taphonomic factors, such as scavenging, deliberate attempts to hide evidence, and varied and poor excavation methods. Natural dispersion occurred in many cases when individuals were not buried, which included scattering by weather conditions, rivers, and animal scavenging. Unfortunately, in many of these cases, the remains may never be recovered, and those that are located tend to be incomplete, fragmentary, and highly commingled.

A few months after the fall of Srebrenica, information came to light indicating the existence of the mass graves; consequently, the perpetrators returned to the sites and attempted to hide the evidence by exhuming the victims from the primary graves and reburying them in secondary locations. This was done using heavy machinery such as backhoes and large trucks, very often driven into the graves themselves. As decomposition had already begun, there was considerable damage to the integrity of complete bodies, which resulted in many cases of individuals divided between two or more graves, both primary and secondary (Fig. 14.2).

In addition to the commingling created by the deliberate movement of bodies, commingling can also inadvertently occur in the field during exhumation. For example, it is possible for the overlapping lower and upper bodies of two different individuals to be collected as one case. Although there are secondary graves and commingling from taphonomic forces elsewhere in the former Yugoslavia, the degree of relocation of the bodies from Srebrenica was exceptional (Fig. 14.3).

During exhumation, cases are assigned numbers in sequential order. A skeletal assemblage collected in one body bag is considered a "case," and each case

Site Links

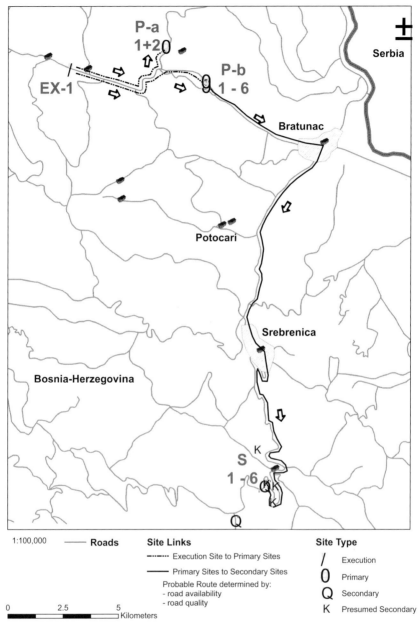

Fig. 14.2 Map showing the spatial relationships among an execution site, two sets of primary graves (P-a and P-b), and secondary graves (S) related to the second set of primaries (P-b). (Map courtesy of Amanda J. Reddick.)

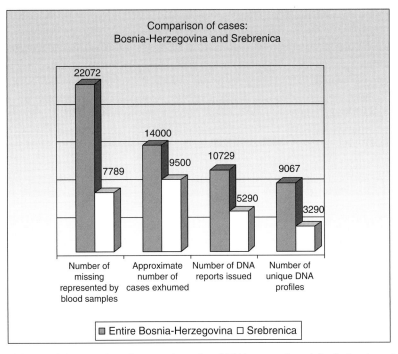

Fig. 14.3 The high proportion of cases exhumed and DNA reports issued for Srebrenica-related cases in relation to the total number of missing for all of Bosnia-Herzegovina reflects the high degree of disarticulation and commingling of remains

is given a designation based on its degree of completeness: "B" for body (>75% of the elements are present), "BP" for body part (<75% of elements are present), and "GBP" for general body part (commingled elements or unarticulated single bones).

Exhumations of victims from Srebrenica have been carried out since the end of the war, beginning in 1996. Unfortunately, there was no coordination of operations, and international teams from many different countries took part. This resulted in different styles of exhumation with different methods of data collection, which were occasionally recorded in different languages; there was no overall coordination to share data. For example, the International Criminal Tribunal for the former Yugoslavia (ICTY) collected data for war crimes prosecutions in The Hague and had no mandate for identification. A forensic team from Finland independently collected surface remains for criminal evidence in 1996, doing its work and issuing official autopsy reports in Finnish. Physicians for Human Rights conducted a Forensic Monitoring Project, monitoring the exhumation of human remains and issuing Findings Reports (Skinner et al. 2002).

In 2001, the local missing persons commissions assumed responsibility for exhumations; in the area of Srebrenica, they are the Republika Srpska Commission for Missing and Detained Persons and the Federation Commission for Missing Persons. Regrettably, these dedicated teams do not employ anthropologists or archaeologists, and a great deal of information is therefore lost during exhumation that could have been helpful later, during the identification process and as evidence at trials.

In light of this, ICMP has fielded teams of international and local anthropologists and archaeologists since 2002 to assist the local commissions as forensic experts in the field. These professionals work under the authority of the local commissions and may fulfill different roles at any given exhumation, ranging from simply being present as a monitor to having significant influence on the excavation procedures. The Excavation and Examination Program within ICMP has developed benchmark operating procedures for both the recovery and examination of remains, which ensure a high standard of practice when they are implemented.

The Missing[2]

During the fall of Srebrenica, the perpetrators targeted a certain cross-section of the population, typically referred to as "men of fighting age"; consequently, the majority of those missing have similar biological profiles (Komar 2003). Out of 3,209 individuals identified to date, only 5 are female, and all belong to a single ethnic group. In addition, although there are individuals as young as 13 and over 80 years old reported missing, most of the victims were between 17 and 45 years old at the time of disappearance. Similarly, though in any population there are very tall and very short individuals, average living stature follows a standard curve, and so the majority of the missing men were between 165 and 185 centimeters tall in life. Dental care had not been regularly available to most individuals living in Srebrenica, and many people had very poor dental hygiene, so what may have ordinarily been a distinctive dental profile with several extractions or severe caries was unremarkable.

Lack of Information

Many of the individuals who went missing in Srebrenica had arrived relatively recently, since it had been declared a UN "Safe Haven." A large number had lived there for up to 3 years with limited access to medical care. Consequently, there is almost no conclusive antemortem information such as dental records, medical records, and hospital X-rays available for comparison with remains. For example,

---

[2] All figures and statistics are accurate as of July 11, 2007, the date of the 12th anniversary of the fall of Srebrenica, and the date of the 7th commemoration ceremony and burial of identified cases at the memorial center at Potočari.

there are only 600 existing dental records for almost 8,000 missing (less than 10%). Additionally, most of the people who sought safety in Srebrenica during the conflict came from rural villages where there was a similar lack of access to medical and dental care.

Because of the lack of institutional records, virtually all antemortem information used in the identification process comes from family members of the missing. This means that many injuries and pathological conditions may have been undiagnosed or untreated, and thus unrecognized. Close family members typically remember major incidents, such as broken bones and severe trauma; however, accuracy depends on when the incident occurred and which family members are queried. For example, a woman may not know about broken bones her husband suffered in childhood or a sister and brother-in-law living abroad may have no information about a recent accident that injured a hand.

Antemortem dental information from relatives can be very vague, as often individuals cannot remember which of their own teeth have been extracted or repaired, much less those of a family member. However, distinctive dental work, such as crowns, bridges, or dentures, is still very useful in the identification process, as most relatives can give good descriptions of such prostheses.

Information about living stature from family members is similarly unreliable, particularly since these are estimates given about someone not seen in the last 10 years. Mothers and grandmothers, especially, may unconsciously add centimeters to a loved one's height when reporting on an antemortem questionnaire.

At the beginning of the identification process, two "Books of Photos" were produced with photographs of clothing recovered with remains. These were shown to families of the missing, and many articles of clothing were recognized. However, subsequent DNA-led identifications showed that only approximately 15% of the clothing recognized by family members in fact belonged to a missing relative. This is due to several factors; for example, several years had already passed since the disappearances; many of the individuals who initially escaped exchanged clothing, especially outerwear; a great deal of clothing was donated and was therefore generic; and there was considerable degradation to organic clothing material. Additionally, the viewing of the photos was a highly emotional and traumatic situation for family members, and in many cases the same clothing was "recognized" as belonging to two or more unrelated missing individuals. Because of this, no identifications were ever closed based solely on clothing recognition.

With the current methods, however, clothing is used as corroboratory evidence once a DNA report provides a potential name for a set of remains. Frequently, unique mending or repair is recognized, which is especially substantiating in the case of underclothes or socks. On occasion, family members shown photographs of clothing and personal effects recovered with the remains adamantly do not recognize anything that was found with that individual. If the anthropological support for the case is weak, it can be cause to take another DNA sample, particularly if commingling is suspected, as all of the remains present may not belong to only one individual.

Techniques

The methods used to produce the biological profile included in the anthropology report for each case are the same as those used by anthropologists working on identifications of unknown remains around the world, and the general reference volumes used are also the same (Bass 2005; Bennett 1993; Buikstra and Ubelaker 1994). Although the vast majority of the remains examined at the Podrinje Identification Project are those of males, sex is determined using conventional criteria: the shape of the pubic bone (Phenice 1969) and sciatic notch (Bruzek 2002). Age at death is estimated using the pubic symphyses (Brooks and Suchey 1990; Katz and Suchey 1986; Todd 1920), auricular surface (Lovejoy et al. 1985), sternal rib ends (Iscan et al. 1984a, b), and teeth (Lamendin et al. 1992) for adults. For subadults and young adults, those between 13 and 20 years old at the time of death, the pattern of epiphyseal fusion is used (McKern and Stewart 1957; Scheuer and Black 2000). Living stature estimates are produced using the Trotter–Gleser standards (Trotter and Gleser 1952). Studies have been done on the suitability of many of these standards to this specific population, which generally report that the existing standards are broadly applicable for the Balkan population (Duric et al. 2005; Slaus et al. 2003), although more accurate standards would be desirable (Donic et al. 2005; Schaefer and Black 2005) and some have been developed (Ross and Konigsberg 2002). Although there are various metric and multifactorial methods for determining sex, age at death, and even to resolve commingling (Byrd and Adams 2003; Giles 1964; Giles and Elliot 1963; Pietrusewsky 2000), they tend to be disproportionately time-

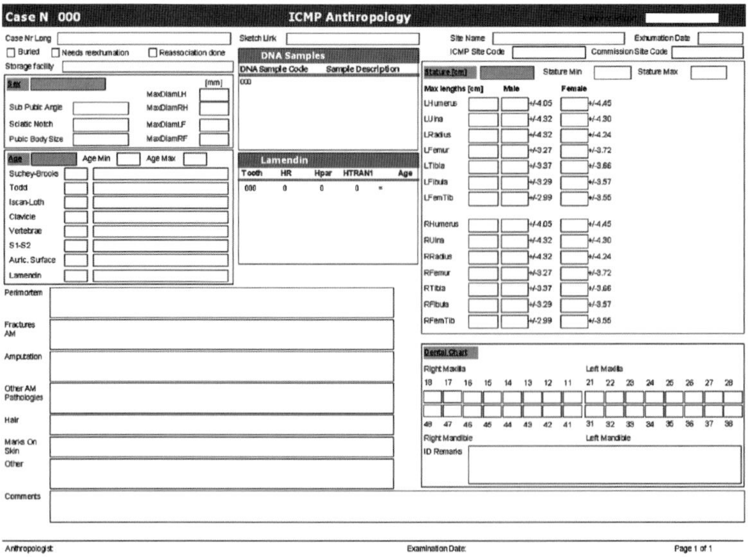
Case N 000
ICMP Anthropology
Case Nr Long
Sketch Link
Site Name
Exhumation Date
Buried
Needs reexhumation
Reassociation done
ICMP Site Code
Commission Site Code
Storage facility
DNA Samples
DNA Sample Code
Sample Description
000
Sex
[mm]
MaxDiamLH
Sub Pubic Angle
MaxDiamRH
Sciatic Notch
MaxDiamLF
Pubic Body Size
MaxDiamRF
Age
Age Min
Age Max
Suchey-Brooks
Todd
Iscan-Loth
Clavicle
Vertebrae
S1-S2
Auric. Surface
Lamendin
Lamendin
Tooth HR Hpar HTRAN1 Age
000 0 0 0 =
Stature [cm]
Stature Min
Stature Max
Max lengths [cm] Male Female
LHumerus +/-4.05 +/-4.45
LUlna +/-4.32 +/-4.30
LRadius +/-4.32 +/-4.24
LFemur +/-3.27 +/-3.72
LTibia +/-3.37 +/-3.66
LFibula +/-3.29 +/-3.57
LFemTib +/-2.99 +/-3.55
RHumerus +/-4.05 +/-4.45
RUlna +/-4.32 +/-4.30
RRadius +/-4.32 +/-4.24
RFemur +/-3.27 +/-3.72
RTibia +/-3.37 +/-3.66
RFibula +/-3.29 +/-3.57
RFemTib +/-2.99 +/-3.55
Perimortem
Fractures AM
Amputation
Other AM Pathologies
Hair
Marks On Skin
Other
Dental Chart
Right Maxilla
Left Maxilla
18 17 16 15 14 13 12 11 21 22 23 24 25 26 27 28
48 47 46 45 44 43 42 41 31 32 33 34 35 36 37 38
Right Mandible
Left Mandible
ID Remarks
Comments
Anthropologist:
Examination Date:
Page 1 of 1

Fig. 14.4 The anthropology report produced by the ICMP Anthropology Database for use in the antemortem-postmortem comparison consuming and, regardless of how accurate the estimates are in this system, they will never be individualizing.

All of the data collected during the anthropological examination are recorded in a database that was designed by ICMP for this purpose (Fig. 14.4). This database ensures that all of the data are collected in a methodical manner and that all analyses are done using the same facts; additionally, the information collected is available to be shared among all parties involved in the identification. A detailed graphical inventory of the skeletal assemblage is also recorded; not only is it used to facilitate reassociation, but it also aids in explaining the condition and completeness of the remains to family members of the missing.

Essential Uses of Classical Methods

In identifying the victims from Srebrenica, there are a number of instances in which traditional methods of identification, including anthropology, are a useful and indispensable part of the identification process: distinguishing between childless siblings (in all such cases, they have been brothers), resolving commingling in a small population, and verifying a DNA match or reassociation.

Because the DNA matches are based on relatives rather than extant samples of the individual's own DNA, they are half-band matches. This means that two or more relatives are needed to provide a match, the best being parents and/or children, as at each locus one allele from each parent or child will be present in the profile of the missing person. In cases where a family is missing two or more brothers who do not have children of their own, this becomes a problem, as it is impossible to determine from the DNA which brother a profile belongs to. Except for identical twins, brothers have different DNA profiles; however, the specific alleles are equally likely to be inherited by each brother, and so their remains can be differentiated only by traditional methods.

The methods used to distinguish between two or more brothers include a biological profile, recognition of clothing and/or personal effects, and circumstantial evidence such as place of disappearance in relation to subsequent exhumation. Most of the sets of childless brothers tend to be quite young, frequently with both of them in their teens or early 20s. This means that the patterns of epiphyseal union can usually be used to determine which is older, even with the amount of interpersonal variation and overlapping age ranges, by examining the remains of all missing brothers together. Unfortunately, older brothers who were close in age are almost impossible to differentiate by age-at-death indicators, and so the other elements of the biological profile become more important, such as status of dentition and antemortem fractures. Accurate and reliable antemortem data from the family on biological characteristics and other information, such as last-worn clothing, personal effects, and place of disappearance, are essential at this stage in the process. With identical twins, even if they have children, there is no way to differentiate between them using DNA, and so the only possibility for clear identification is using these other methods.

It is also possible for an experienced anthropologist to at least partially resolve commingling in a small mixed set of remains; for example, when a few individuals were killed and buried in the same location in a small mass grave, or when it was impossible in the field to separate the cases into discrete bodies and they were collected together. In a case where two or three individuals of varying age and/or size are commingled, pairing antimeres and fitting articulations will resolve the remains into distinct upper and lower bodies, often including many of the smaller and more numerous elements (ribs, vertebrae, feet, and possibly hands).

With a larger number of individuals, it is usually straightforward to group bones by antimeres and articulations, and it is occasionally feasible to separate the outliers, such as the largest, smallest, oldest, youngest, most robust, and most gracile individuals. This not only ensures that each case is as complete as possible, but it also significantly reduces the number of bones that need to be sampled for DNA, from potentially one sample for each pair of long bones and skull, to only one or two samples for each body.

It is not now and may never be possible or feasible to test every single element for identity, and until it is, the expertise of an anthropologist who can associate as many elements as he or she can is invaluable in reducing the cost of DNA analysis and ensuring the return of the correct and most complete remains possible to the victims' families.

Perhaps the most important role the anthropologist plays in a DNA-led system of identification is in the final steps of the official identification. The foremost task is to provide a final check that the individual whose remains belong to a case is actually representative of the individual named on the DNA matching report for that case. Essentially, only the single element that was sampled for DNA can be said to belong unconditionally to the named individual; however, in most cases, the sampled element is associated either with a complete body or with a body part. An experienced anthropologist will detect inconsistencies that may not be noticed by a forensic pathologist during the legal autopsy. In addition to providing a report on the biological profile of the remains for use in the antemortem-postmortem comparison, the anthropologist ensures that the skeleton is consistent, that is, all elements appear to come from one individual (for example, age indicators are similar, all elements reflect the same degree of robusticity) and no extraneous bones are present from other individuals.

Verification of DNA-based reassociations, that is, when two or more DNA matching reports are issued for one individual from different cases of remains, is another vital function of the anthropologist. Unfortunately, due to the high degree of commingling in many cases, it is often not possible to confirm by morphology or articulations that the elements belong together; for example, DNA results indicating a cranium and femur belong to the same individual cannot be verified using anthropological methods, except to state consistency. Of almost 1000 DNA-based reassociations in the ICMP database, fewer than 20% could be confidently confirmed by anthropological methods, predominantly pair matches of long bones or articulations

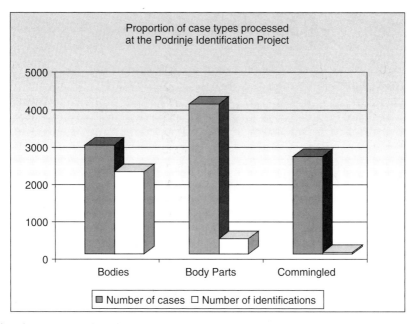

Fig. 14.5 The proportion of bodies (31%) to body parts and commingled cases (42% and 27%) demonstrates how complex the identification process is. As many complete bodies are identified, it becomes more important to be able to confidently identify body parts and sort commingled remains so they may be identified. The categories are based on the case designations assigned during the exhumation

of the vertebral column and/or pelvic girdle. The remainder of the cases represent reassociations of unrelated elements, such as a mandible to a femur, or a humerus to a tibia, which can at most be said to be consistent. Even robust metric techniques do not have the power to validate this type of association to the exclusion of all others among such a large number of missing individuals. It is important that these cases are sorted properly before sampling, however, to ensure that the remains within each case are consistent and belong to the same individual. The importance of a well-designed and thorough DNA sampling strategy cannot be overstated.

Lukavac Re-association Center
Under the umbrella of the Podrinje Identification Project, ICMP established the Lukavac Re-association Center (LKRC) in January 2005 to help overcome the problem of dissociation and commingling of remains in secondary mass graves and to make the process of identification and returning remains to families more efficient. Skeletal remains are put back together at LKRC using a combination of traditional forensic archaeology and anthropology, as well as bone-to-bone DNA matching, which is based on a "mini-amplicon" process. This is less complicated than bone-to-blood matching (used for identification

purposes) as the DNA profiles of different bones of the same individual are identical. This process is extremely important because reassociations using this process could not have been made by way of anthropological analysis alone. The reassociations are of body parts that do not have an anatomical connection (for example, a skull with a leg), and many of the reassociations are from body parts found in separate graves. This innovative approach combining DNA technology and traditional anthropology has proven to be an efficient and effective method in the identification process.

The anthropological data collected during examination can also be used to exclude cases. A biological profile based on anthropological analysis that is significantly different from the antemortem data associated with a DNA link to a missing person is cause to take another DNA sample, as commingling is usually the cause of the discrepancy.

Even the most experienced team of experts cannot identify thousands of individual victims when there are so many with similar biological profiles and so little reliable antemortem information. The persons missing as a result of the fall of Srebrenica in July 1995 would never be identified without the large-scale population-based DNA program that ICMP uses in the Balkans. However, it is a mistake to believe that a DNA profile is the only result that is required to complete an identification. Traditional methods of identification, including anthropology, are not only

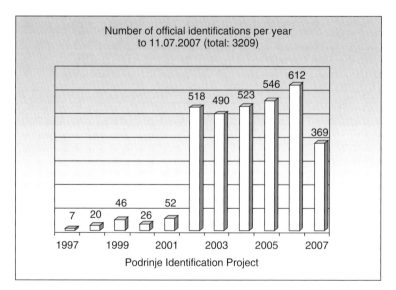

Fig. 14.6 Since the first blind DNA match on November 16, 2001, the Podrinje Identification Project has completed about 500 identifications of the victims from Srebrenica per year. The total for 2007 represents January to July.

useful but also often essential in producing confident and accurate positive identifications. Regardless of how efficient or careful a single line of evidence is, having
a redundant complementary system is the gold standard for high confidence in the
overall process.

Acknowledgments The phenomenal success of ICMP would not have been possible without the
hard work and dedication of all ICMP employees, both past and present: in Sarajevo, the Civil
Society Initiatives, the Government Relations Department, and the Forensic Sciences Department;
within the FSD, the DNA Division, the Identification Coordination Division in Tuzla, and the
Excavations and Examinations Division.

There truly would have been nothing to write about without the incredible team at PIP in Tuzla:
project manager Zlatan Šabanović; team leader Nedim Duraković; case managers Enver Mujagić,
Jasmina Kunosić, Emina Kurtalić, and Senad Hasanbegović; criminologist Amir Hasandjiković;
mortuary technicians Zehrudin Saletović, Jasmin Djulović, and Ermin Numanović; and house-
keeper Denijala Lelić.

References Cited

Bass, W. M. 2005 *Human Osteology,* 5th ed. Missouri Archaeological Society, Columbia.
Bennett, K. A. 1993 *A Field Guide for Human Skeletal Identification*, 2nd ed. Charles C. Thomas,
    Springfield, IL.
Brooks, S. and J. M. Suchey 1990 Skeletal age determination based on the os pubis: A comparison
    of the Acsadi-Nemeskeri and Suchey-Brooks methods. *Hum. Evol.* 5(3):227–238.
Bruzek, J. 2002 A method for visual determination of sex, using the human hip bone. *Am. J. Phys.
    Anthropol.* 117(2):157–168.
Buikstra, J. E. and D. H. Ubelaker (editors) 1994 *Standards for Data Collection from Human
    Skeletal Remains, Proceedings of a Seminar at The Field Museum of Natural History (Arkansas
    Archeological Survey Research Series No. 44).* Spiral ed. Arkansas Archeological Survey,
    Fayetteville.
Byrd, J. E. and B. J. Adams 2003 Osteometric sorting of commingled human remains. *J. Forensic
    Sci.* 48(4):717–724.
Donic, D., M. Duric, D. Babic, and D. Popovic 2005 [Reliability of the individual age assessment
    at the time of death based on sternal rib end morphology in Balkan population]. *Vojnosanit
    Pregl.* 62(6):441–446.
Duric, M., Z. Rakocevic, and D. Donic 2005 The reliability of sex determination of skeletons from
    forensic context in the Balkans. *Forensic Sci. Int.* 147(2–3):159–164.
Giles, E. 1964 Sex determination by discriminant function analysis of the mandible. *Am. J. Phys.
    Anthropol.* 22:129–135.
Giles, E. and O. Elliot 1963 Sex determination by discriminant function analysis of crania. *Am. J.
    Phys. Anthropol.* 21:53–68.
Honig, J. W. and N. Both 1997 *Srebrenica: Record of a War Crime*. Penguin Books, New York.
Iscan, M. Y., S. R. Loth, and R. K. Wright 1984a Age estimation from the rib by phase analysis:
    White males. *J. Forensic Sci.* 29(4):1094–1104.
Iscan, M. Y., S. R. Loth, and R. K. Wright 1984b Metamorphosis at the sternal rib end: A new
    method to estimate age at death in white males. *Am. J. Phys. Anthropol.* 65:147–156.
Katz, D. and J. M. Suchey 1986 Age determination of the male os pubis. *Am. J. Phys. Anthropol.*
    69(4):427–435.
Komar, D. 2003 Lessons from Srebrenica: The contributions and limitations of physical anthropol-
    ogy in identifying victims of war crimes. *J. Forensic Sci.* 48(4):713–716.
Lamendin, H., E. Baccino, J. F. Humbert, J. C. Tavernier, R. M. Nossintchouk, and A. Zerilli

1992 A simple technique for age estimation in adult corpses: The two criteria dental method. *J. Forensic Sci.* 37(5):1373–1379.

Lovejoy, C. O., R. S. Meindl, T. R. Pryzbeck, and R. P. Mensforth 1985 Chronological metamorphosis of the auricular surface of the ilium: A new method for the determination of adult skeletal age at death. *Am. J. Phys. Anthropol.* 68(1):15–28.

McKern, T. and T. Stewart 1957 *Skeletal Age Changes in Young American Males*. Technical Report EP-45. Headquarters Quartermaster Research and Development Command, Natick, MA.

Phenice, T. W. 1969 A newly developed visual method of sexing the os pubis. *Am. J. Phys. Anthropol.* 30(2):297–301.

Pietrusewsky, M. 2000 Metric analysis of skeletal remains: Methods and applications. In *Biological Anthropology of the Human Skeleton*, M. A. Katzenberg and S. R. Saunders, eds. Wiley-Liss Inc., New York.

Rohde, D. 1998 *Endgame: The Betrayal and Fall of Srebrenica, Europe's Worst Massacre Since World War II*. Westview Press, Boulder, CO.

Ross, A. H. and L. W. Konigsberg 2002 New formulae for estimating stature in the Balkans. *J. Forensic Sci.* 47(1):165–167.

Schaefer, M. C. and S. M. Black 2005 Comparison of ages of epiphyseal union in North American and Bosnian skeletal material. *J. Forensic Sci.* 50(4):777–784.

Scheuer, L. and S. Black 2000 *Developmental Juvenile Osteology*. Academic Press, San Diego.

Skinner, M. F., H. P. York, and M. A. Connor 2002 Postburial disturbance of graves in Bosnia-Herzegovina. In *Advances in Forensic Taphonomy: Method, Theory, and Archaeological Perspectives*, W. D. Haglund and M. H. Sorg, eds., pp. 293–308. CRC Press, Boca Raton, FL.

Slaus, M., D. Strinovic, J. Skavic, and V. Petrovecki 2003 Discriminant function sexing of fragmentary and complete femora: Standards for contemporary Croatia. *J. Forensic Sci.* 48(3):509–512.

Todd, T. W. 1920 Age changes in the pubic bone I. The male White pubis. *Am. J. Phys. Anthropol.* 3(3):285–334.

Trotter, M. and G. C. Gleser 1952 Estimation of stature from long bones of American whites and Negroes. *Am. J. Phys. Anthropol.* 10:463–514.

Chapter 15
Marrying Anthropology and DNA: Essential for Solving Complex Commingling Problems in Cases of Extreme Fragmentation

Amy Z. Mundorff, Robert Shaler, Erik Bieschke, and Elaine Mar-Cash

Introduction

On September 11, 2001, 10 terrorists using two planes attacked the World Trade Center (WTC) in New York City. Although this is often thought of as one large event, it was actually four separate disasters (two aircraft crashes and two building collapses) that occurred almost simultaneously and in the same general location. The destruction left 2,749 people dead and more than 20,000 individual pieces of human remains. Jurisdiction fell to the City of New York, and it became the job of the Office of Chief Medical Examiner (OCME) to identify the remains. As might be expected with a disaster of this scale and with such extensive body fragmentation, the identification process was (and is to this day) an extremely complicated endeavor. The goal of this chapter is to highlight some of the challenges and to point out the integral role that both anthropology and DNA played in the process.

This chapter will proceed in two sections. The first section will provide an historical overview of the identification process used to identify victims' remains from the WTC disaster. This was an evolving process that adjusted over time as new techniques were developed to address novel challenges. It focuses on the increasingly complex techniques used to extract DNA, as well as the processes implemented to address identification discrepancies. Specifically, it will discuss the development of a "special projects group" to work on the more complex cases, and the Final Anthropological Review (FAR) program, which was implemented for quality control purposes. The procedures for both the special projects group and FAR highlight the importance of interdisciplinary collaboration in troubleshooting problem cases in any sizable mass fatality incident.

The second section will provide a series of case examples illustrating some mistakes encountered with the identification of WTC victims and how the problems were resolved. Overall, the work of the OCME and ancillary agencies involved in the identifications has been the highest possible quality, given the current restrictions of the technology. Indeed, as will be discussed below, the science of DNA identification was pushed forward by the efforts and expertise of those working on this project. Also, the OCME has embraced an admirable policy of transparency, allowing both successes and setbacks to be discussed openly in a variety of scientific venues. The overriding purpose of this chapter is to provide future practitioners and

From: *Recovery, Analysis, and Identification of Commingled Human Remains*
Edited by: B. Adams and J. Byrd © Humana Press, Totowa, NJ

policy makers a means of learning from the adaptations made over the course of the WTC identification project as they plan and implement programs in response to future events.

Part I: Overview of WTC Identification Process

Victim identification from mass fatality incidents (MFIs) is usually performed by teams of specialists including forensic odontologists, fingerprint examiners, forensic pathologists, and forensic anthropologists. However, since the early 1990s, DNA has become an increasingly common means of identification for mass fatality victims, especially when traditional methods such as fingerprint and dental have been exhausted (Ballantyne 1997; Clayton et al. 1995; Corach et al. 1995; Fernando and Vanezis 1998; Goodwin et al. 1999; Hsu et al. 1999; Kahana and Hiss 1997; Leclair et al. 2004; Ludes et al. 1994; Olaisen et al. 1997). As DNA technology has evolved, its role in the identification of human remains from mass disasters has grown. For example, in the1996 crash of ValuJet Flight 592, the degree of fragmentation as well as logistical and technical limitations were considered to preclude the use of DNA in the identification process (Mittleman et al. 2000). However, just a few years later, DNA was the sole means of identification for the 155 victims of the 2000 Kaprun cable car fire in Austria (Meyer 2003). In the aftermath of events such as the crash of American Airlines Flight 587 in 2001, the Indonesia Tsunami disaster in 2004, and Hurricane Katrina in 2005, DNA has played a primary role in victim identification.

For the WTC disaster in New York City, there was a mayoral mandate to identify as many of the 20,000 remains as possible. This propelled DNA analysis to the center of the WTC identification process. Ultimately, DNA analysis was responsible for identifying the majority of the WTC remains. In fact, of the nearly 11,000 fragments that have been identified to date, over 9,800, or 90%, have been identified using DNA alone. And of the 1,598 victims who have been identified to date, 853 have been identified solely by their DNA. Without DNA technology, more than half of the identified victims would not have been identified.

The Role of DNA in WTC Identifications

Because of the many unique challenges of the WTC disaster, the role played by DNA became even more pronounced while the role of more traditional victim identification methods was comparatively limited. For example, the explosive force of the falling buildings extensively fragmented remains, limiting the application of fingerprint and dental identification, as these methods can only be employed to identify remains that retain either fingers or dentition. With an average victims-to-remains ratio encountered in the WTC disaster (1:7), based on 10,933 identified fragments and 1,598 identified victims, only a small proportion of those remains possess identifying characteristics such as fingers or dentition. With the vast majority of the remains lacking such identifying characteristics, DNA became an essential tool in the victims identification effort. The value of DNA analysis in mass disasters, such as the events of September 11, 2001, results from its ability to identify fragments of human tissue and bone, regardless of the body part recovered or the size of the fragment. DNA identifications were achieved by comparing unknown remains to known references. For example, personal items taken from or used by the missing person, such as stored blood, a toothbrush, or a razorblade, could be used as direct comparison references for victim remains. Concurrently, specimens such as buccal swabs from biological relatives were used to construct kinship pedigrees to compare with victim remains.

Successful DNA analysis also requires a usable sample from the remains. This became increasingly problematic as the WTC remains began showing signs of extensive decomposition caused by the prolonged recovery process and by thermal conditions associated with "hot spots" at the recovery site (Arismendi et al. 2004; Burger et al. 1999; Holland et al. 2003; Imaizumi et al. 2004). As time passed, the likelihood of obtaining intact and usable DNA from soft tissue faded, and those conducting the identifications began to see a growing possibility that DNA degradation might limit identification capabilities, leaving hundreds of individuals unidentified. Struggling to keep pace with the evolving conditions, DNA scientists conducted the process of victim identification in what can now be identified as a series of distinct but overlapping phases.

Phase I utilized standardized DNA tests commonly employed by forensic laboratories throughout the world. During this phase, STR (short tandem repeat) analysis was employed and, minimally, the 13 original loci used in CODIS (Combined DNA Index System) were analyzed. This technology was a logical approach for analyzing the WTC remains because it had been extensively validated and represented a non-controversial choice for analyzing samples that had been exposed to environmental insults. After only three weeks of testing, however, it was clear that a significant percent of the remains were giving either partial profiles (33%) or no profiles (28%) at all. At the conclusion of Phase I testing, nearly 60% of the remains were yielding poor DNA results that were not adequate for meeting the requirement for matching and identification.

While a significant percentage of remains did not yield DNA, 33% yielded partial profiles; in other words, while not sufficiently robust to satisfy STR identification protocols, nearly one-third of the cases provided usable DNA for the purposes of identification. In response, analysts devised strategies for extracting additional genetic information from the compromised remains. Phase II involved reexamination of the original samples and additional research aimed at increasing the yield of analyzable DNA. This effort was successful, as soft tissue and bones originally yielding only partial profiles now yielded either full profiles or partial profiles with additional loci being observed. However, even following this process, some remains still did not yield a sufficient amount of usable DNA for valid identifications. This necessitated another testing strategy, which began Phase III of the victim identification effort.

Phase III began in November 2001 after it became clear that these partial DNA profiles would fall short of the threshold of statistical robustness established for identifications. Three DNA techniques previously unused in the WTC identification process were applied. First, building on a technique that was being developed prior to 9/11, a mini-STR test panel was created. Initially, a study was started with John Butler at NIST (National Institute of Standards and Technology) to investigate using mini-STR analysis for the WTC samples. This study culminated with the development of a mini-STR test panel by Bode Technology Group, which was used successfully on thousands of remains. Second, mitochondrial DNA sequencing for thousands of remains and reference samples was performed. Third, a 70-loci SNPs (single nucleotide polymorphisms) panel was established and used for testing thousands of remains and reference samples. Each of these approaches supplemented traditional STR analysis, leading to new identifications that would not have been possible otherwise.

Additional Challenges to the DNA Identification Effort

In addition to ongoing concerns regarding degraded DNA samples, other issues that could compromise identification efforts continually surfaced, such as commingling and DNA contamination. Anthropologists and DNA analysts collaborated to address these problems at all stages of the victim identification effort. The first few days following many mass fatality incidents have been characterized by overwhelming chaos (Biesecker et al. 2005; Fernando and Vanezis 1998; Moody and Busuttil 1994). Because of the confusion and bureaucracy surrounding a mass fatality incident, mistakes are most likely to occur during the first few days of processing, although they may go unnoticed for days or weeks. However, these mistakes can have a significant impact on the overall identification effort. In order to detect and address these mistakes during the WTC victim identification effort, DNA analysts and anthropologists collaborated to focus on quality control measures throughout the identification project (Budimlija et al. 2003).

In the DNA laboratory, a "special projects group" was formed to handle various sample processing issues, including commingling, contamination, as well as other "questionable identifications" resulting from these core problems (Budimlija et al. 2003). Also within the DNA laboratory, a "WTC data analysis group" was already in place to bridge the gap between anthropologists and the "special projects group" in detecting and troubleshooting these core problems. In general, these problem cases were revealed by illogical DNA test results, such as two left feet identified to the same individual. The most frequent causes for these types of errors were DNA contamination or transcription mistakes. Once a problem case had been identified, the DNA laboratory along with the anthropologist and a medicolegal investigator (MLI) reviewed the case file and examined the remains, often resampling for new DNA analysis. This cooperative effort among DNA analysts, anthropologists, and MLIs resolved numerous errors, such as mislabeling and sampling problems in the mortuary, DNA contamination, lab contamination, transcription errors, data entry mistakes, and also problems with early antemortem sample collection. Many of the problems the special projects group addressed were initially revealed during a quality control procedure called the Final Anthropological Review (FAR) process. FAR was designed in May 2002 in response to a single case in which commingling had been discovered after the remains had been identified, but prior to their release to the funeral home. The purpose of the FAR was to verify and cross-check each fragment of identified human remains prior to approving its release.

Final Anthropological Review

By early April 2002, the use of traditional identification methods, such as fingerprint and dental matching, began to slow. It became clear that the majority of identifications would come through DNA. No identification project to date had attempted to identify so many fragments by DNA alone, and DNA provided the ability to potentially link dozens of pieces of human remains to a single individual (Biesecker et al. 2005). As the pace of DNA identifications began to increase, it became apparent that contamination and commingling had occurred in some of the samples. Additionally, mistakes made during the initial collection of antemortem information from families complicated the identification process. At the family assistance center, the New York Police Department (NYPD) collected personal reference and kinship samples and interviewed victim's families to collect data for the "VIP" victim information forms. These forms recorded antemortem information about the victim that could later be used to assist identifications. Hundreds of federal temporary workers from the Disaster Mortuary Operational Response Teams (DMORT) performed the data entry for thousands of these VIP forms. Unfortunately, one-sixth of the initial information collected had to be corrected because of missing data, incorrectly recorded data, improper kinship sampling, or data entry errors (Biesecker et al. 2005; Cash et al. 2003). These challenges, along with others that occurred during the mortuary and laboratory stages, led to inevitable identification problems. Discovering and rectifying these problems became the main focus of both the DNA laboratory and the Final Anthropological Review.

At the height of the identification efforts, the OCME identified dozens of victims per day using DNA, and many of these individual identifications involved numerous small fragments. Every identification was finalized according to an established routine. First, the DNA lab matched a reference or kinship pedigree to human remains and sent this "DNA match report" to the identification unit. Then, two medicolegal investigators further investigated the case information, checking, among other information, if any remains had been previously identified to the victim or if this was a new identification. They were also responsible for verifying all of the data in the case file, including the victim's antemortem information. In the early months of the recovery and identification effort, the process simply stopped at this point and the identified remains were released to the family. However, in order to catch the potential errors, policy makers determined that the process should include a final measure of quality control; thus, the Final Anthropological Review was added just prior to releasing remains to funeral homes.

The medicolegal investigator and the anthropologist developed a new form for the FAR procedure that included specific information pertinent to a final verification of the remains. This information included the case number, the name of the attending medical examiner, the date of recovery, a brief description of the remains and what was sampled for DNA (bone, muscle, tooth, etc.), the date of identification, and the means of identification. If identified fragments were linked to a previously identified individual, this information was also included on the form. The form also indicated whether or not the previously identified fragments were still curated at the OCME and could be reexamined, or if they had already been released to a funeral home. Every time a new piece or aggregate of pieces was identified, this form was filled out by the medicolegal investigator reviewing the new DNA match.

After the form had been generated, it was then reviewed by the anthropologist to identify any inconsistencies that could indicate a problem with the identification. Potential problems were then flagged on the FAR form before the final examination of the remains. Take, for example, the circumstances in the following hypothetical case. First, the individual in question has already been successfully identified through several pieces of remains, including a partial right foot. Next, a new fragment is linked to that same individual and the paperwork indicates that this new piece is also a partial foot, but the report lacks detailed information indicating which foot, right or left. Under these circumstances, the paperwork would be flagged so that during final examination, the anthropologist could determine if this new piece was an additional fragment of the previously identified right foot, if it was a left foot fragment, or if this was a duplicate body part (the same anatomical elements as the previously identified right foot), indicating a problem with the identification.

Once the paperwork had been reviewed and potential problem cases flagged, the anthropologist reexamined the human remains. Both the newly identified pieces as well as the previously identified pieces that were still curated at the OCME went through a final examination. In cases where fragments had previously been identified and released to funeral homes, the anthropologist relied on the information from the original case file recorded on the FAR form and photographs. During the final examination, the anthropologist initially confirmed that the case number on the outside of the body bag matched the case number and remains inside the bag. Once this information was confirmed, the anthropologist then looked for inconsistencies between the physical remains and the paperwork, duplicated elements, or other discrepancies. This included confirming that the biological profile of the victim matched the remains. If the victim identified was a female, did the remains appear to be from a female of the same approximate age? If there were any disagreements between the documentation and the remains being evaluated, duplication of body parts, conflict between the biological profiles, or any other questions regarding the validity of the identification, the identification was placed on hold. The problems would be investigated by the special projects group, the WTC data analysis group, and an anthropologist until the issue was rectified. Often this investigation included an examination of the chain of custody and antemortem information collected to establish the identification, review of the postmortem information on the remains, and possibly resampling and retesting DNA. Taken as a whole, these quality control measures revealed overwhelming accuracy within the system and very few problems were found.

Part II: WTC Case Examples

Defining Case

This example is paradigmatic of all issues faced in subsequent problem cases and illustrates the importance of a holistic approach to troubleshooting identifications. It is also the case that alerted OCME staff to the need for more rigorous quality control procedures before final release of remains and that led to significant procedural changes, specifically the implementation of the Final Anthropological Review process. The discussion of this paradigmatic case will be followed by a series of short case examples demonstrating the multidisciplinary teamwork among DNA specialists, medicolegal investigators, and anthropologists in detecting and solving complex commingling and contamination problems, transcription and data entry mistakes, and antemortem collection errors from the WTC disaster identification project.

After a disaster such as WTC, the decision regarding when to have a funeral and bury the remains can be wrenching. Families had been informed that because of the extreme fragmentation and the on-going identification process, it was likely that victim remains would continue to be identified days, weeks, months, or even years later. Many were forced into a waiting game as they balanced the desire for a speedy funeral against the desire to lay to rest as much of the decedent's remains as possible. Often, families waited until a "significant amount" of remains had been identified before deciding to claim a loved one's remains. Therefore, it was not uncommon that, upon being notified of an identification, families would request that OCME personnel provide them with an estimate of the percentage of identified remains from that victim.

In May 2002, the OCME notified a family that their missing family member's remains had been identified. In this particular case, the forensic anthropologist examined the remains in collaboration with a medicolegal investigator, at the family's request, to determine the percentage of identified remains. The victim's remains had been excavated from Ground Zero fairly early in the recovery process and were stored in a refrigerated unit for months pending identification. The remains consisted of two major portions: the top portion of a torso down to the fourth lumbar vertebra, and the lower portion of a torso, from the sacrum down. There was no fifth lumbar, which could have articulated the two halves together. At the time, it was not clear whether or not these two portions had been previously articulated by skin or soft tissue and had become disarticulated over time due to decomposition, or whether they had never been physically attached but were grouped together because they were assumed to be from the same individual at the time of recovery. It was not uncommon for two disparate portions of remains to be held together by skin only. For example, although a portion of hip might be attached to a foot by skin, all of the connecting leg bones and other soft tissue in between might be absent. In this case, the original medical examiner's notes stated that the body was in two separate portions (both of which were sampled for DNA) but made no mention of whether or not the remains were connected by skin or soft tissue. Of the two DNA samples, one was used to identify the remains, while the other sample failed to yield viable DNA.

During the interim between the time this body was recovered and the time it was identified, mortuary personnel had learned a great deal about the extent of the devastation at the disaster site. Complicated excavation procedures at Ground Zero combined with enormous fragmentation of the human remains produced far more commingling than had been initially recognized (Mundorff 2003). In response, more rigorous triage standards and examination techniques had been introduced after the first few weeks of recovery. However, this body had been processed through the mortuary during the earliest stages and was not subjected to these more rigorous standards (MacKinnon and Mundorff 2006). The secondary examination revealed that these two pieces were not (or were no longer) attached by tissue, and possibly would not have been grouped together under the more rigorous triage and exam standards. The anthropologist and the medicolegal investigator recommended that the identification be placed on hold until both body portions had been retested for DNA.

Subsequent DNA analysis confirmed the identification on the top portion of the torso but also revealed that the bottom portion belonged to a previously unidentified individual. As a result of this inquiry, new quality control measures were implemented, which included an additional examination of the identified remains prior to family notification and release (MacKinnon and Mundorff 2006). The Final Anthropological Review became a critical quality control measure aimed at identifying mistakes from a variety of sources, many of which were unanticipated when the project began.

Additional Case Examples

This section will highlight WTC case examples in which various problems with identified fragments were encountered and solved using a multidisciplinary approach between anthropology and DNA. Several of the examples are simple, such as mislabeling, and others involve complex DNA investigations. Often, tracing the root of the problem was more complicated than solving the problem itself. However, understanding how the problems occurred allowed for new protocols to be designed and implemented, avoiding future identification errors.

Example #1: Mislabeling in the Mortuary

When processing over 20,000 cases and their corresponding DNA samples, there is a likelihood of labeling errors. Two bone and two tissue samples were submitted to the DNA laboratory from the mortuary labeled with the case number 30776. The two bones were tested and yielded DNA profiles matching two different individuals. The tissue samples had not yet been tested. Based upon the conflicting DNA results from the bones, all four samples were tested as part of the DNA investigation. A sample audit was performed in parallel, and it was determined that case number 30777 (the next consecutive number) did not have any DNA sample submitted. As a result, a bone sample from 30777 was taken independently of the DNA investigation. DNA results confirmed that the four samples originally labeled as case 30776 originated from two different individuals, one of which matched the DNA results from the recently sampled case 30777. Since case numbers were assigned consecutively in the mortuary, it was theorized that two of the four samples submitted as case number 30776 actually belonged to the next case, 30777, and the wrong bar code label was affixed during examination. The curated remains for cases 30776 and 30777, as well as their corresponding DNA samples from the lab, were pulled from storage and inspected by the anthropologist and a DNA analyst. One of the DNA bone samples labeled as 30776 could be conjoined with the case labeled 30777, confirming that this sample had been mislabeled as 30776 in the mortuary.

Example #2: Clerical Error in Case File

A partial body had been identified by dental comparison. The mortuary paperwork for this partial body indicated that there was a left arm, including the hand, present. Months later, DNA matched a left hand to that same individual. While assessing the final anthropological review form, it was obvious that a left hand was being linked by DNA to an individual who apparently already had a left hand attached to a previously identified partial body. However, the body had already been released, so there was no way to confirm that the hand attached to the body was indeed a left and not mistakenly a right. It was not uncommon to encounter right/left mix-ups on the paperwork from examination, and it was also not uncommon to encounter data entry errors where the form stated "right," but "left" was entered into the database. Anthropology confirmed during reexamination that the newly matched hand was left (and not mistakenly a right) and the DNA match was solid. However, during the reanalysis of the paperwork in the case file from the original partial body identification, a note was discovered from the police officer responsible for fingerprinting the "left" hand attached to the body. The note indicated that the hand was actually a right, not a left as previously described by the medical examiner. However, this information was not picked up during data entry, and therefore the information was never corrected in the database to illustrate that the hand attached to the original body was actually a right. Consequently, the newly matched left hand was not a duplicate part, as it originally appeared, but merely a clerical error that was eventually sorted out during the review process.

Example #3: DNA Sample Contamination

A DNA report was sent to the medicolegal investigators indicating that three fragments had been identified to the same individual. During the FAR documentation review, it was noted that all three newly matched fragments were humeri and, specifically, two were described as proximal left while the third fragment was the shaft from the right side. The two proximal left fragments could have both been small fragments of different portions from the same bone or they could have been duplicate body parts; only a visual inspection of the remains could clarify this. The reexamination would also ensure there was not a transcription error, for example, recording "left" for "right" or a "distal" for "proximal." However, this was not the case. In fact, upon examination, based on the fragment's size, it was apparent that the three humeri fragments were from at least two different individuals (Fig. 15.1). Additionally, there were indeed two overlapping proximal left fragments. One of the proximal fragments was robust, possibly indicating male, while the other appeared gracile, possibly indicating female. All three cases were placed on hold until a resampling strategy was devised.

The DNA analyst responsible for quality assurance was concurrently investigating the possibility of contamination during the high-throughput DNA testing process. Due to the extreme fragmentation of the remains, it was common for multiple remains to be linked by DNA to the same individual. In fact, many victims had dozens of fragments identified to them, with one individual having 176 fragments. During this investigation, a pattern was noticed. Samples in the same well position, in sequentially numbered or processed trays, were giving the same DNA profiles (for example: Tray 1 position A4 and tray 2 position A4 yielded the same profile). Many of these remains on the affected trays gave conflicting results when compared to other samples from the same case number. Laboratory procedures were

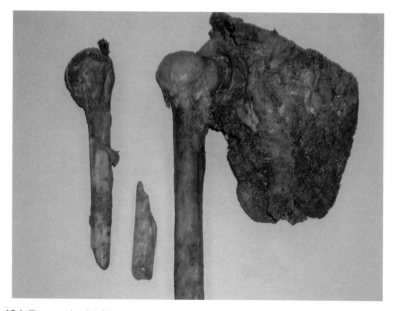

Fig. 15.1 Two proximal left humerii and right humeral fragment (*Source*: Office of Chief Medial Examiner, New York City.)

reviewed, and it was concluded that a robotic pipetting instrument was the cause of the contamination. Insufficient washing of the pipette tips between processing of trays led to sample transfer from one tray to the next. A common characteristic of this phenomenon was high amounts of DNA in the donor tray and a lower amount of the same DNA in the recipient tray.

Once this systematic error was detected, the DNA quality assurance analyst collaborated with a representative from the vendor laboratory in order to resolve the issue. The first step taken in the corrective action was to remove the pipetting robot from the sample processing flow and replace it with a disposable tip system. The second measure taken was to perform a thorough examination of the existing data in search of potentially affected samples. Samples that were deemed to be affected were retested. After subsequent retesting, a determination was made as to the reliability of the original results. Also, DNA profiles that were proven unreliable were invalidated and therefore no longer used for comparison. However, not all potentially affected samples were detected during the DNA investigation; several cases were instead detected during the FAR process such as the previous example presented. Based upon the recommendations of the anthropologist, all three humeri were retested. DNA results confirmed that two of the fragments were consistent with their original results while the third fragment originated from a different individual.

Example #4: DNA Sample Contamination

The mistake in the previous example was noted prior to a visual examination of the actual remains, specifically because the information in the paperwork conflicted. In that case, there were two proximal left humeri fragments. The next example illustrates a similar problem; however, the mistake could not have been seen simply by looking at the paperwork, as the case descriptions did not conflict with each other or any other identified remains. This problem could only be detected by looking at the remains themselves. Two fragments were matched to one individual by DNA. The documentation review of these two fragments made sense—one was a distal right femur and the other was a distal left femur. There was no overlap between these elements, and the victim had not previously had any distal femora identified. However, when the fragments were visually examined, it was noted that, morphologically, these two pieces were very different from each other; one was very large and the other was very small (Fig. 15.2). Hence, there was little possibility that they belonged to the same individual. The two pieces in question were placed on hold and both resampled. Results from the DNA retesting confirmed that the two cases originated from two different individuals. As the original DNA results were investigated further, it was determined that the mistake also resulted from the systematic robotic pipetting error described in the previous example. By only reviewing the documentation and not having looked at the remains, this mistake would not have been discovered, because the identification made sense on paper.

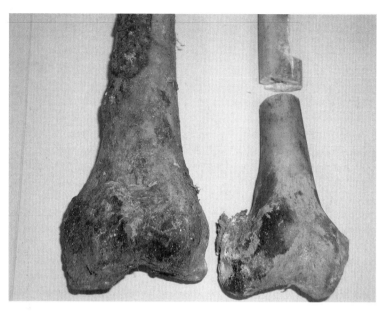

Fig. 15.2 Right and left distal femora (*Source*: Office of Chief Medical Examiner, New York City.)

Example #5: DNA Case Number Mix-up

Two innominate fragments, case numbers 30709 and 85571, were identified by DNA as belonging to the same individual. Both were innominate fragments, specifically recorded as ilium with a significant amount of adhering soft tissue. Because both pieces were listed only as "fragment of ilium" in their case files, they were flagged during the documentation review, indicating a need to ensure the fragments did not overlap. It was not uncommon for case descriptions to lack specifics such as right/left. Over 30 anthropologists from around the United States rotated through the OCME during the processing of remains from WTC. Proficiency levels, especially when it came to experience with decomposed soft tissue obscuring bony landmarks, varied greatly. Therefore, while these pieces may have been easily recognized as ilium fragments, other specifics such as side may have been more challenging for the individual first examining the remains. The final examination revealed that the pieces overlapped; therefore, both cases were placed on hold and resampled (Fig. 15.3). Retesting results for case 30709 confirmed the original data; however, case 85571 results matched a different individual. In general, two separate reactions had to be performed to obtain a full STR DNA profile. The first reaction in the original test result for case 85571 yielded no DNA profile; however, the second reaction yielded the maximum result. This combination of data is unusual, as an analyst would expect to see consistent results from one reaction to the next. In conjunction with the DNA results, a review of the chain of custody led the DNA analysts to theorize that case 85571 had been mixed up with case 8571. Case 8571 matched the original, and the retest results for case 30709 and case 85571 were indeed from a different individual.

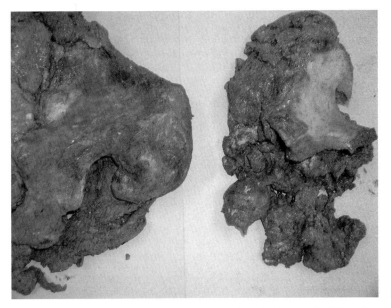

Fig. 15.3 Overlapping innominate fragments (*Source*: Office of Chief Medical Examiner, New York City.)

Example #6: Element Siding Mistake During Examination

Two separate right hands were recovered in February 2002, five months into the recovery process. When they arrived at the Medical Examiner's Office, both cases were fragmentary and in an advanced state of decomposition. Months later, both right hands were linked by DNA to the same individual. This was immediately flagged during the documentation review portion of the FAR. Reexamination proved that one of the hands was actually a left, and so no additional DNA testing was warranted. This mistake could have happened at a few different points in the process, but it is impossible to pinpoint when it occurred. There may have been a communication problem between the examiner and their scribe; this may also have been a transcription error in which case the scribe wrote one thing when he meant to write another; or similar to the previous case, the decomposition and fragmentation could have been so extensive that it was not clear to the examiner processing the case whether the hand was right or left. However, adding in a final verification of the remains can ensure one last level of assurance before identification.

Example #7: DNA Sample Switch

During the Final Anthropological Review, it was discovered that a left distal femur (case number 308230) was matched by DNA to an individual who had already been identified by multiple remains, including a left distal femur (case number 308232). Because of the duplicate body part, the anthropologist initiated an investigation.

During the course of this investigation, the DNA results and the sample handling process were evaluated and it was hypothesized that a sample switch had occurred between these two cases. Case 308232 had already been retested and had confirmed the initial results. Case 308230 was resampled and subsequently matched a different individual. Thus, the new DNA results confirmed the hypothesis of sample mix-up that was noted during the final anthropological review because of duplicate elements.

Conclusion

In summary, because of its scope and complex characteristics, ongoing interdisciplinary collaboration proved vital in the process of identifying victim remains from the WTC disaster. Through various examples, it has been shown that this collaboration should include those who collect and interpret scientific and nonscientific information at both the antemortem and postmortem levels. This continuing collaboration allowed mistakes to be detected and rectified. It also allowed systems to be adjusted to prevent the same mistakes from being repeated. This dynamic process pushed forward both the science of DNA identification and our understanding of the complexities inherent in managing the identification process in a disaster of this magnitude.

References Cited

Arismendi, J. L., L. E. Baker, and K. J. Matteson 2004 Effects of processing techniques on the forensic DNA analysis of human skeletal remains. *J. Forensic Sci.* 49(5):930–934.

Ballantyne, J. 1997 Mass disaster genetics. *Nat. Genet.* 15(4):329–331.

Biesecker, L. G., J. E. Bailey-Wilson, J. Ballantyne, H. Baum, F. R. Bieber, C. Brenner, B. Budowle, J. M. Butler, G. Carmody, P. M. Conneally, B. Duceman, A. Eisenberg, L. Forman, K. K. Kidd, B. Leclair, S. Niezgoda, T. J. Parsons, E. Pugh, R. Shaler, S. T. Sherry, A. Sozer, and A. Walsh 2005 Epidemiology. DNA identifications after the 9/11 World Trade Center attack. *Science* 310(5751):1122–1123.

Budimlija, Z. M., M. K. Prinz, A. Zelson-Mundorff, J. Wiersema, E. Bartelink, G. MacKinnon, B. L. Nazzaruolo, S. M. Estacio, M. J. Hennessey, and R. C. Shaler 2003 World Trade Center human identification project: Experiences with individual body identification cases. *Croat. Med. J.* 44(3):259–263.

Burger, J., S. Hummel, B. Hermann, and W. Henke 1999 DNA preservation: A microsatellite-DNA study on ancient skeletal remains. *Electrophoresis* 20(8):1722–1728.

Cash, H. D., J. W. Hoyle, and A. J. Sutton 2003 Development under extreme conditions: Forensic bioinformatics in the wake of the World Trade Center disaster. *Pac. Symp. Biocomput.,* pp. 638–653.

Clayton, T. M., J. P. Whitaker, and C. N. Maguire 1995 Identification of bodies from the scene of a mass disaster using DNA amplification of short tandem repeat (STR) loci. *Forensic Sci, Int,* 76(1):7–15.

Corach, D., A. Sala, G. Penacino, and A. Sotelo 1995 Mass disasters: Rapid molecular screening of human remains by means of short tandem repeats typing. *Electrophoresis* 16(9): 1617–1623.

Fernando, R. and P. Vanezis 1998 Medicolegal aspects of the Thai Airbus crash near Kathmandu, Nepal: Findings of the investigating pathologists. *Am. J. Forensic Med. Pathol.* 19(2):169–173.

Goodwin, W., A. Linacre, and P. Vanezis 1999 The use of mitochondrial DNA and short tandem repeat typing in the identification of air crash victims. *Electrophoresis* 20(8):1707–1711.

Holland, M. M., C. A. Cave, C. A. Holland, and T. W. Bille 2003 Development of a quality, high-throughput DNA analysis procedure for skeletal samples to assist with the identification of victims from the World Trade Center attacks. *Croat. Med. J.* (44):264–272.

Hsu, C. M., N. E. Huang, L. C. Tsai, L. G. Kao, C. H. Chao, A. Linacre, and J. C. Lee 1999 Identification of victims of the 1998 Taoyuan Airbus crash accident using DNA analysis. *Int. J. Legal Med.* 113(1):43–46.

Imaizumi, K., S. Miyasaka, and M. Yoshino 2004 Quantitative analysis of amplifiable DNA in tissue exposed to various environments using competitive PRC assays. *Sci. Justice* 44:199–208.

Kahana, T. and J. Hiss 1997 Identification of human remains: Forensic radiology. *J. Clin. Forensic Med.* 4(1):7–15.

Leclair, B., C. J. Fregeau, K. L. Bowen, and R. M. Fourney 2004 Enhanced kinship analysis and STR-based DNA typing for human identification in mass fatality incidents: The Swissair Flight 111 disaster. *J. Forensic Sci.* 49(5):939–953.

Ludes, B., A. Tracqui, H. Pfitzinger, P. Kintz, F. Levy, M. Disteldorf, J. M. Hutt, B. Kaess, R. Haag, B. Memheld et al. 1994 Medico-legal investigations of the Airbus A320 crash upon Mount Ste-Odile, France. *J. Forensic Sci.* 39(5):1147–1152.

MacKinnon, G. and A. Z. Mundorff 2006 World Trade Center—September 11th, 2001. In *Forensic Human Identification: An Introduction*, T. J. U. Thompson and S. M. Black, eds., pp. 485–499. CRC Press, Boca Raton, FL.

Meyer, H. J. 2003 The Kaprun cable car fire disaster—Aspects of forensic organisation following a mass fatality with 155 victims. *Forensic Sci. Int.* 138(1–3):1–7.

Mittleman, R. E., J. S. Barnhart, J. H. Davis, R. Fernandez, B. A. Hyman, R. D. Lengel, E. O. Lew, and V. J. Rao 2000 *The Crash of ValuJet Flight 592: A Forensic Approach to Severe Body Fragmentation.* Miami-Dade County Medical Examiner Department.

Moody, G. H. and A. Busuttil 1994 Identification in the Lockerbie air disaster. *Am. J. Forensic Med. Pathol.* 15(1):63–69.

Mundorff, A. Z. 2003 The role of anthropology during the identification of victims from the World Trade center disaster. Paper presented at the American Academy of Forensic Science, Chicago.

Olaisen, B., M. Stenersen, and B. Mevag 1997 Identification by DNA analysis of the victims of the August 1996 Spitsbergen civil aircraft disaster. *Nat. Genet.* 15(4):402–405.

Chapter 16
Sorting and Identifying Commingled Remains of U.S. War Dead: The Collaborative Roles of JPAC and AFDIL

Franklin E. Damann and Suni M. Edson

Introduction

In 1995 the Defense Science Board Task Force was established with the aim of addressing "key issues arising from efforts to identify skeletal remains using new DNA testing technologies" (Lederberg et al. 1995). A report was issued in response to an inquiry regarding identification techniques for the remains of missing soldiers. The authors of that report summarized that DNA technology should continue to be used for identification of ancient remains repatriated to the United States. Mitochondrial DNA (mtDNA) analysis was emphasized as a tool to be used in conjunction with osteological, archaeological, and dental analyses.

This chapter demonstrates how ongoing collaboration among molecular biologists, archaeologists, physical anthropologists, and dentists is vital for achieving individuation from commingled remains. In this effort a combination of specialties is necessary, each controlling and validating the other and ensuring mitigation of potentially erroneous results. To this end, we discuss recent casework that highlights the combined efforts among professional staff at the Joint POW/MIA Accounting Command's Central Identification Laboratory (JPAC-CIL) and the Armed Forces DNA Identification Laboratory (AFDIL). In this combined effort, the identification of once-missing U.S. service members currently averages 100 individuals a year, nearly two persons a week; and over half of these cases involve DNA sequence data generated by AFDIL.

Joint POW-MIA Accounting Command (JPAC)

The JPAC is the agency responsible for recovery and identification of unaccounted-for U.S. service personnel from previous conflicts. Originating during World War II as Central Identification Points that were responsible for the consolidation and identification of war dead throughout Europe, the identification process of U.S. service members has evolved into JPAC. Today the JPAC headquarters and laboratory are located at Hickam Air Force Base, Hawaii. The mission of the JPAC is to search for, recover, and identify remains of U.S. service members associated

From: *Recovery, Analysis, and Identification of Commingled Human Remains*
Edited by: B. Adams and J. Byrd © Humana Press, Totowa, NJ

with World War I, World War II, the Korean War, the Cold War, and the Vietnam War. Excavations are conducted worldwide in order to recover skeletal remains and material evidence, such as dog tags and rank insignia. These items are repatriated to the United States and accessioned into the JPAC-CIL for analysis by the scientific staff, and the findings are reported to the CIL Scientific Director. The majority of the scientific staff are civilian anthropologists (forensic anthropologists and archaeologists). Part of this staff includes a small number of employees responsible for sampling remains for DNA analysis, maintaining communication with AFDIL, and providing external control for associating remains with DNA evidence. Finally, there are forensic odontologists (military dentists) who are responsible for analyzing teeth and for sampling them for DNA when appropriate. The Scientific Director bears the responsibility of compiling all lines of evidence including the results of skeletal, dental, artifact, and DNA analyses in order to make an identification.

Armed Forces DNA Identification Laboratory (AFDIL)

Located in Rockville, Maryland, the AFDIL is attached to the Armed Forces Institute of Pathology and the American Registry of Pathology; it falls under the command of the Armed Forces Medical Examiner System (AFMES). The laboratory was established in 1990 with the primary goal of working with the CIL and the AFMES to identify the remains of U.S. service members using the latest techniques in DNA analysis. There are two main sections of AFDIL performing casework, the Nuclear Section and the Mitochondrial Section. The Nuclear Section is involved with recent death investigations where remains and organic material tend to be well preserved. This section has assisted with the identification of victims from the September 11, 2001, attack on the Pentagon, the U.S. Embassy bombing in Nairobi, Kenya, and NTSB investigations of aircraft crashes including U.S. Airways Flight 427 and American Eagle Flight 4184. The largest section of the AFDIL is the mitochondrial group. This section is devoted to the analysis of mtDNA obtained from remains recovered by JPAC. Remains recovered by JPAC are in an historic context, often in harsh environments, and they are not as well preserved as those typically encountered by the Nuclear Section; thus, the mitochondria have been the standard source of genetic material for JPAC skeletal cases, and last year the AFDIL processed over 800 skeletal and dental samples for the CIL.

Between these two sections at AFDIL, there are three different types of DNA analysis being used in forensic casework. The first originates from the mitochondria, and the other two analyses originate from nuclear DNA. The different analyses include sequencing of the mitochondrial hypervariable regions, nuclear DNA autosomal STR profiling, and non-recombining Y-chromosome STR profiling. Y-chromosome analysis is currently under validation at AFDIL and not yet actively used, although the technology promises to be highly valuable in instances where there are no maternal relatives (e.g., mtDNA references) available. Given the myriad of taphonomic processes that negatively affect preservation of skeletal material, mtDNA has proven to be the most reliable means for obtaining molecular data since there are many more mitochondrial genomes per cell than nuclear genomes. Recent improvements in nuclear DNA analysis such as the introduction of mini-STRs (Coble and Butler 2005) and research into low copy number (LCN) STR analysis, however, are finding a place alongside mtDNA in CIL casework.

MtDNA Sequencing

The circular mitochondrial genome consists of approximately 16,569 base pairs (bp) and is inherited as a single locus through the maternal line with no paternal recombination. There are multiple copies of the mitochondrial genome within each mitochondria and hundreds of copies per cell. The number of mitochondria per cell makes them a good target for difficult samples such as delaminated and friable skeletal samples that are often recovered by the JPAC-CIL.

Within the genome, the region of interest is an approximately 1,100-bp fragment called the control region (CR). This region is treated as a single locus with haplotype variants consisting of unique polymorphisms of point mutations, insertions, and deletions (Torroni et al. 1996, 1998). Within the control region, the two hypervariable regions (HV1 and HV2) are targeted because they tend to be more diagnostic (i.e., have more mutations) than the rest of the mtDNA genome. These regions, along with the rest of the CR, are noncoding and as such are not subject to recombination and natural selection. The remainder of the mitochondrial genome encodes various enzymes, transfer RNA, and ribosomal RNA genes.

In a survey of the samples in the AFDIL population database, 41.1% of the variation in the CR is found in HV1 and 33.7% in HV2 (Edson et al. 2004). Fig. 16.1 shows the distribution of polymorphic sites among HV1, HV2, and mini-variable regions one and two (mVR1 and mVR2).

After sequencing the mtDNA regions, AFDIL compares sequence data with the revised Cambridge Reference Sequence (rCRS) (Andrews et al. 1999) and records only the base-pair differences from the rCRS. These polymorphisms are then reported as the mtDNA profile. In order to distinguish one mtDNA profile from another, the base-pair polymorphisms are compared. If more than two differences are present between those being compared, the two sequences are excluded from one another, indicating that the sequences represent two individuals. AFDIL's current reporting protocol requires a minimum of two single nucleotide differences between sequences to exclude. Those differences must be in addition to any point heteroplasmies or length heteroplasmy resulting from variation in either of the two "c-stretch" regions. C-stretch regions are polycytosine stretches at base-pair positions 16182 to 16193 in HV1 and 302 to 315 in HV2. Amplification and sequencing of these repeat regions may be affected by strand slippage and a mixture of length variants within

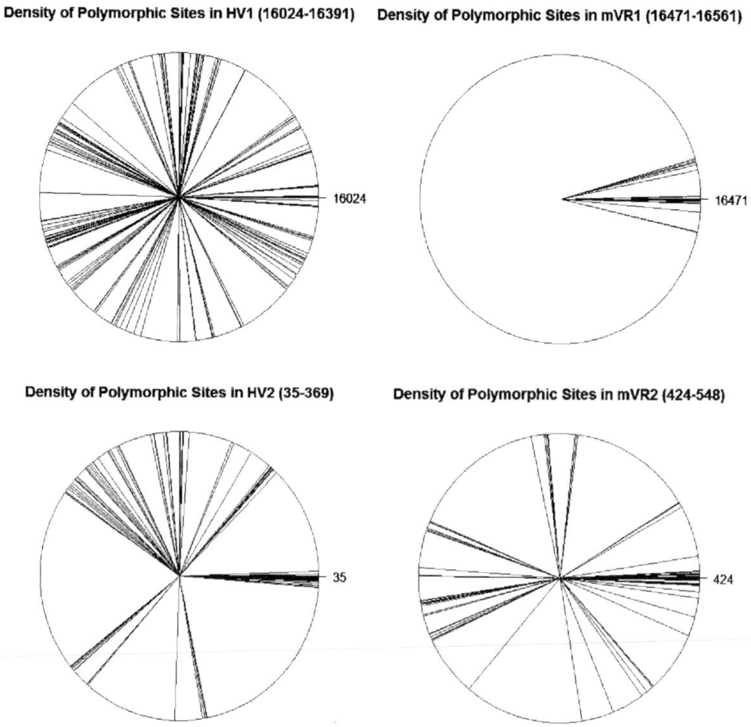

Fig. 16.1 Frequency plots of polymorphisms among the two hypervariable regions (HV1 and HV2) and the two mini-variable regions (mVR1 and mVR2) (redrawn from Edson et al. 2004). Each slice represents a specific polymorphic base-pair location, and each chart is read counterclockwise from the listed base pair. Larger slices are interpreted as those polymorphic positions that appear with greater frequency in the database than the smaller slices, which indicate less common polymorphic sites ($n = 4021$). Note that while there are more polymorphic sites present in HV1, HV2 contains sites that are more common across all populations

an individual, thus generating a sequencing result of an indeterminate number of cytosine repeats in either HV1 or HV2 that cannot be accurately reported. Although typically a predominant length species can be determined, variability within these regions is not considered accurate enough for exclusionary purposes. Advances in mtDNA testing such as single nucleotide polymorphisms (mtSNP) that identify point mutations throughout the entire circular genome and additional sequencing in the mVRs have assisted in distinguishing similar HV1/HV2 sequences (i.e., by locating additional polymorphisms and thereby meeting current reporting protocol).

While the greatest amount of variation exists within the two hypervariable regions and sequences can be differentiated based only on two polymorphic positions, mtDNA profiles can still be quite common in certain populations. When samples are consistent with one another, there is a certain probability that the consistency resulted from a random match within the population at large. In order to determine how common a sequence is, the profile is always compared to a population database of mtDNA sequences. In an analysis of mtDNA diversity from North American populations, Melton and Collegues (2001) reported that the most frequent mitotypes were observed in approximately 15% of the European-American population using single-stranded oligonucleotide typing. Drawing from the AFDIL database of HV1/HV2 sequences, the most common haplotype is present in just over 7% of individuals within the U.S. Caucasian population (Coble et al. 2004). Despite the disparity between these two findings, most likely the result of the use of different typing methods, the important point is that seemingly unrelated individuals could share the same mtDNA sequence across hypervariable regions (Fig. 16.2). However, the majority of mtDNA sequences are unique, having never been seen in the population database (represented by the long, low tail in Fig. 16.2).

Mitochondrial DNA data provide putative evidence for identification since the power of forensic mtDNA analysis is mainly through exclusion. Barring any other line of evidence, it is the non-individuating characteristic of mtDNA, or the possibility that two unrelated people share the same sequence, that prohibits mtDNA from being used as evidence of positive identification. When a consistency exists between two mtDNA sequences, this evidence is used in conjunction with other lines of forensic evidence, such as physical anthropology, archaeology, and odontology, thereby increasing the likelihood of individuation and identification as the independent lines of evidence are taken together.

Nuclear DNA STR Profiling

Short tandem repeats (STRs or microsatellites) are sections of nuclear DNA within genes that have repeating motifs of four to six nucleotides in length. Because STRs originate from nuclear DNA, an individual's genotype consists of pairs of alleles, one allele from each parent. Excluding amelogenin, which has only two alleles related to sex determination—X or Y—the number of alleles at each locus varies

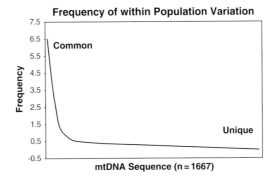

Fig. 16.2 Distribution of common mtDNA sequences within the Caucasian data set ($n = 1667$). There is a subset of individuals within the Caucasian database that has a similar sequence, approximately 7%. As single-event polymorphisms are introduced, the number of unique sequences increases dramatically (redrawn from Coble et al. 2004)

greatly; thus, the number of *possible* genotypes (combination of alleles) at a single locus is always greater than the number of alleles. When multiple loci are added, genetic variability increases and the number of possible genotypes increases dramatically. The majority of commonly tested loci are located on different chromosomes, and the repetitive elements that are passed from parent to offspring are inherited independently from those of the next locus. Because each locus is inherited independently, the multiplication rule of probability applies and as such a probabilistic statement can be calculated across all loci given the appropriate population frequency data (National Research Council 1996).

Recent death cases obtained from AFMES tend to have better tissue preservation than those cases received from the CIL, allowing AFDIL to perform STR testing. PowerPlex16® (Promega Corp., Madison, WI), a kit comprised of the 13 core CODIS (Combined DNA Index System) loci plus amelogenin, Penta E, and Penta D, can be used to generate an STR profile that identifies allelic variation at each of these specific heritable loci. By using these independently inherited alleles, consistency among all alleles evaluated between the unknown and the reference samples permits strong evidence for positive identification.

Y-Chromosome STR Profiling

Y-chromosome STR profiling is a relatively new type of DNA testing that observes heritable loci on the Y-chromosome. New heritable sites are constantly being identified, and a core set of testable loci has not yet been defined by the forensic DNA community. However, this type of testing is very useful for the identification of both recent and skeletal remains, as it provides yet another pool of references from which to draw. Y-DNA analysis is similar to STR testing in that it examines variation at specific loci; however, these loci are not independent of each other as they are all located on the same gene. Thus, there is a certain possible lack of independent assortment, although testing kits are being developed with specific loci to avoid this issue. Y-chromosome testing increases the pool of individuals that can be used as references, given that the variation within the Y is paternally inherited and remains fairly stable between generations. Like mtDNA testing, Y-STRs are a putative identification since multiple individuals can have the same profile. When combined with other types of DNA analysis and other evidence, Y-STRs will prove to be a strong analytical tool in the future.

Family Reference Samples

In addition to processing CIL skeletal samples where mtDNA is used most frequently, AFDIL processes mtDNA reference material collected from living relatives of the deceased for comparison with sequences derived from unknown skeletal samples. These reference materials are most often whole uncoagulated blood received in potassium EDTA-treated tubes, but it is becoming more common to submit buccal swabs, a noninvasive collection method that causes little to no discomfort.

Since nuclear DNA is acquired from both parents and is recombinant, it is best to get a direct self-reference from the suspected unknown individual or from the presumed parents of the unknown decedent for comparison. For recent deaths of military personnel, nuclear DNA is a common means of identification. Today this is possible because all service members are required to submit a blood sample that is archived at the Armed Forces Repository of Specimen Samples for the Identification of Remains (AFRSSIR). In the event of a service member's death, DNA is extracted from their archived blood card, which is then used as a reference for comparison to DNA extracted from the decedent.

In contrast to nuclear DNA analysis, Y-STR profiles are from the non-recombining Y-chromosome; thus, the potential references are identified through the paternal line and include only male relatives. Mitochondrial DNA, on the other hand, is inherited strictly from the mother, as the father contributes no mitochondria to the child. In contrast to Y-chromosome inheritance, both males and females of the maternal line are appropriate references for mtDNA analysis.

Additional sources of reference material include items belonging to the victim (i.e., direct self-reference) or a relative. In the past, alternative references submitted to AFDIL for processing included hair from hairbrushes and razors; hats; sealed envelopes and stamps; nail clippings; clothing; or even archived medical biologi-cal material, such as paraffin blocks from a hospital. Positive interactions with the public and families can often produce items acceptable for analysis.

Skeletal Sample Selection

The process for selecting the best possible bone samples from commingled remains follows a few simple steps. First, remains from a single incident should be sorted as best as possible following anthropological techniques, which include evaluation of archaeological provenience and identification of duplicating elements, skeletal age indicators, size and shape differences among elements, articulating elements, and conjoining skeletal fragments. Metric sorting of skeletal elements is also applied (Byrd and Adams 2003). If two or more anatomically identical elements are present within a single assemblage, then sampling of those duplicated elements is preferred as they clearly represent distinct individuals and permit their possible identification. If several elements are associated by articulation, such as teeth to a mandible or a series of conjoining vertebrae, then only one element should be sampled. This not only minimizes the cost of analysis and destructive sampling, but it also identifies potential samples for additional testing should the first not produce a sequence.

If commingling of skeletal remains results in poorly associated cranial and postcranial remains, by either missing or poor articulation of the first cervical ver-tebra with the cranial base, then it is recommended to procure at least one cranial or dental sample and one sample from the postcranial remains. This strategy will allow the majority of remains to be segregated from the grouped assemblage and reassociated into individuals, creating the potential for positive identification based on DNA and dental evidence.

Samples are also selected based on their potential for preserved endogenous DNA. Preservation depends highly on the environment from which the remains were recovered, and the persistence of DNA is correlated loosely with the same taphonomic processes that affect the micro- and macroscopic structure of skeletal material (Damann et al. 2002; Hagelberg et al. 1991; Herrmann and Hummel 1994; Parsons and Weedn 1997). Experience demonstrates that the best nondental samples are those from long bones with thick cortices, such as the femur, tibia, and humerus (Edson et al. 2005), whereas elements typically preferred when creating a biological profile such as the os coxae and crania are relatively poor DNA candidates due to their thin cortices (Fig. 16.3).

Generally, dense skeletal elements provide protection of endogenous DNA from deleterious taphonomic agents that destroy bone and its constituent parts. It should also be stated that the desire for samples with thick cortical tissue is due partly to pre-extraction laboratory processing that attempts to remove any exogenous contamination by sanding and washing. While destructive to the sample, it has been

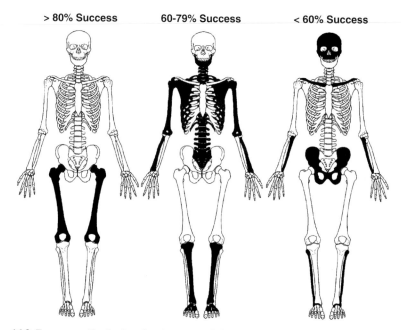

Fig. 16.3 Frequency distribution for the successful amplification and sequencing of mtDNA from human remains recovered by the CIL and processed by the AFDIL (redrawn from Edson et al. 2005). This distribution is based on 3,721 skeletal samples. Success is defined as a sample that yielded at least two identical sequences greater than 100 base pairs in length. Statistics pertain to elements shaded black. Elements with fewer than 30 samples such as the patella, sternal body, manubrium, carpals, and metacarpals are not included in this distribution

found that without these mitigating steps, many samples are unusable as sequences often contain mixed DNA sequences or the endogenous "ancient" target DNA is outcompeted by relatively new and more viable DNA from contaminating sources such as soil organisms from the area where the remains were recovered or analysts that handled the case.

When mtDNA results are obtained from multiple samples in a commingled case, matching sequences may be attributed to the same individual, they may represent more than one individual because of the non-unique properties of mtDNA, or they may represent an exogenous contaminate. In order to ensure the highest quality in the DNA sequence results, AFDIL analysts employ stringent protocols. This includes independent duplication of sequence results prior to reporting and their use of appropriate internal controls throughout the extraction, amplification, and sequencing processes.

Since the CIL submits samples to AFDIL free of provenience and incident-related information, the anthropologist must interpret the DNA results to determine if the mtDNA sequence originates from a single individual or if multiple people are represented by the same sequence. One easy way this is accomplished is by following a sound sampling strategy. If two samples are determined to have the same sequence, then the anthropologist must check to see if the shared sequence is from duplicating elements or elements that are excluded from one another based on differences in morphological and metric analyses.

Without the mitigating steps of the anthropologist's initial segregation and subsequent review of sample sequences and skeletal data, the potential exists for making erroneous skeletal associations based on accurate mtDNA sequence data. One recent case exemplifying this potential error occurred with an assemblage of remains recovered from a U.S. bomber crash in Papua New Guinea that was carrying a crew of nine service members. In late 1943, the crew took part in a night reconnaissance mission and an attack on Japanese ships in the vicinity of New Ireland. After reporting a successful attack, the aircraft and crew never returned to their airbase and were presumed lost at sea. Subsequent search efforts provided no useful information regarding the whereabouts of the bomber and crew. In 2002, a representative of the Morobe Provincial government provided information to the U.S. Embassy regarding the location of aircraft wreckage and remains. The following year JPAC-CIL deployed to the site and recovered remains and aircraft information correlating the recovery site to that of the bomber lost in late 1943. As part of the skeletal analysis, mtDNA sequences were obtained. A shared sequence between two individuals soon became evident to the anthropologist reviewing the case since the same sequence was reported for two duplicated fragments of right femur. With this information, the AFDIL analysts used the DNA extracts from the two femora fragments and obtained a partial nuclear STR profile for each sample. This additional information was sufficient to genetically distinguish the two individuals. Without the anthropologist's recognition that the two samples could not have originated from the same individual (duplication of skeletal elements), these bones might have been erroneously associated to the sample decedent. Following a well-planned sample selection process, the appropriate steps are in place to recognize potential problems of shared sequences.

A careful sampling strategy also prohibits unnecessary and excessive sampling that leads to stresses on the DNA laboratory workload and inflated costs to the submitting agency.

Kiska Island, Alaska

The following case example details the recovery and identification efforts of the JPAC-CIL and AFDIL for a World War II aircraft crash on Kiska Island, one of the largest islands in the Aleutian Island chain off the coast of Alaska.

Weinberg (1994) and Morison (2001) provide descriptions surrounding the events taking place in the North Pacific in June 1942. According to their descriptions, Japanese aircraft attacked islands of the Aleutian chain in order to draw U.S. attention away from the ongoing Battle of Midway and to keep the United States from staging an attack on Japan from the North Pacific. In this effort, the Japanese secured and deployed troops to Kiska and Attu Islands. Three days later, U.S. forces in the Pacific became aware of the Japanese movement into the Aleutian Islands and ordered U.S. Naval aircraft to attack. Over the next several days, U.S. aircraft continued bombing missions. On June 14, 1942, a U.S. Navy PBY-5, carrying a crew of seven, took part in the bombing of Japanese ships moored in Kiska Harbor, when "it [the PBY-5 aircraft] was last seen plunging into a cloud bank over Kiska Harbor" (Commander Fleet Wing Four to the Judge Advocate General 10 September 1943). Since the aircraft never returned to its unit, it was believed to have been shot down by enemy activity and subsequently lost in the vicinity of Kiska Island, Alaska.

After U.S. forces recaptured the island from the Japanese in August 1943, the bodies of seven crewmembers were found. A review of military records indicated that seven crewmembers of the PBY-5 were buried in a common grave on the northwest side of Kiska Volcano. At the head of the grave, a cross was placed with the words *Seven U.S.N. Airmen*. The bodies stayed at this location for nearly six decades before an attempt was made to recover and identify them.

In 2001, an associate professor of wildlife biology at the Memorial University of Newfoundland, Canada, was conducting research within the Alaska Maritime Wildlife Refuge where he encountered aircraft wreckage. In late 2002, the JPAC-CIL was made aware of the site and researchers at the CIL were able to correlate serial numbers on wreckage to the PBY-5 that was last seen in 1943. During the summer of 2003, a CIL archaeologist led a team of U.S. service members and civilians to recover the skeletal remains buried in a single mass grave on the side of Kiska Volcano. For several days the team lived on a ship in Kiska Harbor and flew from the ship to the site via helicopter. Once at the site, the team began their recovery effort by pedestrian reconnaissance on the northwest side of the volcano at 2,700 feet to locate the crash site. Miscellaneous wreckage was located in a number of erosional gullies along the downslope edge of a snowfield; however, the main wreckage field was discovered upslope at an elevation of 3,027 feet above sea level.

A small rock cairn with wood fragments was identified approximately three meters away from the main concentration of aircraft wreckage. Upon closer inspection, one wooden fragment had the letters "USN AIRMEN" carved on one side (Fig. 16.4).

The main wreckage field (approximately 15 by 15 meters in size) was excavated, including the rock cairn. Throughout most of the excavation, incident-sterile sediment was rather shallow given the erosional formation process of the site. The feature below the rock cairn was the only area where excavation extended in excess of 20 centimeters below ground surface. The rock cairn was mapped; after the initial level of boulders and cobbles was removed, a grave was located and excavated using trowels, brushes, and small bamboo sticks.

Human remains in the grave represented collections of skeletal elements, both articulated and disarticulated, some of which were wrapped in sheepskin flying garments. The commingling of the remains made it difficult, if not impossible, to sort individuals within the feature fill. Consequently, an effort was made to identify and excavate articulating elements (i.e., upper arm to forearm, upper leg to lower leg, etc.) and place the excavated articulations in individual bags. All sediments within the burial feature were screened through $^1/_4$-inch wire mesh, and items recovered from the screen were bagged separately and labeled accordingly. All recovered skeletal, dental, and material evidence was then transported to the CIL for analysis.

Upon accessioning, skeletal analysis segregated seven potential individuals based on duplicated femora. Dental, osteology, and archaeological provenience data were

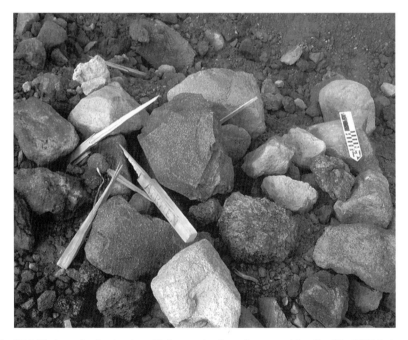

Fig. 16.4 Photograph of rock cairn with fragments of wooden cross at the site of the PBY-5 aircraft crash on the side of Kiska Volcano.

used during the initial sorting to identify a total of 14 clusters, consisting of seven groups of postcranial remains, six clusters of dental remains, and one group of unassociated remains. Separation was possible because provenience was maintained for elements articulating *in situ*; age and size differences were evaluated; bilateral nonmetric traits were recorded and compared; conjoining elements and fragments were refit; preservation factors such as bone deterioration, color, and integrity were evaluated; and metric sorting was applied (Byrd and Adams 2003). After all of the anthropological associations were completed, there were two main challenges: (1) linking the clusters to each other, in essence rebuilding people; and (2) positively identifying the seven airmen.

For this case, antemortem dental records were available for the entire crew from their archived medical records. The level of detail contained in the files, coupled with the diversity of dental treatment observed on the remains, made it relatively straightforward to identify most of the teeth and associated skeletal structures to the seven airmen. Although all of the crew could be identified, this would only pertain to a small amount of the total quantity of remains. As such, a decision was made to use mtDNA to reassociate the dental remains with the clusters of postcranial remains. A well-designed DNA sampling strategy was developed to test specific elements from the anthropologically sorted clusters. In addition to providing a solid means of reassociation, it also provided a confirmatory test of the gross sorting procedures used to group bones together.

Normally, family reference samples (maternal relatives) are needed when comparing mtDNA sequence data. Finding such references generations removed from this case proved difficult, which is becoming normal for cases examined nearly 60 years after the incident. Because this case involves the loss of U.S. Navy service members, correspondence with relatives, including finding the appropriate relatives for reference material, is the responsibility of the U.S. Navy Casualty Office. Given the antiquity of the case, the Navy Casualty Office had difficulty acquiring the maternal references and was only able to obtain one sample from the presumed decedents. Thus, in lieu of reference samples from living relatives, the CIL and AFDIL decided to use direct self-references for six of the seven sets of remains. This means that a decision was made to sample the identified teeth since they could be associated to specific crew members. By doing this, the need for collecting the other six references could be avoided. Congruent sequence matches between the positively identified teeth and the unassociated bone clusters would be conclusive evidence for linking these elements to the same person.

From the 14 groups of separated remains, a minimum of one sample from each of the seven postcranial clusters and six dental groups was taken. The anthropologist identified other elements for sampling in order to test the initial sorting hypotheses as well as associate those elements suitable for estimating a biological profile from the unassociated group. In all, the anthropologist selected 32 samples for mtDNA analysis, which included teeth from the grouped cranial remains and duplicated femora from the postcranial groupings.

Sampling of remains at the CIL always occurs in sterile hoods where a wedge of bone or a pulverized dental sample is packaged and then sent to AFDIL for analysis.

Of the 32 samples submitted to AFDIL, 29 generated full reportable sequences. From those 29 samples, seven distinguishable mtDNA profiles were obtained (i.e., there were at least two or more polymorphisms between any two sequences). The MNI as determined by osteology coincided with that determined by mtDNA. The seven separate mtDNA sequences supported the initial segregation into seven individuals; however, minimal rearrangement of a few elements among clusters was warranted. Due to some postmortem damage, some associations contained in the initial sort were considered to be tentative (i.e., they appeared to be more consistent with one set of remains than others, but the association was not to the exclusion of all other possibilities). The DNA sampling strategy was specifically designed to test some of these associations. Once the DNA results were available, it was found that there were some minor adjustments needed with some of the postcranial clusters. While the initial segregation needed more work, the well-thought-out sorting and sampling plan established by the anthropologist was able to resolve any discrepancies and make the appropriate associations.

The seven crewmembers aboard the U.S. Navy PBY-5 that crashed in early summer 1943 were able to receive an identification based on consistency with antemortem dental records, historical records documenting the reported loss location and flight manifest, archaeology, osteology, and mtDNA evidence. In this case, initial separation of commingled remains was accomplished using archaeological provenience and osteological techniques. Subsequent mtDNA sequence results allowed a confirmation of the initial sorting procedures (with minor adjustments) and were essential for linking the numerous clusters of bones and teeth into seven distinct individuals. The success of this case resolution was due in large part to the implementation of a systematic DNA sampling approach.

Conclusion

Applying DNA analysis to sort and identify commingled human remains requires the anthropologist to choose the type of DNA test that will best address their question. In so doing, it is important to understand the population dynamics and the inherent resolution power for the different types of DNA tests. When skeletal and soft-tissue preservation is good, nuclear STR data can be used. By generating full STR profiles, positive identification is possible because of the unique properties of nuclear DNA due to recombination. At the same time, STR profiles will allow for the segregation of remains based on observed differences in DNA profiles. For many anthropologists, mtDNA is an appropriate genetic tool given the relative ease for obtaining mtDNA sequences from cases with poor skeletal preservation. However, mtDNA only provides putative evidence due to the non-unique nature of mtDNA profiles in the population at large and, as such, requires additional information to support a positive identification. When there is a need to separate commingled remains, mtDNA is often sufficient, especially when an anthropologist institutes the appropriate control mechanisms to her sampling strategy so that potentially shared sequences can be resolved.

Not only is it important to determine the type of DNA that would be most effective for testing, but it is also important to determine whether or not reference materials are available for the desired testing. DNA testing is generally only useful as long as there is a reference sequence to compare to the sequence from the unknown remains. For the individuals recovered from certain circumstances, such as Kiska Island, an mtDNA self-reference obtained from dental remains is appropriate because the anthropologists and dentists are able to group remains prior to DNA analysis.

When selecting samples for DNA analysis, the anthropologist's assessment of the skeletal assemblage and development of initial sorting into potential individuals is imperative to determine a thoughtful sample strategy and to prevent future errors of associating remains based solely on a shared profile. An appropriate strategy should consist of sampling duplicated elements and/or elements that can be associated through other techniques (e.g., articulation, pair-matching, etc.). Key elements to sample are also those that display characteristics useful in estimating a biological profile. By establishing testable hypotheses of those associations, an appropriate sampling strategy reduces the potentials for oversampling and unnecessarily increasing the cost of analysis.

Finally, it is imperative to develop and maintain rapport with the respective labs in order to reach identification and case resolution from commingled remains. Applying DNA analysis to the segregation of commingled remains can be an expensive and laborious process, but the process becomes efficient through collaboration among team members. Communication between the different groups of scientists on a regular basis is essential to the identification process. A successful relationship between laboratories will lead to rapid resolution of most casework issues, more targeted sampling of remains, and a more efficient identification process overall. Over the past 15 years, the combined efforts of the JPAC-CIL and AFDIL have identified hundreds of individuals from commingled settings, such as battlefield mass graves and aircraft crashes. The individuation and identification of the seven crewmembers recovered from a commingled grave on the slopes of Kiska Volcano is just one example of the interaction among anthropologists and molecular biologists that leads to the successful resolution of a complicated scenario.

References Cited

Andrews, R. M., I. Kubacka, P. F. Chinnery, R. N. Lightowlers, D. M. Turnbull, and N. Howell 1999 Reanalysis and revision of the Cambridge reference sequence for human mitochondrial DNA. *Nat. Genet.* 23(2):147.

Byrd, J. E. and B. J. Adams 2003 Osteometric sorting of commingled human remains. *J. Forensic Sci.* 48(4):717–724.

Coble, M. D. and J. M. Butler 2005 Characterization of new miniSTR loci to aid analysis of degraded DNA. *J. Forensic Sci.* 50(1):43–53.

Coble, M. D., R. S. Just, J. E. O'Callaghan, I. H. Letmanyi, C. T. Peterson, J. A. Irwin, and T. J. Parsons 2004 Single nucleotide polymorphisms over the entire mtDNA genome that increase the power of forensic testing in Caucasians. *Int. J. Legal Med.* 118(3):137–146.

Commander Fleet Wing Four to the Judge Advocate General 10 September 1943 Serial 1108, "Administrative report on loss of PBY-5 Airplane, Bureau No. 04511."

Damann, F. E., M. D. Leney, and A. W. Bunch 2002 Predicting Mitochondrial DNA (mtDNA) Recovery by Skeletal Preservation. Paper presented at the American Academy of Forensic Science, Atlanta, GA.

Edson, S. M., J. P. Ross, M. D. Coble, T. J. Parsons, and S. M. Barritt 2004 Naming the dead— Confronting the realities of rapid identification of degraded skeletal remains. *Forensic Sci. Rev.* 16:63–90.

Edson, S. M., H. A. Thew, F. E. Damann, C. A. Boyer, S. M. Barritt-Ross, and B. C. Smith 2005 Success Rates for Recovering Mitochondrial DNA (mtDNA) from 4,000 "Ancient" Human Skeletal Remains. Paper presented at the 17th Meeting International Assocociation of Forensic Scientists.

Hagelberg, E., L. S. Bell, T. Allen, A. Boyde, S. J. Jones, and J. B. Clegg 1991 Analysis of ancient bone DNA: Techniques and applications. *Philos. Trans. Roy. Soc. London B Biol. Sci.* 333(1268):399–407.

Herrmann, B. and S. Hummel 1994 *Ancient DNA: Recovery, Analysis of Genetic Material from Paleontological, Archaeological Museum, Medical and Forensic Specimens.* Springer-Verlag, New York.

Lederberg, J., J. Bashinski, B. Budowle, P. Gill, M. Stoneking, D. Wallace, B. Weir, and G. White-sides 1995 *Report of the Defense Science Board Task Force on the Use of DNA Technology for Identification of Ancient Remains.* Office of the Under Secretary of Defense for Acquisition and Technology.

Melton, T., S. Clifford, M. Kayser, I. Nasidze, M. Batzer, and M. Stoneking 2001 Diversity and heterogeneity in mitochondrial DNA of North American populations. *J. Forensic Sci.* 46(1): 46–52.

Morison, S. E. 2001 *History of United States Naval Operations in World War II: Coral Sea, Midway and Submarine Actions, May 1942–August 1942,* Vol. 4. Castle Books, Edison, NJ.

National Research Council 1996 *The Evaluation of Forensic DNA Evidence.* National Academy Press, Washington, DC.

Parsons, T. J. and V. W. Weedn 1997 Preservation and recovery of DNA in postmortem specimens and trace samples. In *Forensic Taphonomy: The Postmortem Fate of Human Remains,* W. H. Haglund and M. H. Sorg, eds., pp. 109–138. CRC Press, Boca Raton, FL.

Torroni, A., H. J. Bandelt, L. D'Urbano, P. Lahermo, P. Moral, D. Sellitto, C. Rengo, P. Forster, M. L. Savontaus, B. Bonne-Tamir, and R. Scozzari 1998 mtDNA analysis reveals a major late Paleolithic population expansion from southwestern to northeastern Europe. *Am. J. Hum. Genet.* 62(5):1137–1152.

Torroni, A., K. Huoponen, P. Francalacci, M. Petrozzi, L. Morelli, R. Scozzari, D. Obinu, M. L. Savontaus, and D. C. Wallace 1996 Classification of European mtDNAs from an analysis of three European populations. *Genetics* 144(4):1835–1850.

Weinberg, G. L. 1994 *A World at Arms: A Global History of World War II.* Cambridge University Press, Cambridge.

Chapter 17
Resolving Commingling Issues During the Medicolegal Investigation of Mass Fatality Incidents

Elias J. Kontanis and Paul S. Sledzik

By definition, mass fatality incidents result in numerous deaths occurring over a relatively narrow time frame. These events produce complex multidisciplinary investigative challenges (Labovich et al. 2003; Ludes et al. 1994; van den Bos 1980). From a medicolegal perspective, investigators seek to identify decedents, resolve cause of death, and assist with determining the cause of the event (Wagner and Froede 1993). Oftentimes, severe fragmentation and commingling of human remains are the byproducts of the causative forces and pose significant challenges to investigators (Sledzik and Rodriguez 2002). In a mass fatality context, the overarching tenet regarding commingling is that human remains with no anatomical/physical connection *must* be considered to be commingled. This principle also applies to remains that are spatially associated but present no valid anatomical connection. From the perspective of the forensic investigator, resolving commingling, and ultimately decedent identification, requires careful management of both the human remains and the data generated during recovery and postmortem examination. This chapter examines effects of fragmentation and commingling on the identification process and discusses the role of triage during the postmortem data collection process as a means to facilitate recognition and reassociation of commingled remains.

Identification

Identifying human remains is a primary investigative objective for legal, cultural, and scientific reasons. Family members of the deceased require identification for insurance, wills/probate, child guardianship, and remarriage (Wagner and Froede 1993). From an investigative perspective with aircraft incidents, aircrew identification and injury pattern analysis are often instrumental for determining and evaluating actions of the aircrew at the time of the accident (Midda 1974; Read and Pillay 2000; Taneja and Wiegmann 2003). In addition, correlating passenger injuries with seating assignments may aid incident reconstruction and evaluation of safety equipment (Armstrong et al. 1955; Cullen and Turk 1980; Li and Baker 1997; Vosswinkel et al. 1999). More broadly, the humanitarian and moral obligations to

From: *Recovery, Analysis, and Identification of Commingled Human Remains*
Edited by: B. Adams and J. Byrd © Humana Press, Totowa, NJ

identify the dead are nearly universal. State, national, and international laws govern the status of decedents, the need to identify the dead, and the status of unidentified remains (PAHO 2004).

Mass fatality investigators often rely on a combination of positive and presumptive methods during the identification process. Ultimately, positive identification requires comparing the unique biological attributes that are a component of the decedent's antemortem record with those biological characteristics observed during postmortem analysis. Fingerprints, odontological evidence, the presence of surgical implants, anatomical anomalies, and, most recently, DNA methods, are utilized for positive identification. Presumptive identifiers such as associated personal effects and the biological profile (i.e., sex, age, ancestry, stature, and characteristics of individuation) often provide an identification hypothesis that can be accepted or rejected based on a comparison of unique biological attributes. Presumptive identifiers can also permit identification by exclusion in closed populations when all decedents in a definable category are accounted for.

Closed population mass fatality incidents are typified by commercial aircraft accidents, where relatively accurate passenger manifests are available soon after the accident. In a closed population event, the goal is to account for all potentially identifiable remains for each decedent. Often, this approach does not require analysis of all remains, just those that have a potential to be identified. With open decedent populations, typified by natural disasters, neither the number of victims nor their names are known. Under these circumstances, general practice is to analyze and, if possible, identify every fragment recovered. This is the only way to provide an accurate accounting of decedents. Such an approach requires more time and cost, as DNA methods are often the only way to provide this information.

Fragmentation, Reassociation, and Identification: Influencing Parameters

The condition of human remains, particularly the fragmentation severity, will have a substantial effect on fatality management, decedent identification, and reassociation of commingled remains. In this chapter, fragmentation severity is described using the "fragmentation index," which is simply the ratio of recovered remains to the number of decedents. Table 17.1 demonstrates the range of fragmentation severities observed during the investigation of several recent aviation accidents. Fragmentation severities range from a low of 1.3 remains per decedent resulting from the crash of the Executive Air BAE J-31 turboprop on approach to landing, at an estimated speed of approximately 174 feet per second and an impact angle of 60 degrees nose-down (NTSB 2002). The other end of the fragmentation severity spectrum is represented by the ValuJet Flight 592 DC-9 jet that impacted terrain at a 70–80 degree angle traveling approximately 675 feet per second (Mittleman et al. 2000). A total of 4,282 fragments was recovered, representing 38.9 remains per decedent.

Table 17.1 Fragmentation Severity Data from 11 Aviation Crashes That Occurred Between 1994 and 2004

Incident (Year)	Aircraft/Type	# of Decedents	# of Remains Recovered	Fragmentation Index	Months Dedicated to Identification
USAir 427 (1994)	B-737/Jet	132	1,771	13.4	2
ValuJet 592 (1996)	DC-9/Jet	110	4,282	38.9	3.5
Swissair 111 (1998)	MD-11/Jet	229	2,500	10.9	3.5
Egyptair 990 (1999)	B-767/Jet	217	6,000	27.7	6
Alaska Air 261 (2000)	MD-83/Jet	88	950	10.8	4
Executive Air (2000)	BAE J-31/Prop	19	25	1.3	0.17
American 77/Pentagon (2001)	B-757/Jet	188	2,000	10.6	3
United 93 (2001)	B-757/Jet	44	1,500	34.1	3
American 587 (2001)	A-300/Jet	265	2,077	7.8	1
USAirways 5481 (2002)	B-1900/Prop	21	43	2.1	0.23
Corporate Airlines 5596 (2004)	BAE J-32/Prop	13	30	2.3	0.5

While the fragmentation index presents a coarse perspective on incident dynamics, it is broadly influenced by recovery strategies and postmortem data collection protocols. Recoveries executed by highly experienced personnel using systematic scene processing strategies will result in a realistic approximation of the fragmentation severity, whereas inexperienced personnel can introduce recovery biases that depress the fragmentation severity index. Morgue protocols can also influence the fragmentation index. Managers responsible for postmortem data collection may decide that fragments classified as common tissue will not be part of the tally, which will also depress the fragmentation index. Nevertheless, the fragmentation index is a useful concept for comparing the fragmentation severity between incidents with varying numbers of decedents.

As the number of decedents and the number of recovered human tissue fragments increase, forensic identification experts must make decisions about how best to use the limited resources of personnel, time, and funds. Data from 11 aviation mass fatality incidents suggest that there is no significant relationship between the number of decedents and the amount of time dedicated to the identification process when the effect of the number of recovered remains has been removed ($r = -0.0760$, $p = 0.835$) (Fig. 17.1, Table 17.1). The relationship with time becomes significant when the number of recovered remains per decedent (i.e., the fragmentation index), controlling for the number of decedents, is examined ($r = 0.6944$, $p = 0.026$) (Fig. 17.2, Table 17.1). While fragmentation severity appears to have a significant influence on investigative resources, the number of individuals cannot be neglected. For example, the investigative effort and consequently the amount of time required to obtain antemortem records will undoubtedly increase as the numbers of decedents increase. Even though the correlation between the fragmentation index and time is significant, the coefficient of determination (i.e., R^2-value) suggests that fragmentation severity is responsible for less than 50% of the change in the amount of time dedicated to the identification process. This finding emphasizes the confounding influence of additional variables on the identification process that have not

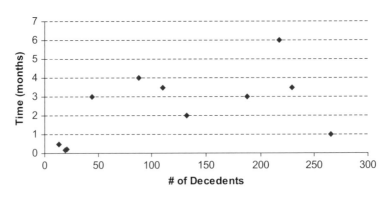

Fig. 17.1 Data from 11 aviation incidents demonstrating the relationship between the number of decedents and the amount of time dedicated to the identification process

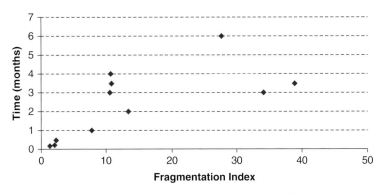

Fig. 17.2 Data from 11 aviation incidents demonstrating the relationship between the fragmentation index (i.e., the ratio of recovered remains to the number of decedents) and the amount of time dedicated to the identification process

been quantified, such as antemortem and postmortem data management practices (Kontanis et al. 2001; Tyrrell et al. 2006).

In addition to time, fragmentation severity will influence the utility of traditional and molecular (i.e., DNA) identification methods. Traditional identification methods, such as fingerprint and odontological analysis, are based on the physical examination of remains and do not rely on molecular identification strategies. Figs. 17.3 and 17.4 describe the relative contributions of molecular and traditional identification modalities as a consequence of incident dynamics. In these figures, the dependent variable is the number of identifications generated using either molecular or conventional modalities expressed as a percentage of the total number of identifications. Figure 17.3 demonstrates that with increasing fragmentation (controlling for the number of decedents) there is increasing reliance on DNA to produce identifications ($r = 0.9064$, $p = 0.002$). Conversely, as the fragmentation severity increases, the utility of traditional identification methods diminishes ($r = -0.9064$, $p = 0.002$; Fig. 17.4). In other words, relatively complete remains will have a

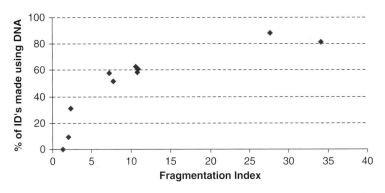

Fig. 17.3 Data from 10 mass fatality incidents demonstrating the relationship between the percent of identifications made using DNA technologies and the fragmentation index (i.e., the ratio of recovered remains to the number of decedents)

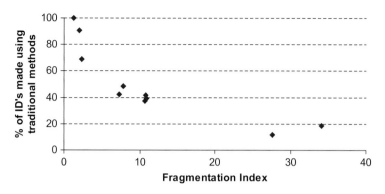

Fig. 17.4 Data from 10 mass fatality incidents demonstrating the relationship between the percent of identifications made using traditional methods (i.e., dental, fingerprint, medical comparisons) and the fragmentation index (i.e., the ratio of recovered remains to the number of decedents)

greater chance of bearing the unique physical identifiers necessary for traditional identifications. However, as fragmentation severity increases, the possibility of recovering fragments lacking fingerprints, dental remains, or other unique identifiers increases. Consequently, the lack of unique anthroposcopic features results in an increased reliance on DNA identification methods. These figures also demonstrate that the relationship between identification modality and fragmentation severity is asymptotic. Simply stated, even in cases of extreme fragmentation, some of the remains will bear anthroposcopic features of a high enough value to render a traditional identification possible. Furthermore, even with the liberal application of DNA technologies, a small percentage of the human remains may not be identified. Some remains will be too small to test, or testing may result in consumption of the entire specimen. Perimortem and postmortem factors such as thermal modification, contact with amplification inhibitors, and decomposition will destroy DNA or render it of a low quality that is unsuitable for identification purposes.

Managing the Identification Process: Applying Human Remains Triage Principles

An effective identification process hinges largely on the application of appropriate morgue management principles. Incident morgue designs must allow for rapid yet thorough examination of decedent remains while meeting incident-specific investigative goals. This is especially imperative when the fragmentation index is high. In disaster medicine, triage is used to successfully manage the initial care of mass casualty patients by sorting patients into predefined categories based on injury severity and treatment urgency (Auf Der Heide 1989; Bowen and Bellamy 1988; Nijman 1980). In order to perform this task, medical personnel are trained to rapidly and effectively assess and classify patients in a systematic fashion (Janousek et al. 1999; Kennedy et al. 1996; Robison 2002). The concept of triage is readily applicable to the mass fatality morgue management system, where systematic decisions concerning the potential of fragmented remains to lead to an identification will facilitate postmortem data collection and, consequently, identification.

Establishing Human Remains Triage Guidelines

Before postmortem examinations can begin, personnel responsible for data collection need to (1) develop a tracking system that takes fragmentation severity and commingling into consideration, (2) determine the need for, and specifically define, a common tissue classification, (3) develop a triage probative indexing system, and (4) establish DNA sampling guidelines. Morgue personnel must also establish personal effects and evidence chain-of-custody stipulations with the appropriate controlling agencies. Personnel responsible for establishing evidence processing guidelines must understand that decisions made early in the process will have long-lasting and very significant consequences for the families of the decedents and for the agencies involved with the investigation.

Evidence Tracking Systems

An effective human remains tracking system must account for the number of decedents and the condition of remains, specifically the hypothesized fragmentation severity. The system should also consider search and recovery methods, which can profoundly affect commingling and the accuracy of provenience information (Dirkmaat et al. 2001). While provenience data can clarify the levels of commingling, this line of evidence cannot be used as the sole method of reassociation. Recovery tracking systems are applicable in the morgue only if they account for potentially commingled remains, a circumstance that is rare because most search and recovery numbering systems are designed to record coarse provenience information for complete bodies or large fragments and do not always discriminate individual remains in severe fragmentation events. When commingling is apparent, an effective morgue tracking system captures information that can be used to potentially associate fragmentary remains and assist with reconstruction of incident causation. The tracking system should not be revised once morgue operations have begun. Modifications during an active operation will result in confusion and an increased risk of error. Furthermore, the human remains tracking system must not interfere with systems used for other incident operations such as antemortem records or evidence tracking. Also, the system should not interfere with the tracking system utilized by the presiding medical examiner or coroner office to handle non-incident cases.

Common Tissue Classification

Identifying fragmented and commingled human remains from mass disasters involves both scientific and ethical considerations. Before processing remains, investigators must decide whether the focus will be on identifying all victims or on identifying all remains. Advances in DNA technology provide forensic scientists with powerful tools to identify and reassociate remains that would have been previously considered unidentifiable. However, the existence of these tools does not argue for their exhaustive application. The term "common tissue" is often used for remains that are not identified or that are not examined further beyond the initial triage. Common tissue is tissue that, under the highest scientific standards, is judged to be devoid of all potential identifiable characteristics attributable to a specific individual and/or yields no information useful to death investigation and the determination of incident causation. From a scientific perspective, the need for a common tissue category is dictated by the condition of remains (i.e., fragmentation severity, degree of thermal modification, and decomposition severity), whether the decedent population is open or closed, and the availability of antemortem information (Fig. 17.5). Additional considerations include family and public expectations and the availability of investigation resources. Even though a policy may dictate attempts to identify all fragments, this may not be possible, and thus the common tissue category would still be necessary. Common tissue classification guidelines must be clearly defined if remains are severely fragmented and if identification of all decedents, but not all fragments, is the ultimate goal. Common tissue guidelines are incident-dependent and, once established, should not be changed.

Fragmentary Remains ⟶ Complete Remains		
• Reported missing vs. actual missing • Increased reliance on DNA IDs • Lesser role for conventional ID • Re association required *World Trade Center*	• Reported missing vs. actual missing • Conventional IDs • Minimal DNA required/ corroborative role • Re association not required *Hurricane Katrina*	Open population ⟶
• Decedent list known • More rapid acquisition of antemortem data • Increased reliance on DNA IDs • Lesser role for conventional IDs • Re association required *United 93, Egyptair 990*	• Decedent list known • More rapid acquisition of antemortem data • Conventional IDs • Minimal DNA required/ • Re-association not required *Mass transit MVA (e.g. tour bus)*	⟶ Closed Population

Fig. 17.5 Fragmentation severity and population status matrix

The Probative Index System

A probative index system that allows triage personnel to systematically and objectively classify human remains according to their identification potential or investigative value is essential. Table 17.2 provides a template for the development of such a system. The system relates the presence of positive and presumptive identifying features to the potential for a DNA, fingerprint, dental, or medical identification. Numeric values are assigned and tallied for each fragment based on the presence of attributes useful to the identification process. Remains with high probative scores are most likely to be identified or aid in the determination of incident causation, and thus are the highest priority for detailed examination.

In principle, antemortem information drives the identification process, which makes it essential for the antemortem and postmortem data sets to be both relevant and congruent (Tyrrell et al. 2006). Consequently, the probative index must be designed as an incident-specific sorting tool, since factors such as the condition of remains, the decedent population demographic parameters, and the availability and accuracy of antemortem information will impact the value of postmortem data. Investigative goals also need to be considered. For instance, if tissue samples for DNA analysis are collected from all remains, the indexing system can be modified to denote sampling priority. Systematic evaluation and prioritization ensures optimal use of available resources, which is an important consideration for high-volume morgue operations.

DNA Sampling Guidelines

Triage personnel must collaborate with DNA specialists to develop an appropriate sample nomination strategy, which is reflected in the probative index score. Important considerations include differential DNA preservation and the potential for sample contamination when evaluating the identification potential of fragmentary remains. The current state of forensic DNA science has proven very effective in resolving identifications and reassociating fragmentary remains in mass fatality contexts (Ballantyne 1997; Brenner and Weir 2003; Goodwin et al. 1999; Leclair et al. 1999). However, sample contamination still poses a substantial challenge, especially when degradation and commingling are apparent (Alonso et al. 2005; Budimlija et al. 2003). During the postmortem data collection process, the primary sources of contamination are other remains and investigators that have come in contact with the samples (Lygo et al. 1994). It is therefore essential to implement sample contamination mitigation procedures prior to recovery and postmortem data collection operations. At the morgue, triage personnel must also consider whether tissue sampling will hinder subsequent morphological analysis. In such cases, the probative value of morphological analysis must be weighed against the potential for further DNA contamination or degradation. If the fragment is

Table 17.2 A Template of the Triage Probative Index System

	Fingerprint	Dental	DNA	Morphology/Medical	Associated P.E.
HIGH (2)	Full prints attainable	Dental remains present with extensive restorations	Numerous high quality samples that will yield a complete STR profile or mtDNA sequence	Biological profile, prosthesis, tattoo, etc.	Personal effects possessing unique identifying information associated with remains (e.g., ring with inscription)
LOW (1)	Partial prints attainable	Dental remains with no restorations	Decomposed, thermally modified, and/or low mass sample, that will most likely yield partial STR profile or mtDNA sequence	Nothing unique, fragment descriptive as to portion only	Personal effects with no unique identification information associated with remains (e.g., shoe and sock associated with foot)
NONE (0)	No printable tissue (hands/feet missing)	No dental remains	Inappropriate sample (e.g., calcined bone, fibro-fatty tissue)	Unidentifiable fragment	No associated personal effects

considered a good candidate for tissue sampling but is of minor morphological value, sampling prior to invasive examination is recommended. Morphological analysis must, however, take precedent if tissue sampling will compromise anthroposcopic characteristics useful for individuation. Simply stated, there is seldom any good reason to destroy important morphological indicators prior to formal analysis.

Mass Fatality Morgue Operations

Once morgue operations commence, investigators use the probative index to systematically examine, categorize, and route human remains and material evidence to the pertinent morgue sections and agencies (Fig. 17.6). Decedent remains are brought from the scene to the morgue and placed in refrigerated storage until examined. The examination process begins with radiographic screening of each container holding remains. Radiographs provide triage personnel with an overview of the container contents and can be referenced to locate human remains and evidentiary material potentially obscured during the external examination (Lichtenstein and Madewell 1982; Lichtenstein et al. 1980). Radiographic screening has also been used to locate live ordnance prior to examination of the 1992 Persian Gulf War dead (Lichtenstein 1998), and more recently during the 2001 Pentagon attack investigation (Rodriguez 2003).

Material is then physically examined and items relevant to the investigation are identified. Material evidence and unassociated personal effects are documented and

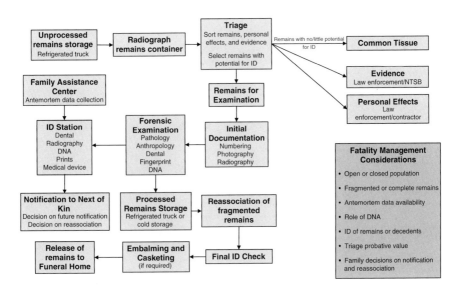

Fig. 17.6 A flow diagram of mass fatality morgue operations

routed to the appropriate controlling agencies after the material has been photographed and described (McMeekin 1980). Personal effects that are physically
associated with remains (e.g., jewelry on a finger) should not be separated at
triage. Removal of such items should be conducted at the pathology station by
personnel trained in documenting and describing personal effects associated with
remains.

Forensic personnel at the triage station then begin to sort human remains according to their potential for identification using preestablished criteria. Investigators
begin resolving commingling issues by separating the various fragments and portions of human remains. Once separated, each fragment can be assessed using the
probative index. Remains that are considered to be common tissue are removed from
the morgue flow based on previously established guidelines. Remains meeting the
criteria for potential identification or investigative value then enter the morgue flow
for documentation and postmortem analysis. Decisions concerning tissue sampling
for DNA analysis are also made at triage. If applicable, a triage form is completed to
indicate specific routing of individual tissue fragments. Individually bagged remains
are then directed to the initial documentation station, where sequential accession
numbers are assigned. Remains are then routed to the applicable postmortem data
collection stations. If, during the course of subsequent examinations, additional
commingling is noted, the remains will be routed back to triage and evaluated using
the established decision-making process. Upon completion of all examinations and
fulfillment of the investigative goals, remains are released from morgue custody for
final disposition.

Case Study: United Airlines Flight 93

The United Airlines Flight 93 investigation presents a recent example of how
the triage concept was utilized to facilitate the identification process. Flight 93
crashed on September 11, 2001, in Shanksville, Pennsylvania, killing all 44 passengers and crew. Approximately 1,500 fragments were recovered, weighing approximately 600 pounds, which represents 8.5% of the estimated passenger and crew
weight.[1] Fragmentation and commingling were significant issues that required
personnel to develop a morgue operations plan that included a triage protocol

---

[1] The low percentage of the total estimated passenger weight recovered during the United 93
investigation is probably due to a variety of factors including impact forces and environment. A
comparison of the United 93 and ValuJet 592 incidents illustrates the importance of the recovery
environment on the weight of recovered remains. The fragmentation indices are similar for the two
crashes (United 93 = 34.09, ValuJet 592 = 38.93); however, United 93 crashed into a field, whereas
ValuJet 592 crashed in a swamp. Approximately 4,000 pounds of human remains, representing
23% of the estimated passenger weight, were recovered from the ValuJet 592 crash site (Mittleman
et al. 2000), compared with 600 pounds from the United 93 site. Passenger weight is largely comprised of body fluids. Upon impact, particularly at high speed in a terrestrial environment, most
of the body fluids will be dispersed into the surrounding environment. It is plausible that in an

(Sledzik et al. 2003). Prior to commencing morgue operations, triage personnel were briefed on the basic triage protocol and DNA tissue sampling guidelines to assure proper handling and routing of human remains.

Recovered material came to the incident morgue and went through a slightly modified version of the aforementioned postmortem data collection process. In this case, radiographs of the disaster pouches were unavailable prior to examination at triage. At times, ubiquitous soft tissue obscured embedded bone or evidentiary material, which made sorting remains based solely on visual inspection difficult. Investigators palpated tissue to determine the presence of bone or evidentiary material. Radiography would have allowed for more rapid and less intrusive examination. Selection criteria for remains that entered the postmortem data collection operation were based on size and tissue type of individual specimens. When commingling was discovered post-triage, remains were returned to the triage station for assessment; if commingling was confirmed, one fragment would retain the original accession number and the other fragments would go through the triage evaluation process independently.

Processing remains took approximately 11 days. During this time, 12 individuals were identified using dental and fingerprint methods. In the following 2 months, DNA analysis resulted in the identification of the remaining 32 decedents and additional remains from those previously identified. Subsequent quality assurance, retesting, and remains reassociation were completed by six months after the event. On average, 12 specimens were identified per decedent (Fig. 17.7). Of the approximately 1,500 fragments recovered, 1,000 (67%) yielded no information leading to identification and were therefore categorized as common tissue at the conclusion of

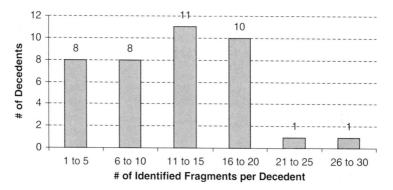

Fig. 17.7 The number of identified fragments per decedent for United Airlines Flight 93. These are minimum estimates since approximately 1000 fragments (67% of recovered remains) were not identified

---

aqueous environment remains will maintain their weight; however, there is no empirical evidence that supports this hypothesis.

the investigation. These remains, along with those not selected for analysis during triage, were categorized as common tissue at the conclusion of the investigation.

Additional Triage Considerations: Staffing, Quality Assurance, and Quality Control

Successful morgue operations are contingent upon collaboration with numerous agencies representing a vast range of investigative interests (Jensen 2000). Understanding their respective roles will mitigate improper handling and/or misrouting of personal effects and evidence during triage. Triage staff must also possess a solid understanding of human anatomy and the multidisciplinary human identification process in order to accurately assess the probative value of each set of remains. Pathologists and anthropologists with prior mass fatality investigation experience are ideal triage station staffing candidates. Triage should also be staffed by evidence specialists and personal effects specialists to evaluate non-human material, and photographers to document material. Odontology, fingerprint, and DNA specialists should assess remains if the primary triage staff is unable to interpret the remains according to preestablished guidelines.

Triage is a dynamic process, requiring constant reevaluation during subsequent phases of examination. Analyses by the various forensic disciplines can reveal potential problems with initial commingling assessments and the probative index. Instituting formal quality assurance reviews will detect any potential inconsistencies in these areas. Common tissue must be reexamined at regular intervals to ensure that potentially identifiable tissue has not been improperly classified. Ideally, reexamination should include radiographic and visual assessment of common tissue. Indirect and direct review should reveal inconsistencies with the triage decision-making process.

Triage brings an additional benefit for understanding taphonomic processes related to the incident. Since it is the only morgue section staffed by a multidisciplinary team, the triage personnel can observe patterns in the types of remains and evidence as they relate to search and recovery operations. Decisions made in the field can compromise the medicolegal investigation if recovery personnel fail to recognize human remains or draw the wrong conclusions regarding the spatial relationships of remains and other material. Brannon and Morlang (2002) and Brannon and Kessler (1999) discuss how improper recognition and recovery of dental remains can negatively impact the identification process. Also, spatial relationships among human remains, personal effects, and evidence can be misinterpreted, leading to erroneous field decisions concerning unassociated personal effects and remains found in close proximity (Wolcott et al. 1980). Recognizing these patterns at triage could suggest improper recovery techniques and thus assist in guiding search and recovery efforts. Effective triage can serve as a communications link between field and morgue operations, one that can minimize the potential for recovery-induced commingling.

Family Assistance Considerations

In the past several years, the term "family assistance" (as it applies to mass fatality situations) has come to define a standard of care and services provided to the family members of decedents. In the United States, the Aviation Disaster Family Assistance Act of 1996 (U.S. Public Law 104-264, Title VII) establishes important rights for families of passengers who die or are injured in major aircraft accidents. The law specifies the National Transportation Safety Board as the lead federal agency to coordinate the resources of other federal agencies, the airline, the American Red Cross, and local agencies in supporting family members (NTSB 2000). The support families receive encompasses travel to and from the accident site, lodging, informational briefings (including information on victim recovery and identification), mental health counseling, accident scene visits, memorial services, and long-term information sharing. The number of family members in attendance at family assistance functions varies greatly depending on the family organization of the passenger population, the accident location, and the ability of family members to travel to the accident site.

Victim identification is a critical aspect of the family assistance process (Levin 2004; OVC 2000; Slater and Hall 1997). Families are involved in the identification process by providing antemortem information and, when appropriate, DNA reference samples. The medical examiner or coroner, as the primary authority responsible for the identification process, works closely with individual family members or in groups at family briefings to inform them about the various identification methods being implemented (Robb 1999) and to reassure families that morgue personnel treat all remains with respect. During these meetings families often ask for, and receive, specific information regarding the particulars of identification.

The issues seen with commingled remains also impact the family members of the decedents. Families often presume that the remains from disasters are complete and that they can be visually recognized. Families must be informed of the general condition of remains because the condition dictates the time needed to complete identification. It is also necessary to explain that, even with the use of DNA technology, there is a chance that all remains will not be identified.

Families are also asked to make decisions about death notification, final disposition of remains, and other concerns. In cases of fragmentation, where multiple fragments from one individual are identified over a lengthy period, families choose when and how often they wish to be notified about identification (i.e., initially, each time an identification of the decedent is made, or never). Families also choose if and when remains will be released to them: as they are identified or when they are reassociated at the end of the identification process. Family preference regarding the disposition of remains is optimally determined prior to the start of the identification process.

Because not all fragmented remains are identifiable, the medical examiner or coroner must decide, in conjunction with the families, about the final disposition of common tissue. Families are informed of the presence of these unidentifiable remains and preferably work as a group to decide upon the final disposition. If families cannot decide, the medicolegal authority takes action under the jurisdiction's laws to dispose of the remains.

Ethical Perspectives on Identification

The need to identify the disaster dead creates a set of unique ethical questions arising from the interplay of three very different worlds: the condition of remains, the expectations of family members, and the tools and technical limitations of identification scientists. The questions, asked by scientists, family members, and society, delve into concerns about how remains are identified, the extent of resource allocation to conduct identifications, and expectations about what is returned to the family for final disposition. These questions are not unique to disaster work; forensic scientists involved in human rights investigations have raised similar concerns (Williams and Crews 2003).

- Should the limited resources available to conduct identification be used to identify all fragmentary remains or all decedents?
- Why does the identification process take so long?
- How large does a specimen need to be for DNA testing?
- Why isn't every specimen analyzed and tested?
- What if a specimen is consumed entirely in testing and yields DNA that leads to an identification?
- At what point does the identification process end?
- Should remains recovered years after a disaster be processed for identification?
- What should be done with unidentifiable remains?

As the agents of society's wishes for the dead, scientists endeavor to use all applicable techniques and technology in the identification process. Despite this, and because of taphonomic factors, science often comes up short. When families expect that identifications will happen quickly and that whole bodies will be returned, scientists must readjust the families' expectations to make them more consistent with the taphonomic reality of the disaster. This difficult but necessary readjustment helps families truly understand the reasons behind the answers to the aforementioned questions. Answers depend on the particulars of the disaster, desires of the family members (individually and as a disaster-specific group), cultural beliefs about death and final disposition of remains, societal expectations about what science can provide, and the availability of appropriate forensic identification tools and techniques (PAHO 2004).

The ethical dilemmas are tempered somewhat by the condition of the remains. For complete remains, since the identifiable features (dental structures, fingerprints, etc.) are directly associated with the body itself, once the body has been identified, the individual has been identified. However, when fragmentation exists, there is no "body" to identify. Rather there are individual anatomical structures that may or may not contain identifiable features or reveal a probative DNA profile. When a specimen contains a unique physical feature that is identified as belonging to a decedent, the presumption is that that decedent is "identified." However, multiple "identifications" can take place as more specimens with individual anthroposcopic features and high-fidelity DNA profiles are identified for that decedent. Because not all fragments are identifiable or provide a DNA profile, these unidentifiable remains (i.e., common tissue) must be managed as an assemblage of remains representing all decedents. Consequently, family members need to be informed of the presence of these remains and participate in the decision-making process governing their final disposition.

One of the more complex decisions is whether to identify all remains or all decedents. The approach to identification efforts varies depending on the answer to this question. In the case of an open population (where not all decedents are known) and fragmented remains, all remains must be analyzed for DNA so that profiles on all decedents can be obtained. Certainly, scientists are aware that not all DNA testing will lead to profiles, but the work must proceed so that all obtainable profiles are available for identification. In a closed population where the decedent information is known, a focus can be placed on identifying the maximum number of remains for each decedent. In these cases, there is no scientific need to test very small fragments since the decedent population is known. A probative index developed with an understanding of these factors is a critical method in ensuring that the needs of the science and those of the family members are considered.

Resolving these ethical quandaries is not often done through public dialogue, given the sensitivities of discussing the horrific details of the event. But, for these questions to be answered appropriately, informed public discussion is essential. Family members of the disaster dead want and deserve frank yet compassionate discourse on these questions. The discussion is difficult, and yet it helps families navigate the complex grief process wrought by a disaster. It also helps society appreciate that even in death, their fellow citizens are considered and cared for. Forensic scientists must do this work for legal reasons, yet they choose to do it because it provides solace to those in need. As Mate Reyes (2003), Spanish philosopher and Holocaust researcher, reflected: "For a civilization to deserve that name, all of life must be valued, including the absent life of the dead."

Conclusions

In order to develop a capable investigative strategy, personnel responsible for establishing mass fatality morgue operating guidelines must have a fundamental understanding of the variables that produce fragmentation and commingling and their effects on the identification process. Before the identification process begins, investigators should decide how best to manage fragmented and commingled remains and establish human remains and evidence processing guidelines. These guidelines must address human remains and evidence tracking procedures, common tissue classifications, the probative index system, and DNA sampling issues. The aforementioned information is then synthesized and a comprehensive triaging system is developed. Triage facilitates the investigative process by detecting and separating commingled remains and by directing human remains, personal effects, and evidence to the relevant morgue examination stations or agencies. Decedent identification success is not necessarily limited by the aforementioned variables, but the speed and effort involved are affected. Keeping family members informed about the progress of identification, and the ways in which commingling and fragmentation impact the process, is a critical aspect of the medicolegal investigation of mass fatality events.

References cited

Alonso, A., P. Martín, C. Albarrán, P. García, L. Fernández de Simón, M. J. Iturralde, A. Fernández-Rodríguez, I. Atienza, J. Capilla, J. García-Hirschfeld, P. Martínez, G. Vallejo, O. García1, E. García, P. Real, D. Álvarez, A. León, and M. Sancho 2005 Challenges of DNA profiling in mass disaster investigations. *Croat. Med. J.* (46):540–548.

Armstrong, J. A., D. I. Fryer, W. K. Stewart, and H. E. Whittingham 1955 Interpretation of injuries in the Comet aircraft disasters; an experimental approach. *Lancet* 268(6875):1135–1144.

Auf Der Heide, A. 1989 *Disaster Response: Principles of Preparation and Coordination*. CV Mosby, St. Louis.

Ballantyne, J. 1997 Mass disaster genetics. *Nat. Genet.* 15(4):329–331.

Bowen, T. E. and R. F. Bellamy (editors) 1988 *Emergency War Surgery*, 2nd ed. Department of Defense, Washington, DC.

Brannon, R. B. and H. P. Kessler 1999 Problems in mass-disaster dental identification: A retrospective review. *J. Forensic Sci.* 44(1):123–127.

Brannon, R. B. and W. M. Morlang 2002 Jonestown tragedy revisited: The role of dentistry. *J. Forensic Sci.* 47(1):3–7.

Brenner, C. H. and B. S. Weir 2003 Issues and strategies in the DNA identification of World Trade Center victims. *Theor. Popul. Biol.* 63(3):173–178.

Budimlija, Z. M., M. K. Prinz, A. Zelson-Mundorff, J. Wiersema, E. Bartelink, G. MacKinnon, B. L. Nazzaruolo, S. M. Estacio, M. J. Hennessey, and R. C. Shaler 2003 World Trade Center human identification project: Experiences with individual body identification cases. *Croat. Med. J.* 44(3):259–263.

Cullen, S. A. and E. P. Turk 1980 The value of postmortem examination of passengers in fatal aviation accidents. *Aviat. Space Environ. Med.* 51(9 Pt 2):1071–1073.

Dirkmaat, D. C., J. T. Hefner, and M. J. Hochrein 2001 Forensic Processing of the Terrestrial Mass Fatality Scene: Testing New Search, Documentation, and Recovery Methodologies. Paper presented at the 53rd Annual Meeting of American Academy of Forensic Science, Seattle, WA.

Goodwin, W., A. Linacre, and P. Vanezis 1999 The use of mitochondrial DNA and short tandem repeat typing in the identification of air crash victims. *Electrophoresis* 20(8): 1707–1711.

Janousek, J. T., D. E. Jackson, R. A. De Lorenzo, and M. Coppola 1999 Mass casualty triage knowledge of military medical personnel. *Mil. Med.* 164(5):332–335.

Jensen, R. A. 2000 *Mass Fatality and Casualty Incidents: A Field Guide*. CRC Press, Boca Raton, FL.

Kennedy, K., R. V. Aghababian, L. Gans, and C. P. Lewis 1996 Triage: Techniques and applications in decision making. *Ann. Emerg. Med.* 28(2):136–144.

Kontanis, E. J., F. A. Ciaccio, D. C. Dirkmaat, and M. I. Jumbelic 2001 Variables Affecting the Success of Victim Identification in Mass Fatality Events. Paper presented at the 53rd Annual Meeting of the American Academy of Forensic Science, Seattle, WA.

Labovich, M. H., J. B. Duke, K. M. Ingwersen, and D. B. Roath 2003 Management of a multi-national mass fatality incident in Kaprun, Austria: A forensic medical perspective. *Mil. Med.* 168(1):19–23.

Leclair, B., C. J. Frégeau, K. L. Bowen, S. B. Borys, J. Elliott, and R. M. Fourney 1999 Enhanced Kinship Analysis and STR-based DNA Typing for Human Identification in Mass Disasters. Paper presented at the 8th International Society of Forensic and Haemogenetics Congress, San Francisco, CA.

Levin, B. G. 2004 Coping with traumatic loss: An interview with the parents of TWA 800 crash victims and implications for disaster mental health professionals. *Int. J. Emerg. Ment. Health* 6(1):25–31.

Li, G. and S. P. Baker 1997 Injury patterns in aviation-related fatalities. Implications for preventive strategies. *Am. J. Forensic Med. Pathol.* 18(3):265–270.

Lichtenstein, J. E. 1998 Radiology in mass casualty situations. In *Forensic Radiology*, B. G. Brogdon, ed. CRC Press, Boca Raton, FL.

Lichtenstein, J. E. and J. E. Madewell 1982 Role of radiology in the study and identification of casualty victims. *Radiologe* 22(8):352–357.

Lichtenstein, J. E., J. E. Madewell, R. R. McMeekin, D. S. Feigin, and J. H. Wolcott 1980 Role of radiology in aviation accident investigation. *Aviat. Space Environ. Med.* 51(9 Pt 2): 1004–1014.

Ludes, B., A. Tracqui, H. Pfitzinger, P. Kintz, F. Levy, M. Disteldorf, J. M. Hutt, B. Kaess, R. Haag, B. Memheld et al. 1994 Medico-legal investigations of the Airbus A320 crash upon Mount Ste-Odile, France. *J. Forensic Sci.* 39(5):1147–1152.

Lygo, J. E., P. E. Johnson, D. J. Holdaway, S. Woodroffe, J. P. Whitaker, T. M. Clayton, C. P. Kimpton, and P. Gill 1994 The validation of short tandem repeat (STR) loci for use in forensic casework. *Int. J. Legal Med.* 107(2):77–89.

McMeekin, R. R. 1980 An organizational concept for pathologic identification in mass disasters. *Aviat. Space Environ. Med.* 51(9 Pt 2):999–1003.

Midda, M. 1974 The role of dental identification in mass disasters. *J. Irish Dent. Assoc.* 20(2):51–62.

Mittleman, R. E., J. S. Barnhart, J. H. Davis, R. Fernandez, B. A. Hyman, R. D. Lengel, E. O. Lew, and V. J. Rao 2000 *The Crash of ValuJet Flight 592: A Forensic Approach to Severe Body Fragmentation.* Miami-Dade County Medical Examiner Department.

Nijman, J. 1980 Triage: The evaluation of disaster casualties. In *Disasters, Medical Organization*, J. D. Boer and T. W. Baillie, eds., pp. 79–83. Pergamon Press, Oxford.

NTSB 2000 Federal Family Assistance Plan for Aviation Disasters. National Transportation Safety Board, Washington, DC.

2002 *Aircraft Accident Brief, Accident No. DCA00MA052.* National Transportation Safety Board, Washington, DC.

OVC 2000 Responding to Terrorism Victims: Oklahoma City and Beyond. U.S. Department of Justice, Office for Victims of Crime, Washington, DC.

PAHO 2004 *Management of Dead Bodies in Disaster Situations: Disaster Manuals and Guidelines Series, No. 5.* Pan American Health Organization, Washington, DC.

Read, C. A. and J. Pillay 2000 Injuries sustained by aircrew on ejecting from their aircraft. *J. Accid. Emerg. Med.* 17(5):371–373.

Reyes, M. 2003 *Memoria de Auschwitz.* Editorial Trotta, Madrid.

Robb, N. 1999 229 people, 15,000 body parts: Pathologists help solve Swissair 111's grisly puzzles. *CMAJ* 160(2):241–243.

Robison, J. L. 2002 Army nurses' knowledge base for determining triage categories in a mass casualty. *Mil. Med.* 167(10):812–816.

Rodriguez, W. C. 2003 Attack on the Pentagon: The Role of Forensic Anthropology in the Examination and Identification of Victims and Remains of the '9/11' Terrorist Attack. Paper presented at the 55th Annual Meeting of the American Academy of Forensic Science, Chicago.

Slater, R. E. and J. E. Hall 1997 *Final Report: Task Force on Assistance to Families of Aviation Disasters.* Department of Transportation and National Transportation Safety Board, Washington, DC.

Sledzik, P. S., W. Miller, D. C. Dirkmaat, J. L. de Jong, P. J. Kauffman, D. A. Boyer, and F. N. Hellman 2003 Victim Identification Following the Crash of United Airlines Flight 93. Paper presented at the 55th Annual Meeting of the American Academy of Forensic Science, Chicago.

Sledzik, P. S. and W. C. Rodriguez 2002 Damnum fatale: The taphonomic fate of human remains in mass disasters. In *Advances in Forensic Taphonomy: Method, Theory, and Archaeological Perspectives*, W. D. Haglund and M. H. Sorg, eds., pp. 321–330. CRC Press, Boca Raton, FL.

Taneja, N. and D. A. Wiegmann 2003 Analysis of injuries among pilots killed in fatal helicopter accidents. *Aviat. Space Environ. Med.* 74(4):337–341.

Tyrrell, A. J., E. J. Kontanis, T. L. I. Simmons, and P. S. Sledzik 2006 Restructuring Data Collection Strategies and Investigation Priorities in the Resolution of Mass Fatality Incidents. Paper presented at the 58th Annual Meeting of the American Academy of Forensic Science, Seattle, WA.

van den Bos, A. 1980 Mass identification: A multidisciplinary operation. The Dutch experience. *Am. J. Forensic Med. Pathol.* 1(3):265–270.

Vosswinkel, J. A., J. E. McCormack, C. E. Brathwaite, and E. R. Geller 1999 Critical analysis of injuries sustained in the TWA Flight 800 midair disaster. *J. Trauma* 47(4):617–621.

Wagner, G. N. and R. C. Froede 1993 Medicolegal investigation of mass disasters. In *Medicolegal Investigation of Death: Guidelines for the Application of Pathology to Crime Investigation*, 3rd ed., W. U. Spitz and R. S. Fisher, eds., pp. 567–584. Charles C. Thomas, Springfield, IL.

Williams, E. D. and J. D. Crews 2003 From dust to dust: Ethical and practical issues involved in the location, exhumation, and identification of bodies from mass graves. *Croat. Med. J.* 44(3):251–258.

Wolcott, J. H., R. Menzies, E. Donahue, and N. Hoffa 1980 Use of personal effects in the Canary Island accident investigation. *Aviat. Space Environ. Med.* 51(9 Pt 2):1019–1020.

Chapter 18
Data Management and Commingled Remains at Mass Fatality Incidents (MFIs)

Michael Hennessey

Introduction

Commingling occurs when the remains of more than one victim become intermixed. A thorough review of fragmentary remains during triage at the morgue should resolve most instances of commingling, but in some cases commingling may be detected only when separate examinations yield contradictory results. For example, at the World Trade Center (WTC), multiple DNA tests on the same set of remains sometimes yielded different profiles. In other cases, dental X-rays and DNA from the same set of remains were linked to different victims. Conflicting antemortem and postmortem data can also indicate commingling. In another case from WTC, the DNA from a victim's reference sample (known personal effect) matched a set of remains, yet the jewelry on the remains was contrary to the description provided by the spouse. After further review, the identification was reassigned. In each of these cases, visual examination had not initially detected the presence of commingled remains.

A key lesson learned from mass fatality incidents (MFIs) is that one cannot rely on a single identification method to detect commingling. All postmortem results for a case need to be reviewed for consistency. Then all of the postmortem data must be reconciled against all of the antemortem information associated with the identification. This administrative review process ("admin review") relies on being able to locate all of the case information in a timely fashion. Unfortunately, gathering all of the case information is error-prone as missing data are not always obvious. For example, if there is a matching DNA result, one might not think to ask if there is a *second* DNA test extant.

The main point of this chapter is that even if great care is exercised in the recovery and analysis of remains, the identification process may be compromised if the data are not managed correctly and an investigator misses an inconsistency. This chapter will examine the most common challenges in this regard and suggest some solutions. The framework presented here is that admin review is a data management process that spans the antemortem and postmortem information gathering systems and unites the various identification methods (anthropology, DNA,

From: *Recovery, Analysis, and Identification of Commingled Human Remains*
Edited by: B. Adams and J. Byrd © Humana Press, Totowa, NJ

fingerprint, dental, pathology, property, and X-ray). In this way, the detection and resolution of commingled remains is a multidisciplinary effort.

Unless otherwise noted, the examples in this paper are real cases. The names and identifying numbers have been anonymized to protect the privacy of the families.

MFI Data

In response to an MFI, a family assistance center (FAC) is usually established to provide services to the families of the victims. In addition, interviewers at the FAC will collect missing persons reports. Employers will provide information about staff presumed lost at the scene, and other organizations (tour agencies, airlines) may also have data to contribute regarding the victims. Anyone filing a report is an *informant,* and this antemortem (AM) information can be divided into three categories:

1. Primary data for identifications: Fingerprints, X-rays (primarily dental), and DNA are the principal methods of identification. Although other techniques can be used, such as tracing the serial number from a surgical implant, they are not applicable in most cases. While families do not always bring the X-rays or fingerprint cards to the FAC, they do provide the contact information for the custodians of this data. DNA reference materials (such as a razor or toothbrush), on the other hand, are usually provided directly by the family.
2. Secondary data for identifications: Although not sufficient to make a positive identification on its own, descriptive information about the victim's jewelry, clothing, tattoos, surgical histories, or distinctive anatomical features can be used to generate investigational leads that can point to the correct primary data for an identification. Secondary data can also be used to return property to the families of the victims.
3. Administrative data for case management: The victim's contact information (name, date of birth, address, phone number, etc.) and demographic data (age, race, gender, stature, etc.) are used to create and manage the case file. The demographic data can also contribute to the creation of investigational leads as well as the detection of potential problems (e.g., a male DNA profile associated with female remains). In addition, a case number is usually established at this time. Information about the interview itself belongs in this category: the informant and interviewer's name, their contact information, date and time of the interview, etc.

When remains are received in the morgue, they will generate postmortem (PM) data that are also primary, secondary, and administrative. In many ways, the identification process at an MFI is a function of integrating the AM and PM information. This chapter will specifically review the principal challenges an investigator faces in reconciling such data.

Identification Errors at an MFI

The remains of victims at disasters are sometimes fragmented, so a victim's primary AM data will often match the primary PM data from multiple sets of partial remains. The reverse, however, is problematic: Primary PM data from a set of remains linking to more than one AM file should undergo further review. Such cases are usually the result of commingling, investigative mistakes, or administrative error.

MFIs are often associated with severe physical traumas (plane crashes, earthquakes, explosions, etc.) that can result in the fragmented remains of one victim becoming embedded in the tissue of another victim. Such cases are not always apparent to the naked eye and may not be recognized during triage at the morgue. The tissue of person A may become fused with the bone of person B such that it appears to be articulated to it. Open wounds can suffer DNA contamination from the blood of other victims. Furthermore, recovery workers may place multiple sets of remains in one body bag. It is standard practice to separate such remains into different cases during mortuary intake (e.g., triage), but this is sometimes missed in the initial chaos of the disaster response. Finally, commingling can sometimes occur *during* the autopsy. This happened on occasion in Thailand after the 2004 Asian Tsunami (hereafter referred to as "Tsunami") when fingers or hands removed for prints were returned to the wrong body bag.

Investigative Mistakes

Investigative mistakes can happen in two ways. First, errors may occur during the analysis of the remains or reference items, resulting in flawed primary data. Second, an analyst may make a fortuitous match between primary AM and PM data due to incomplete test results or, with DNA, make a mistake keying in a kinship equation. A complicating factor is that the analysis and matching activities may be performed in different locations by different personnel.

Administrative Error

Administrative error is where the information is accurate but is in the wrong case. This can happen with AM or PM data, but AM records are more at risk, as victims with similar names can have their case files confused. This potential increases if they share other information such as an address or DNA donor. Victims from the same family are especially vulnerable in this regard. But AM or PM files with nothing in common can be erroneously combined if case numbers are confused or tracking numbers transposed.

Example: Commingling

In one case at WTC, two separate remains with matching DNA profiles were linked to John Smith. The anthropology review showed that the first set of remains was an upper torso with a complete mandible and limbs, while the second set of remains was a complete mandible. The case file for the disarticulated mandible stated that it had been recovered from the chest cavity of the remains to which it was matching by DNA.

Odontologists matched the disarticulated mandible to the AM records of Walter Jones. They also confirmed that the mandible attached to the torso was consistent with the dental chart for John Smith. When the second mandible had been recovered from the chest cavity, a tissue sample was taken for DNA testing. Apparently, the force of the impact affixed tissue from the torso so firmly to the mandible that it appeared to be articulated to it and it was sampled for DNA. As a result, the DNA profile for the loose mandible matched the torso and the personal effects of John Smith. At this point, a tooth was taken from the disarticulated mandible and DNA testing showed it was consistent with the reference samples for Walter Jones. Both identifications were finalized.

Example: Investigative Mistakes

Investigative mistakes usually do not result in false matches because two victims would need to have nearly identical profiles, the analyst would have to make a mistake only at that single point of difference, and the error would have to be such that it transforms the data from the first victim to match the second victim. Given the underlying frequency distributions of DNA, fingerprint, and dental profiles (which are all highly heterogeneous), it is more likely that an investigative error would result in a false exclusion. That said, there are two situations where the potential for a false match increases: DNA testing on degraded remains and DNA matching using partial profiles. These are related issues in that degraded remains often produce partial DNA profiles, but they lead to investigative mistakes in different ways.

DNA Testing on Degraded Remains

DNA samples are often tested in batches, with samples placed into wells on a tray. A well can contaminate an adjacent well on the same tray, and tray-to-tray contamination can occur if robotic pipettes carry trace sample from a well in one tray to the corresponding well in the following tray. Two DNA profiles in one well will be flagged during the technical review, but a well with sample from remains too degraded to yield DNA will only show the profile from the *contaminating* well. In this way, the DNA profile of one set of remains can be incorrectly assigned to a second set of remains.

In one WTC case, DNA linked two remains to the same victim, but an anthropology review showed that they could not be from the same person. The anthropologist noted that one of the remains was badly burned, suggesting its DNA was compromised. This remain was retested, it failed to give a DNA result, and it was removed from the identification. A review of the laboratory process located the source of the contamination and it was fixed. This illustrates the need for a multidisciplinary approach: Anthropology not only caught a mistake, but it alerted the DNA laboratory to an operational problem.

Partial DNA Profiles

A second scenario where an investigative mistake can result in a false match is when working with partial DNA profiles. An error at a single point of comparison will usually not be enough to make the full profiles of two different people appear to be the same, but degraded remains may yield only a handful of genetic markers. When compared to the AM data, it is possible that the difference between this limited PM data set and the complete AM profile is so small that a single error of interpretation may be sufficient to lead an analyst to make a fortuitous match.

Example: Administrative Error

In the spring of 2002, a whole body was recovered from WTC's Ground Zero with personal effects for "Jason Arturo." An arm had already been identified as Arturo's by DNA in the fall of 2001. The whole body was tested for DNA, and it had a different profile than the arm. The laboratory file for Arturo showed that six separate DNA reference collections were received from the FAC in the fall of 2001. But an audit of the collection logs from the FAC showed that only *five* DNA collections had taken place for Arturo (this log had not been available to the laboratory when the arm was identified as Arturo).

At the FAC, victims were given case numbers while each DNA collection received a tracking number. The extra collection number in Arturo's laboratory file was 453. The log at the FAC listed collection 453 as belonging to Nathan Riley, victim number 227. One of Arturo's DNA collection numbers was also 227. The author reviewed the errant package and noted that numbers 453 and 227 were present, but with no label to indicate which was the victim number and which was the collection number. Riley's name was also missing, a failure of the standard operating procedure at the FAC. The log showed that collections 453 for Riley and 227 for Arturo took place on the same day, so there was an overlap in their handling. Based on the review, it was apparent that Riley's victim number had been confused with Arturo's collection number and that his reference samples had gone in the wrong folder. After the error was recognized, Riley's samples were given their own case file. All of Arturo's reference samples were tested, and they matched the whole body recovered in the spring of 2002.

It has been pointed out to the author that if all the reference items had been tested, then a conflict among Arturo's samples might have been noticed much earlier. While true, this ignores the fact that thousands of reference items were pouring into the laboratory, some of dubious quality. Testing everything would have delayed the identification process by months, without appreciably improving the chances of an identification. In order to spot conflicts within a case (or suspicious matches between unrelated cases), all of the AM testing would have to be completed first. Refusing to release the first DNA match until the last reference item has been tested is probably not a viable policy given the urgency of releasing identifications as soon as possible. However, it *is* possible to compare the FAC collection logs to the case files in the DNA laboratory when a match is made, and an audit of this kind would have flagged Arturo's case. Once the FAC collection log was available to the DNA laboratory at WTC, such audits became a routine part of the admin review.

Likewise, while conflicting PM results from a single set of remains will be discovered during a case review, this assumes that remains will not be released until all primary methods are complete. Again, pressure to release identifications in a timely manner may trump such a policy, and many fragmented remains are simply not amenable to multiple examination techniques. For these reasons, one cannot rely on conflicting primary data to flag commingling, investigative mistakes, or administrative errors. However, an investigator can review the secondary and administrative data for matches, as inconsistencies at this level would suggest that further review is needed. For example, with WTC, the husband of Donna Parker donated his wife's hairbrush as a source of DNA. The profile matched several sets of fragmented remains, including a hand wearing an engagement ring and wedding band with multiple diamond settings. A review of the property report filed by the husband listed only a single gold wedding band. An investigator called the husband and confirmed that Donna did not have a diamond ring and wore only the plain wedding band. Meanwhile, a search of the jewelry descriptions in the AM records found a match to both rings in the file of an unidentified victim. The hand was removed from the Parker identification and placed under separate investigation.

Summary of Identification Errors at an MFI

At an MFI, an investigator should not treat a match between primary AM and PM data as an identification, but as the start of the investigation. The next step is to reconcile all of the AM and PM data (primary, secondary, and administrative). This admin review can catch commingling, investigative mistakes, and administrative errors that would otherwise go undetected. To audit a match, however, an investigator needs to review all of the information related to a case. As it turns out, locating all of the relevant data can be a challenge, especially with the AM files. The next section in this chapter will examine why this is so difficult.

AM Information Intake Dynamics

At an MFI, numerous people will file missing persons reports for the same victim, but will not do so as a single group. The spouse may file a report the day of the disaster, a sibling may go to the FAC the next day, and the parents might fly into town later. It is unrealistic to expect that they will go to the FAC together. Some informants may have to travel a significant distance, while others are nearby and want to file a report immediately. People in different stages of grief may not be ready to visit the FAC at the same time. And some family members may be estranged and prefer to make separate visits.

In addition to family intakes, employers will provide AM data for staff that perish at an MFI, either as victims or as responders. Because the WTC were office buildings, most of the victims were at work when the attack took place, and their employers provided a great deal of information. Several employers played a liaison role, transferring DNA reference samples from families abroad to the FAC. The Fire Department of New York (FDNY) played a similar liaison role on behalf of the firefighters lost at WTC.

This dynamic of staggered intakes was also quite pronounced after the Tsunami. Survivors filed reports in Thailand for missing family members. At the same time, friends and family in the home countries went to their local FACs to do the same, sometimes mistakenly reporting individuals as missing who had survived and were themselves providing AM data in Thailand on other victims.

If an informant is not aware that a file already exists for a victim, the interviewer will create a duplicate file. Even when the informant knows that a case has already been opened, the interviewer may have to start a fresh intake if he does not have access to the existing file, or he may elect to start a new form, recognizing that different informants sometimes provide conflicting information.

In addition to multiple informants, a single informant may initiate multiple intakes. In the time between a disaster and the establishment of the FAC, an informant may file a report with her local police and then again with the police department in the jurisdiction of the disaster. These reports are usually forwarded to the FAC. An informant may call the FAC to open a report before visiting in person. Once there, she may not be able to complete the intake on the first visit as most people do not know their mother's shoe size or the phone number of their brother's dentist. They may need to gain access to their son's apartment to retrieve a toothbrush for DNA testing. Finally, they may be too grief-stricken to finish the interview in one sitting. At WTC, it was not unusual for a case file to contain several intakes from the same informant. After the Tsunami, tourists filed missing persons reports in Thailand and then again in their home country. After Hurricane Katrina, not only did officials collect AM data in the Gulf, but some municipalities where survivors were relocated also collected redundant missing persons reports.

All of the interviews for a victim need to be integrated at some point. But since most intake forms are quite long, they are rarely completed in full. When looking at files that might be for the same victim, a file manager is usually working with data that only partially overlap. This is especially true for updates from returning

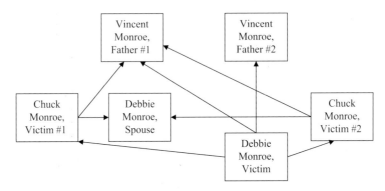

Fig. 18.1 Chuck, Vincent, and Debbie Monroe: one case or three?

informants since the very purpose of a follow-up intake is to provide information that was not available during the previous interview. If different informants give conflicting answers (or if different interviewers record similar answers in a disparate manner), the records manager may hold intakes apart until clarifying information can be gathered. On the other hand, just as comparing partial primary PM data to full AM data can lead to a fortuitous match, so can comparing two partial AM intakes lead to two files being wrongly combined.

Figure 18.1 represents the file from WTC for Chuck Monroe. It contained several intakes from the father, Vincent, and the spouse, Debbie. Not only did the intakes from Debbie and Vincent disagree on some basic issues, but the different intakes from each informant were not internally consistent. Eventually, it was determined that there were *two* victims named Chuck Monroe and that their files had been mistakenly combined. One was unmarried and had a father named Vincent, while the other was married to Debbie. Complicating the matter was the fact that there was also a victim named Debbie Monroe and some of her information wound up in the file for Chuck Monroe because the informant and victim name were transposed. As if that were not enough, the informant for Debbie was her father, a gentleman named Vincent Monroe. At this point it appeared that Debbie and one of the Chuck Monroes might be siblings. Their reference DNA was analyzed to establish that they were unrelated, their files were reorganized, and their identifications went forward.

Case Numbers

Issuing a Missing Person (MP) number for each victim can reduce many problems associated with victim names since it can be used like a case number to manage the files. When returning to the FAC, the MP number can be used to link an update to the correct case, but it is not foolproof:

- An informant may be related to more than one victim and have several MP numbers. If he gets the numbers mixed up, then the data will be linked to the wrong case.

- Different agencies (FEMA, Red Cross, the police, etc.) will issue their own case numbers, which an informant may confuse with the MP number.
- The MP number can be corrupted. At WTC, telephone intakes were given T Numbers (example: T-138) while personal interviews at the FAC got P Numbers (example: P-138). T Numbers were accidentally converted to P Numbers in some databases so that T-138 became P-138. This meant that P-138 was in the system twice, linking to two different victims. As a result, some of the DNA reference samples and AM intakes were misfiled. Eventually, a Reported Missing (RM) number replaced both the P and T Numbers and the errant cases were reconciled.
- Reading MP numbers is error-prone. MP 1221 may get confused with MP 1212. If the victim list is alphabetized and assigned consecutive MP numbers, then victims with the same last names will have nearly identical case numbers: Lee (133), Lee (134), Lee (135). Barcodes can make case numbers more reliable but cannot eliminate these problems. Their initial assignment can be incorrect, subsequent intervention in the tracking database can introduce errors, and incompatible barcode systems in a multi-agency response is almost a guarantee. Finally, even with barcodes, some file handling will still be conducted manually.

Summary of AM Intake Dynamics

Multiple informants per victim and multiple intakes per informant can lead to AM files that are consolidated incorrectly. As a result, a victim's information may be spread out over several unlinked files, each lacking the data necessary to make an identification. And if one file does contain primary data that match a PM case, an investigator may not realize that crucial information exists in another folder. Conversely, if data for victim A are placed in the folder for victim B, then a PM match to victim A will be identified as victim B. To better understand how these two outcomes occur and what an investigator can do in response, we need to examine the AM interview process in detail.

Challenges in the AM Interview Process

There are at least six possible points of failure in the AM interview process:

1. Incorrect information from the informant
2. Informant misunderstands the question
3. Lack of standardized answers
4. Typos and transpositions
5. Handwriting
6. Data in the wrong field

Incorrect Information from the Informant

It is possible that the informant will provide incorrect information. In fraud cases, this is intentional. Once in the system, such information (and reference items) can become mixed with legitimate cases. For this reason, even fraudulent case files must be audited.

At WTC, one fraud case had the same name as a real victim and a personal effect from the legitimate case was accidentally filed in the fraudulent case folder. Even though no DNA testing was scheduled for the fraud case, its file was audited. The errant personal effect was discovered and used in the identification of the legitimate case.

Informants will also unintentionally provide incorrect information. Given the variety of people who go to the FAC (parents, siblings, spouse, children, co-workers, employers, etc.) and the range of questions asked, it is to be expected that a given informant may be mistaken in some of her answers. This results in intakes with conflicting information that an investigator needs to reconcile. Because names and dates are often used to manage case files, they merit special consideration.

- Anglicized names: Foreign nationals often adopt Anglicized names while living in English-speaking countries. Friends, co-workers, and employers may refer to the adopted name while parents and siblings use the birth name. Won Park went by John Park at work, and his AM records at WTC included both names.
- Nicknames: An informant may provide the victim's nickname, such as Katie or Jack, while others provide the full name Catherine or John.
- Alias: Some people use an alias or go by their middle name. "Carl James Anderson" might be reported as such, while others refer to him as "Jim Anderson."
- Incomplete surnames: If a surname has multiple terms, one informant may give just the last term while others provide the full surname. This happened regularly at WTC with Hispanic, Arabic, Asian, and African names. For instance, AM intakes for Hector Tirado Jimenz included both Hector Tirado Jimenz and Hector Jimenz.
- Maiden names: A woman may retain her maiden name at work for business reasons. The employer, co-workers, and old friends may report her missing by the maiden name while immediate family members will provide the married name.

Some of these examples may appear trivial at first. After all, anyone looking at the files for Catherine Bigsby and Katie Bigsby can see the likely connection. But this relies on some cultural familiarity. An American might know that Jack is a common nickname for John, but is that widely known abroad? The popular Southern nickname "Bubba" can substitute for any first name, a fact that may not be widely known abroad. Conversely, how many Americans know that the Russian diminutive for Alexander is Sasha? Or that Jay can be short for Sanjay?

Spotting the similarities between the names on two case files also relies on their being in close proximity to each other. But when the victim list at WTC was sorted by surname, Carl Anderson and Jim Anderson were separated by several entries

(Clyde Anderson, Dave Anderson, etc.), diluting the apparent connection. And a search for "Tirado Jimenez" failed to retrieve this victim's folder, which was filed under "Jimenez." Only after the victim list was sorted by date of birth did these records cluster together.

Another problem can occur because adult children don't always know the year of their parent's birth and may be too embarrassed to admit it, so they estimate. And couples can marry privately and have a public wedding later. In such cases, the wedding date provided by the parents will not match the date given by the spouse. This is important when trying to link the date inscription on a ring to an AM file.

Informant Misunderstands the Question

"What is your relationship to the victim?" An informant at WTC answered "Father," but his DNA profile did not fit the family pedigree. A review of the intake showed that his date of birth was after the victim's, which meant that the victim was *his* father. The pedigree was revised and it worked. This shows how administrative data (the donor's date of birth) can resolve problems. Other questions that can be misinterpreted by the informant include "Address?" (the informant's or the victim's?), "Parents of the victim?" (biological or legal?), and "Where did they work?" (location or employer?).

Lack of Standardized Answers

If interviewers use different terms to record the same information, then a search of the AM database by one term will only find a portion of the relevant records. And if the AM and PM nomenclature is not consistent, then searching either database for investigational leads becomes problematic. Most intakes use checkbox answer menus where possible, but some concepts are not so easily categorized and the interviewer has to manually record the data, leading to more nonstandardized answers.

Jewelry descriptions in the Tsunami database included "YM," "yellow metal," and "gold." All are accurate, but a search by one term will fail to find the records using the other term. A PM report at WTC for the top half of a head read "male, hair = none." A search of the AM database for men where hair was "none" failed to return the records for bald men. While all manually recorded data are subject to this problem, names, dates, and object descriptions are particularly vulnerable.

Names

There are three main standardization issues with regards to names: generational identifiers, multi-termed names, and word order.

Generational identifiers such as Junior, Jnr., and Jr. are all accurate, but if inter-viewers use all three, then separate intakes for the same victim will often lack matching names. A search for "Smith, Jr." will not find "Smith, Junior," and vice versa.

Multi-termed surnames present two challenges. The first is determining where the surname begins. The second is deciding how to handle hyphens. In a case from WTC, a woman named Alice Mayhew-Jones had separate AM intakes filed under

- Alice Mayhew-Jones
- Alice Mayhew Jones
- Alice Jones
- Alice Mayhew (filed by the parents, who were estranged from their son-in-law)

Sorting the records by last name meant that Mayhew-Jones and Jones did not cluster together. Searching by "Jones" or "Mayhew" retrieved only half the records. And searches by "Mayhew Jones" failed to return Mayhew-Jones.

Word order: In English, it is typical to address people by their forename and list names alphabetically by surname. But some cultures do the opposite. If an American interviewer is told that the victim's name is "Kim Won Duk," he may reverse the terms to correspond to the "surname, forename" format, as in "Won Duk, Kim." But if the informant gave the name in the Korean style (surname first), then Kim is the surname, not Won Duk. Other informant-interviewer pairs may generate different combinations for the same victim.

Dates

The European format is Day/Month/Year while in the United States it is Month/Day/Year. Since many disasters in the United States have an international dimension, both date formats will likely appear in the AM records, especially if foreign employers, embassies, or police agencies are involved in collecting information from the home countries. A wedding date on a foreign-sourced intake may read 7/3/75 while a PM report on wedding band from a set of remains may be recorded as 3/7/75. Complicating the matter is that some common software programs format numeric dates as text. In this way, it is not immediately apparent that March 7, 1975, and July 3 could be the same date.

Objects

Certain objects associated with a victim can be useful to an investigator, such as jewelry, clothing, and tattoos. Unfortunately, it is very difficult to standardize their descriptions, as the "YM vs. yellow metal vs. gold" jewelry example illustrates. For the Tsunami, AM reports came in from around the world, and there was a multinational presence in the morgue. As a result, AM and PM descriptions often reflected national variations in describing the same object. For example, swimwear was alternatively described as swimsuits, bathing suits, bathing costumes, bikinis, swim trunks, or Speedos.

A final example illustrates how widespread nonstandard entries can be. At WTC, searching the AM database for employees of "Cantor-Fitzgerald" would not retrieve records for "Cantor Fitzgerald" (no hyphen), "Cantor Fitz," or "Cantor." Each entry is accurate and clear to anyone reading it, but these variations made it challenging to find all of the cases related to the company.

Typographical Errors and Transpositions

All manual intake systems are prone to typographical errors, and MFI data are no exception. For example, in the clothing descriptions of the AM files at WTC, there were 26 variations on the spelling of "khaki." Transpositions can occur in phone numbers, addresses, and birth dates. Even names can be transposed. An intake for "Andrew Clarke" was filed under "Clarke Andrew." In more than a few cases, the informant and victim names were transposed. Not only did this make it harder to find the AM data for a victim, but it put a living person on the list of the reported missing.

Handwriting

Many intake systems are handwritten. Not only is handwriting hard to read, but it encourages the use of abbreviations and acronyms, which may not be obvious to the reader. These forms often provide only limited space to record answers, forcing one to write smaller (reducing legibility) and use more abbreviations. When later entered into a database, there is the possibility of transcription errors. For example, the number 4 can look like a 9, the letter a can be confused with the letter o and so on. The victim list at WTC had an entry for AHOV, but no AM intake could be found for this person. Eventually, the file was found under the correct name, Attov. The two lowercase ts had been read as an uppercase H.

Data in the Wrong Field

If an AM tattoo description is logged in the field for clothing descriptions, it is effectively hidden from an investigator searching for a match to a tattoo on a set of remains. A more common problem is that data can often be recorded in more than one place. For example, many forms have fields for describing a wallet and its contents. Most intakes also have a section for the driver's license. Because these are often found in the wallet, it is not unusual to see them documented in the wallet section instead.

The generic instance of this dynamic is the intake question with checkbox answers where the last choice is "Other," accompanied by a blank text field. While this design has obvious merit, it means that the answer may reside in the text field or the checkbox. In addition, most forms have a section at the end for "Other Information." Data are often entered here despite the existence of a dedicated section elsewhere on the form. As a result, searching the answer checkboxes to a dedicated question will often miss relevant records.

Error Rates in the AM Records

The Disaster Mortuary Operational Response Team (DMORT) is an agency of the U.S. government that assists local medical examiners at MFIs. They have an AM/PM data collection system called the Victim Identification Program (VIP); the AM form is 7 pages long with nearly 300 data fields for about 200 questions. There are more fields than questions because some questions ask for several pieces of information, such as addresses (street, city, state, and zip code). The author's experience in working with VIP at WTC was that an average intake completed about 200 data fields.

If there are six variables in capturing information correctly (detailed above), then we can estimate the accuracy of an intake with the formula ($\%^N$), where $\%$ is the chance that a variable is executed correctly and N is the number of variables. This assumes the variables are independent and that the chance of success for each is constant. If an AM interview is 99% accurate at each of the 6 possible points of failure, then an answer is estimated to be correct 94% of the time ($.99^6$). The estimated error rate is 1 minus the estimated accuracy rate, or $1 - 0.94 = 0.06$. With 200 data fields, a 6% error rate yields an estimated 12 errors per interview.

But 99% accuracy may be too much to expect. Consider sitting in the comfort of your home buying books on the Internet. You are providing a small amount of personal information that is well known to yourself. There is no handwriting and no interviewer, just you entering data into the computer. Yet, it is not uncommon to make mistakes in this setting, suggesting that the accuracy rate may realistically fall below 99%. Now imagine you are at an FAC in a distant city being interviewed by a complete stranger regarding a loved one presumed dead in a disaster. The interviewer asks numerous personal questions, such as your wife's bra size or whether your brother was circumcised. Was he ever arrested? Who is his dentist? The interviewer is polite but hastily writes down your answers. Later they will be entered into a computer by someone else who has already read dozens of intakes that day.

In this context, 99% accuracy might be optimistic. If we lower it to a more realistic 95%, then the estimated accuracy of a data field is ($.95^6$) = 75%, or an error rate of 25%. For 200 data fields, this is 50 problems per intake. A plane crash with 150 victims and 3 informants per victim would have about 22,500 data problems ($150 \times 3 \times 200 \times 0.25$). If each informant has a follow-up interview during which she completes another 50 data fields ($150 \times 3 \times 50 \times 0.25$), that is another 5,625 problems, for an estimated total of 28,125.

It is worth stressing here that this does not mean the data are wrong (although that is possible). Problem data in this context can mean that a correct answer is in the wrong field or was recorded in an irregular manner (Jr. vs. Junior, hyphens in the surname, European date format, etc.). It may have a minor typo or transposition or answers a different question than the interviewer intended. As a result, the record will not be found by a search or sort of the files using these criteria. Linking updates can also be challenged by such problem data.

Assume that there is one informant per victim and each makes an initial visit to the FAC, creating a case file. Each informant then returns a few days later to provide a DNA sample. With 150 victims, that is 150 updates that have to be linked to the correct case. If this process is 95% accurate, then 5% of the follow-ups are at risk. If these 7 or 8 updates are added to the wrong folder, then about 15 cases would be impacted, or 10% of the total. One can see how this number increases with each successive round of updates and if more than one informant is involved.

At WTC, there was a victim named Henry Niles and another named Henry Niles, Jr. They were unrelated. The son of Henry Niles made several trips to the FAC, as did many members of the family, resulting in numerous intakes and case numbers. The son was named Henry Niles, Jr., and on one visit to the FAC his update was accidentally placed into the file for the victim named Henry Niles, Jr., because the person handling the file confused the informant name with the victim name. Unfortunately, this update contained DNA reference samples. Eventually, these profiles linked to a set of remains that were incorrectly identified as Henry Niles, Jr. The error was only discovered during the admin review.

Error Rates in the PM Records

PM records are vulnerable to (1) lack of standardization in recording data, (2) handwriting issues, (3) typographical errors, and (4) storing data in the wrong field. Assuming 99% accuracy at each possible point of failure means a record is 96% accurate (.99^4). PM forms often mirror the AM intakes in organization and can run several pages with hundreds of data fields. Not every topic will be relevant for each set of remains, so assume that only 200 data fields will be completed. That is about eight errors per record.

Cases may be reexamined and these updates need to be linked to the correct folder. If 25% of all autopsies are reexamined and 5% of these are incorrectly linked, then there will be about a dozen update errors per 1,000 cases. Since each error affects 2 cases, about 2.5% of all PM cases will have a filing error ($1,000 \times 0.25 \times 0.05 \times 2$).

For example, assume there is an MFI with 200 victims and each body fragments into 7 pieces (at WTC, nearly 20,000 remains were recovered for about 2,750 victims). That is 1,400 PM cases. Eight mistakes per intake and a 2.5% updating error rate mean a PM database with 11,235 problems. Again, this does not mean just errors of fact, but correct data that are recorded in a manner that makes it difficult for an investigator to pursue a match or consolidate records.

Addressing the Problems

While an ounce of prevention is certainly worth a pound of cure, the nature of disaster response seems to guarantee that there will always be problem data. This section will look at prevention first and then address how to work with problem data.

Preventing Problems

There are several steps an agency can take to reduce the data errors at an MFI. First, it should define the AM/PM intake forms it will use ahead of time. Since local authorities will likely receive assistance from DMORT, it is a good idea to preview VIP, available at www.dmort.org. Interpol also has a series of Disaster Victim Identification intake forms that may be helpful (www.interpol.org). An agency could use one of these systems and create supplemental forms to reflect local needs, or it could design its own MFI system based on the missing persons forms already used in its jurisdiction.

Once the intake system has been defined, standardized recording formats should be adopted for names (generational identifiers, multiple-termed surnames, hyphens, etc.) and dates (MM/DD/YYYY or DD/MM/YYYY). The rest of the questions should be reviewed to standardize answers where possible, particularly the abbreviations and acronym for describing objects, concepts, and affiliations. It is critical that both PM and AM intakes use the same nomenclature. This is not a matter of finding the "correct" format so much as having a consistent approach.

Rather than limiting this process to those who will collect the data (mortuary staff and interviewers at the FAC), it should also include the database managers who will administer the system as well as the investigators who will use it to make identifications: medical examiners, pathologists, odontologists, anthropologists, fingerprint examiners, and DNA analysts. DNA is noteworthy here because not only are DNA experts often left out of disaster preparedness planning, but they are sometimes not even included in the immediate disaster response because of the perception that DNA is not timely.

When finally deployed, DNA often inherits policies and systems that do not reflect the needs of forensic biology, impeding their effectiveness. Concerns regarding the pace of DNA testing are often deflected by calling it the method of last resort, and this is dutifully repeated by the media, perpetuating the notion that DNA methods are slow. In many ways it is a self-fulfilling prophecy. A notable exception to this mindset is the close coordination between the Armed Forces DNA Identification Laboratory (AFDIL) and DMORT. Not only are the protocols in place for DNA testing prior to a disaster, DNA teams from AFDIL deploy with DMORT as part of the initial disaster response.

Computer resources should be secured to avoid handwritten intakes. Staffing rotations should be established for the morgue and the FAC. Liaisons at partner agencies should be included in the planning stages and vendors expected to provide services, equipment and consumables should likewise be included to ensure that they have the necessary surge capacity.

Conduct mock AM interviews. Not only is it valuable training, but it will test the efficiency of the intake system and may help flag individuals who really are not suited to interviewing grieving families.

Barcode systems should be established and checked for intra-agency compatibility. Tracking labels based on the barcode numbers should be readable by humans, and a case name/numbering schema should be developed to create a unique identifier for every object in the system. On the PM side, this would include body bags, recovered property, and samples taken for fingerprinting, odontology, or DNA. On the AM side, there are informants, victims, intakes at the FAC, and reference materials submitted for fingerprints, X-rays, and DNA.

There are four general considerations in developing the naming schema. First, it has to contain enough information to allow a human operator to work with the object. A person should be able to tell at a glance if he is holding an AM or PM folder.

Second, toe tags, file folder tabs, X-rays, test tubes, etc. can be quite small. This places a practical limit on the length of the label name. Using a tiny font to make a name fit does not support the first guideline. In these cases it may be prudent to place small items in larger containers that can support larger labels.

Third, the label should not include any information that may be modified or updated. As has been shown, victim data can change with each intake, even for seemingly static concepts like name and date of birth. The problem is that corrections to a label are not backwards-compatible. The old label already exists on boxes, on sample tubes, and in printouts. It resides in spreadsheets and databases that may not be available for updating. An investigator working with a changed label will not be able to trace a reference sample backwards through the system to intake, voiding its chain of custody.

On the other hand, uncorrected label names are a source of confusion. At WTC, a reference sample for Jonas Clare had the prefix BM for Biological Mother. But it had a male profile. A review of the AM intakes for Clare showed that the spouse brought their infant son to the FAC to provide DNA. Mrs. Clare signed a consent form for minors and under "relationship to donor," she wrote "mother." The interviewer entered this as the relationship to the *victim,* and a tracking label was created with the prefix BM. This sample was flagged as a problem by every new analyst who saw it, consuming countless hours of staff time explaining the situation or reinvestigating the matter. But changing it to BS (Biological Son) would have created a different problem: The collection log for Clare at the FAC (maintained by a separate agency) still showed a single DNA donation from the mother and all of the transaction records for this case listed a BM sample. An investigator starting with the BS sample would not be able to work backwards to find a DNA collection from the son of Jonas Clare, and the chain of custody would have been broken for a perfectly viable sample. In the end, it was decided that being able to track the sample through the identification process was more important than a name with the correct relationship code, a decision the author wholly supported. From a data management point of view, it is better to have a name that is flawed but consistent than one that is inconsistent. But the best approach is simply not to embed data about the sample in the sample name, as this information can and will change.

The fourth guideline for creating a naming schema is that it be compatible with systems already in place. Collaborating agencies and vendors will have their own information management systems, complete with accessioning numbers, data fields, reporting tools, and standard operating procedures. The more information one tries to include in the label name, the more likely it is to conflict with these preexisting systems. For instance, one could mandate that label names for property include the letter R if it is a ring. The evidence division at a supporting police agency may already have a protocol of using J for jewelry, followed by a number to indicate the type: 1 = ring, 2 = necklace, etc. Everyone working on property will have to translate R to J1 and back again. And they will have to perform separate translations for each property type. The situation becomes even more cumbersome when the label name attempts to capture information from the internal process at the supporting agency. DNA testing is a complex undertaking with several process steps and the potential for samples to repeat certain steps. While the operating parameters in place at each step may be useful to the analyst interpreting DNA results, there is no need to squeeze this into the sample label. Such data are fully available in the laboratory's information management system (LIMS) and can be linked to the sample name as a supporting file.

Ultimately, labels designed to display information regarding the handling of an object are easily compromised. In Thailand after the Tsunami, body bag numbers were based on the nationality of the autopsy team. Unfortunately, countries rotated staff every few weeks, reducing the specificity of this number. Other autopsy teams were multinational in composition, rendering the number ambiguous. As bodies were reexamined, autopsy teams added new body bag numbers to reflect their nationality. This became a significant source of confusion as many body bags eventually had more than one tracking number.

Solving Problems

In order to audit a proposed identification or create an investigational lead, one must first assemble all of the potentially relevant AM records. First, conduct multiple searches that are broad enough to ensure that no relevant record is missed (this approach accepts that irrelevant files will be also retrieved). Second, compile the searches and cull unrelated cases by sorting the list via a demographic detail and removing the records in clusters that are disqualified. Manually review the remaining cases to consolidate or exclude. For example, search for Employer = Acme and Gender = Male. If the victim lived in New Jersey, sort the results by State and omit all entries except NJ.

Some basic tips for conducting broad searches:

- Use truncated surnames with wildcards to overcome typographical errors: Rama* will find Ramachandran and Ramashandran.
- Phonetic variations can find misspelled names: Lee & Li, Cane & Kane.
- Wildcards can find nonstandard uses of generational identifiers and hyphens: Hernan* will find Hernandez-Tirado, Hernandez Tirado, Sr., and Hernandez, Senior.
- Objects can be described in a variety of ways, so try synonyms like gold & yellow, brown & brunette, or bikini & swimsuit.
- Consider acronyms and abbreviations, such as YM vs. yellow metal or FDNY vs. Fire Department, New York City.
- Try reverse searches: If you are looking for the files on Terry John, try putting Terry in the surname field. If a ring has a date inscription of 11/8/83, query the wedding date fields for that as well as 8/11/83.
- Search related fields such as (wallet/purse and driver's license). Query catch-all summary fields in associated sections of the intake.
- Do not use AND with multiple field searches. Remember that many fields in an intake will be left blank and records lacking data in a field will be excluded by searches that mandate data be present. A search for "Asian" AND "Male" AND "Tattoos = Yes" will not return records for tattooed males where race was left blank.

Again, the key to finding all the potentially relevant records is not to conduct a single, precise search that finds "the" record for a case. In fact, it could be argued that the only thing worse than a search that returns no matches is a search that returns some matches, creating a false sense of success. The search strategy has to exhaust all possible avenues of linking to a relevant file.

The heuristic of conducting several broad searches and then excluding irrelevant records is a tactical approach for researching individual cases. But there is also a need for a comprehensive, systemwide view of the data. First, one should map the AM and PM operations in order to identify the links in the chain where material and/or information is handed off. Once the process has been mapped, then the inventory manifests between each link can be compared to reveal missing or surplus items.

For example, remains will be recovered at the disaster site, moved to a local collection area, transported to the morgue's holding facility, pulled for autopsy, and placed in storage. A different group will carry out each step, the performance of which will generate time and date stamps, employee names, and details specific to the function at hand. Search teams will note the location where remains were found, evidence techs will list the property recovered, pathologists will provide autopsy findings, and mortuary attendants will note where the remains are stored. In addition to the body bag number and a master PM file that travels with the remains, each group may have its own recordkeeping system complete with tracking numbers, barcodes, and databases.

If the morgue accessions a dozen set of remains from the disaster site in a single day and all are autopsied, then mortuary storage should also accession a dozen set of remains that day. If not, that would be a cause for review. At WTC, the accession and inventory numbers did not always match, because as anthropologists reviewed the remains in autopsy, they discovered cases of commingling. The remains would be separated, creating a new postmortem case. In other instances, they determined that the remains were nonhuman and removed them from the system. Both were sound policies and accounted for the disparate numbers at different points in the process.

A critical component of mapping the system and reconciling inventories is defining the terminology used at each link in the chain. The FAC at WTC generated a P Number for each victim and a DNA Case Number for each DNA collection. This information, along with the DNA references, was sent to the New York State Police DNA laboratory. The NYSP database already had dedicated fields for tracking data, so the P Number was filed under their Incident Number and the DNA Case Number went in their Reference field. The Case field in the NYSP database was then populated with a tracking number called the WDI Number. When tracing DNA samples through the system, it was important to clarify which Case Number was being referred to, the one from the FAC or that from the NYSP. It was also critical to know that the P Number at the FAC became the Incident Number at the NYSP and that the DNA Case Number became the Reference Number.

Generic terms like case, file, collection, incident, sample, reference, and item were routinely used by agencies at WTC with different meanings, a phenomenon the author witnessed again in the Tsunami response. While it may not be possible to standardize the usage of these terms across all links in the chain, defining their different meanings can reduce handling errors and facilitate tracing an item's chain of custody.

Summary

Preparing for the information management needs of a disaster ahead of time may not eliminate all of the data management problems that can arise when numerous agencies collaborate on a project, but it can reduce the scope of the problems that will emerge. A sound data management strategy after the disaster will allow for the effective integration of AM and PM records in support of the identification process. The most critical dimension of this process is using the data to create investigational leads and reconcile all of the information (primary, secondary, and administrative) when there is a match between AM and PM data.

Index

Notes on Editors

Bradley J. Adams

Bradley J. Adams received his BA from the University of Kansas and his MA and PhD from the University of Tennessee. He is currently the Director of the Forensic Anthropology Unit for the Office of Chief Medical Examiner in New York City. He is also affiliated with numerous universities in the NYC area. In his present position with the OCME, Dr. Adams and his team are responsible for all forensic anthropology casework in the five boroughs of New York City (Manhattan, Brooklyn, Queens, the Bronx, and Staten Island). Since 2006, Dr. Adams and his team have been undertaking a large-scale effort to recover additional human remains associated with the terrorist attacks on the World Trade Center. Prior to accepting the position in New York City, Dr. Adams was a Forensic Anthropologist and Laboratory Manager at the Central Identification Laboratory in Hawaii.

John E. Byrd

John E. Byrd received his Doctor of Philosophy in Anthropology from the University of Tennessee in 1994. In 1998, he became a Forensic Anthropologist at the Central Identification Laboratory and in 1999 was promoted to Laboratory Manager. Dr. Byrd has led field recovery operations throughout Europe, Asia, and the Pacific as part of his duties in JPAC's CIL. Dr. Byrd has published papers in the *Journal of Forensic Sciences*, *Journal of Field Archaeology*, and *Journal of Anthropological Archaeology* as well as numerous book chapters. He is a Diplomate of the American Board of Forensic Anthropology and currently serves as a member of the Editorial Board of the *Journal of Forensic Sciences*.

Notes on Contributors

Patricia Bernardi

Patricia Bernardi has an advanced degree in Anthropology from Universidad de Buenos Aires. She cofounded EAAF (Equipo Argentino de Antropología Forense) 23 years ago, and since then has acted as expert witness for the judiciary, special commissions of inquiry, and international tribunals. She has worked for EAAF in Argentina and other Latin American countries, the Balkans, Ethiopia, Zimbabwe, Congo (DRC), East Timor, Sierra Leone, Rwanda, and Romania on the application of forensic anthropology and archaeology to the investigation of human rights cases. She has conducted training seminars, presentations, and lectures on the application of Forensic Sciences at both academic and legal venues all over the world.

Erik T. Bieschke

Erik T. Bieschke has earned degrees in biology (BS) and forensic science (MS). He has worked in the field of forensic biology since 1999. From 2002 to 2005, he was responsible for analyzing, interpreting, and troubleshooting DNA test results associated with the identification of victims from the World Trade Center. He has also been involved with criminal casework, as well as research, development, and validation for new testing methods, which have lead to publications and presentations at regional, national, and international conferences.

Emily A. Craig

After earning her master's degree in medical illustration from the Medical College of Georgia in 1976, Emily A. Craig worked at the Hughston Sports Medicine Foundation in Columbus, Georgia for 15 years. In 1994 she earned a Ph.D. in physical anthropology from the University of Tennessee in Knoxville. That same year she accepted a position with the Kentucky Medical Examiner's Office and she now works full-time as that state's forensic anthropologist. Her responsibilities include field recoveries, laboratory analysis, and identification of decomposed, fragmented, and skeletonized human remains. She is an associate coordinator of Kentucky's Mass Fatality Response Team and she serves as gratis Assistant Clinical Professor in the University of Louisville School of Medicine's Department of Pathology & Laboratory Medicine.

Sharna Daley

Sharna Daley is a Forensic Archaeologist for the International Commission on Missing Persons (ICMP), based in Sarajevo—Bosnia and Herzegovina. She received her BSc in Zoology from Queen Mary and Westfield Collage, University of London and her MSc in Forensic Archaeology from Bournemouth University. For the past 5 years she has been employed by ICMP within the Forensic Science Division, providing technical assistance to the local national authorities—assisting with and directing excavations of complex mass grave sites and other complex site types. In her current role as Supervisory Forensic Archaeologist/Field Operations Manager, she is responsible for the implementation of ICMP's guidelines and policies at excavations sites, as well as for the training of local and international staff and development of the division.

Franklin Damann

Franklin Damann is a graduate of Louisiana State University, Baton Rouge with an MA in anthropology. He is currently a PhD candidate in anthropology at the University of Tennessee, Knoxville. He worked as a forensic anthropologist at the JPAC Central Identification Laboratory prior to his current position as Curator of the Anatomy Department, National Museum of Health and Medicine AFIP, Washington, D.C.

Joanne Bennett Devlin

Joanne Bennett Devlin is a faculty member in the Department of Anthropology at The University of Tennessee, Knoxville. She is a skeletal biologist broadly trained in bioarchaeology and forensic anthropology. She received both her MA and Ph.D. degrees from UTK, where a focal point of much of her research was upon the impact of taphonomic processes upon bone. Current research foci include deducing particular signatures of heat alteration and establishing models of fire behavior in automobiles.

Mercedes Doretti

Mercedes Doretti has an advanced degree in Anthropology from Universidad de Buenos Aires. She cofounded EAAF (Equipo Argentino de Antropología Forense) 23 years ago, and since then has acted as expert witness for the judiciary, special commissions of inquiry, and international tribunals. She has worked for EAAF in Argentina and other Latin American countries, the Balkans, Ethiopia, South Africa, Zimbabwe, the Ivory Coast, Congo (DRC), East Timor, Iraq, and the Philippines on the application of forensic anthropology and archaeology to the investigation of human rights cases. She has coordinated EAAF's New York office since 1992, has recently published in forensic anthropology anthologies, and has conducted training seminars, presentations, and lectures on the application of Forensic Sciences at both academic and legal venues all over the world.

Suni Edson

Suni Edson is a graduate of the State University of New York College of Environmental Science and Forestry in Syracuse, New York with an MS in environmental and forest biology. She is currently employed as a supervisory DNA analyst at the Armed Forces DNA Identification Laboratory in Rockville, MD, where she has been employed since 1999.

Sofía Egaña

Sofía Egaña has an advanced degree in Anthropology from Universidad Nacional de Rosario. Since she joined the staff of EAAF (Equipo Argentino de Antropología Forense) 5 years ago, she has acted as expert witness for the judiciary, special commissions of inquiry, and international tribunals. She has worked for EAAF in Argentina, East Timor, El Salvador, Brazil, Mexico, and South Africa on the application of forensic anthropology and archaeology to the investigation of human rights cases. She has conducted training seminars, presentations, and lectures on the application of Forensic Sciences at both academic and legal venues all over the world.

Laura C. Fulginiti

Laura C. Fulginiti is a board-certified forensic anthropologist working in the Phoenix metropolitan area. She provides service to the Medical Examiners for the northern and western counties in Arizona, as well as the National Park Service, the FBI, and other agencies as necessary. Dr. Fulginiti maintains an office and laboratory at the Maricopa County Forensic Science Center in downtown Phoenix. She provides training for the law enforcement communities in Arizona, Nevada, Ohio, Colorado, and at FLETC in Georgia. She is an adjunct professor at Arizona State University, a Visiting Assistant Professor at The Colorado College and an Instructor at Northern Arizona University. Dr. Fulginiti is a member of DMORT, Region IX, a federal disaster response team. She has responded to multiple mass fatality events including airline crashes in Colorado, Guam, California, and Pennsylvania (9/11), the tri-state crematory incident in Georgia and Hurricanes Katrina and Rita. She is involved in research pertaining to traumata incurred during MVA vs. Pedestrian accidents, age-at-death determination, and the effects of corrosive chemicals on bone and tissue.

Anahí Ginarte

Anahí Ginarte has an advanced degree in Anthropology from Universidad Nacional de la Plata. Since she joined the staff of EAAF (Equipo Argentino de Antropología Forense) 17 years ago, she has acted as expert witness for the judiciary, special commissions of inquiry, and international tribunals. She has worked for EAAF in Argentina and other Latin American countries, the Balkans, Ethiopia, South Africa, Zimbabwe, the Ivory Coast, Congo (DRC), Sierra Leone, and East Timor on the application of forensic anthropology and archaeology to the investigation of human rights cases. She has conducted training seminars, presentations, and lectures on the application of Forensic Sciences at both academic and legal venues all over the world.

Michael Hennessey

Michael Hennessey is the Director of Disaster Response at Gene Codes Forensics (Ann Arbor, MI). Gene Codes Forensics was the principal DNA data management consultant for the World Trade Center victim identification project and Mr. Hennessey was the project lead. In this capacity, he directed the administrative review process for the identification effort and helped develop the Mass Fatality Identification System (M- FISys), which is the DNA matching software that manages the WTC DNA data. In addition to 9/11, Mr. Hennessey's experience includes the crash of American Airlines Flight 587, the Asian Tsunami of 2004, Hurricane Katrina, and missing persons investigations at the Procuraduria General de la Republica in Mexico. In addition, he helped implement an informatics solution for disaster victim identification in the United Kingdom. Mr. Hennessey has a Masters of Business Administration from the University of Michigan.

Nicholas P. Herrmann

Nicholas P. Herrmann serves as a Research Assistant Professor for the Department of Anthropology at the University of Tennessee, Knoxville. He received his Bachelor's and Master's degrees in Anthropology from Washington University in St. Louis. His studies focused on anthropological archaeology and biological anthropology. Dr. Herrmann completed his doctorate at the University of Tennessee, where he concentrated on skeletal biology, GIS applications, and forensic anthropology.

Mike Hochrein

Mike Hochrein received his Bachelor of Arts degree from the University of Pittsburgh. His postgraduate work in anthropology and the administration of justice was also accomplished at the University of Pittsburgh. Since 1988 he has been a Federal Bureau of Investigation Special Agent. He is currently assigned to the Laurel Highlands Resident Agency within the FBI's Pittsburgh Division. There, he investigates a variety of federal violations including violent crimes, computer crimes, public corruption, and financial crimes. Prior to joining the FBI, Agent Hochrein was a field archaeologist and analyst on salvage and research projects. Specializing in historical archaeology, he worked for the Carnegie Museum of Natural History and University of Pittsburgh Cultural Resources Management Program. As an FBI Evidence Response Team member, Agent Hochrein develops and conducts research, teaches, publishes articles, and testifies in areas of geotaphonomy and forensic archaeology, as well as crime scene mapping and general evidence collection. Agent Hochrein has traveled to the Middle East, Africa, and Southeast Asia to assist in crime scene investigation training for national police organizations.

Ute Hofmeister

Ute Hofmeister is the Forensic Advisor of the Assistance Division of the ICRC (International Committee of the Red Cross), based in Geneva. Since 1995 she has worked internationally as forensic specialist in a variety of contexts for international organizations (such as UN, ICTY, ICMP) and for local teams (EAAF, FAFG)—mainly in Latin America and the Balkans—before joining the ICRC in 2005. After studying at the Universities of Heidelberg, Vienna, and Arizona, she has specialized in forensic archaeology, documentation, and management of forensic data. Among other things, she is currently responsible for developing a database for forensic investigations and human identification especially for post conflict and developing country contexts.

Rifat Kešetović

Rifat Kešetović completed his medical studies in Tuzla, Bosnia–Herzegovina in 1987 and worked as a general practitioner in Brcko. He went on to finish a specialization in Forensic Medicine in 1998 also at Tuzla University. He obtained an MSc in Forensic Medicine in 2002, and is currently working on a PhD. Dr. Kešetović

has worked for the International Commission on Missing Persons since 1999 as the
Chief Forensic Pathologist at the Podrinje Identification Project.

Lyle W. Konigsberg

Lyle W. Konigsberg is a Professor of Anthropology at the University of Illinois at
Urbana-Champaign, where he teaches anatomy in the Medical School and anthropology in the Anthropology Department. He received his Ph.D. from Northwestern
University and was a postdoctoral scientist in the Department of Genetics at the
Southwest Foundation for Biomedical Research in San Antomio, Texas. Following
his postdoc, he was Assistant, Associate, and then Full Professor of Anthropology at
the University of Tennessee, Knoxville. He is a past Vice President of the American
Association of Physical Anthropologists. His research focuses on human biological
variation, population and quantitative genetics, human skeletal biology, and paleodemography.

Elias Kontanis

Elias Kontanis received his Ph.D. in 2005 from Cornell University, and is currently
a forensic anthropologist and DNA coordinator with the Joint POW/MIA Accounting Command-Central Identification Laboratory (JPAC-CIL). Dr. Kontanis participated in the investigation of the 2001 attack on the World Trade Center and the
1999 crash of Egypt Air 990 as a member of the Disaster Mortuary Operational
Response Team. He has also worked as an anthropologist in Cyprus with Physicians
for Human Rights and served in Thailand as a JPAC-CIL anthropologist during the
medicolegal investigation of the 2004 South Asian Tsunami. His research focuses
on the medicolegal aspects of mass fatality incident management and the human
identification process. He is an associate member of the American Academy of
Forensic Sciences, a member of the International Association for Identification, and
a registered Medicolegal Death Investigator (D- ABMDI). Dr. Kontanis is an FAA-
certified instrument-rated private pilot for single- engine land, fixed-Wing aircraft.

Elaine Mar-Cash

Elaine Mar-Cash was the lead supervisor of the World Trade Center DNA Identification Unit for the New York City Office of Chief Medical Examiner. During her 4
1/2 years on the project to identify the highly fragmented remains of 2,749 victims,
she oversaw the daily operations of the DNA identification process. This included
comparisons of STR, mitochondrial and SNP profiles, performing kinship analysis,
verification of chains of custodies (for both unknown and exemplars samples), data

management of over 100,000 DNA profiles, and the review of data and Quality Control problems. Her responsibilities also required that she act as liaison between the Forensic Biology Department and other departments regarding WTC issues, frequently working with forensic anthropologists to resolve commingled cases. In addition to her work on the aftermath of 9/11, she worked on the crash of American Airlines Flight 587 as well as over 200 criminal cases, including homicides and sexual assaults. She brought her expertise to Phuket, Thailand as a volunteer after the tsunami. Mrs. Mar-Cash has a Bachelor's degree in Molecular and Cell Biology from UC Berkeley and her Masters in Forensic Science from John Jay College of Criminal Justice in New York.

Amy Zelson Mundorff

From 1999 to 2004, Amy Zelson Mundorff was the Forensic Anthropologist for the Office of Chief Medical Examiner, the City of New York, where she analyzed forensic cases involving unidentified individuals and bone trauma. She also helped direct mortuary operations for several disasters, including the World Trade Center attacks, the crash of American Airlines Flight 587, and the Staten Island Ferry crash. She holds a Master's degree from California State University, Chico. Currently, she is completing her Ph.D. at Simon Fraser University in the Department of Archaeology. Besides forensic anthropology, she also has experience as a field archaeologist in California, Hawaii, Jamaica, and New York, excavating prehistoric and historic sites as well as performing osteological analyses.

Gary Reinecke

Gary Reinecke received his Bachelor of Science Degree from the State University College of New York at Buffalo. Since 1977 he has been involved in crime scene investigations, both as a Police Officer with the Columbus, Ohio Division of Police and as a Special Agent with the Federal Bureau of Investigation. He has been assigned to the FBI Laboratory Division for the past 9 years as part of the FBI Evidence Response Team Unit as a Supervisory Special Agent. He is responsible for the training of ERT members and is mainly focused on operational matters. His experience is in the recovery of human remains and he manages an annual FBI ERT class in the recovery of human remains in conjunction with the University of Tennessee. His operational experience includes death investigations in Kosovo, Mexico, Persian Gulf, Afghanistan, Lebanon, Albania, and he deployed to Thailand during the recent tsunami. He has conducted crime scene training in Europe, the Middle East, and Asia.

Joseph L. Rife

Joseph L. Rife is an ancient historian and archaeologist who investigates social structure, mortuary behavior, and skeletal biology in the Greek world during the Roman Empire and the Early Byzantine period. He received his Ph.D. in Classical Studies from the University of Michigan and he now teaches at Macalester College (St. Paul, Minnesota); he has previously held positions at Cornell University and the Institute for Advanced Study in Princeton. Over the past 18 years Prof. Rife has conducted research widely in the Mediterranean basin. He has directed the Kenchreai Cemetery Project (2002–2006), an interdisciplinary archaeological program at a major port of Roman date in southern Greece, and he is codirector of a large-scale excavation at Kenchreai under the auspices of the American School of Classical Studies and in collaboration with the Hellenic Ministry of Culture.

Maureen Schaefer

Maureen Schaefer is a postdoctoral researcher at the University of Dundee, Scotland, where she is currently working on a lab manual to help with the identification and aging of juvenile skeletal material. Her doctoral research was also conducted at the University of Dundee and focused on the use of epiphyseal union data as a means to help overcome problems associated with the identification process. The idea for her research stemmed from her involvement in Bosnia, while working for the International Commission on Missing persons from 2002 to 2003. She also has an MA in anthropology, obtained from Louisiana State University (2001) and a BS in mortuary science, obtained from the Cincinnati College of Mortuary Science (1995).

Robert C. Shaler

Robert C. Shaler received his doctoral degree from the Pennsylvania State University in 1968. He joined the scientific staff of the Pittsburgh and Allegheny County Crime Laboratory in 1970, where, as a criminalist, he practiced forensic science, testified in court, and investigated crime scenes. He joined the Aerospace Corporation staff in 1977 and managed four Law Enforcement Assistance Administration contracts. In 1978, he joined the staff of the New York City Medical Examiner's Office as the head of its serology laboratory, a position he held until 1987, when he moved to the Lifecodes Corporation, the nation's first forensic DNA typing laboratory. It was there that he introduced "DNA Fingerprinting" to the Nation's legal and law enforcement communities through a series of nationwide, informational lectures. Dr. Shaler returned to the Medical Examiners Office in 1990 where he created a modern Department of Forensic Biology. In the wake of the terrorists' attacks on the World Trade Center, he assumed responsibility for DNA identification effort.

He designed the testing strategy and eventually coordinated the work of six different laboratories in that effort. In July 2005, he retired from the medical examiner's office and accepted professorship at The Pennsylvania State University where he is the director of the university's new forensic science program.

Paul S. Sledzik

Paul S. Sledzik received his MS in Biological Anthropology from the University of Connecticut and has been with the NTSB since 2004. From 1990 to 2003, he served as curator of the anatomical collections at the National Museum of Health and Medicine, Armed Forces Institute of Pathology. In 1998, he was the first forensic scientist to be appointed as a Disaster Mortuary Operational Response Team (DMORT) regional commander. He has worked in different capacities in several major disasters, but always seeks to incorporate forensic anthropological methods to the disaster response. His current position with the NTSB involves coordinating local, state, and federal resources for transportation disaster victim identification.

Frederick Snow

Frederick Snow is the Forensic Anthropologist for the State of Georgia and has been employed with the Georgia Bureau of Investigation (GBI) in Decatur, Georgia since 2002. He has worked in Kosovo excavating mass graves as an agent of the United Nations, and in 2001 he spent 8 months in Bosnia and Herzegovina excavating mass graves and analyzing the remains for the International Commission on Missing Persons. Shortly after returning from Bosnia he was called to Noble, Georgia by the Disaster Mortuary Operational Response Team (DMORT) to serve as an anthropologist during the Tri-State Crematory incident. In 2005 he spent 3 weeks in Thailand serving in an administrative role during a multinational effort to identify the victims of the tsunami as well as 8 days in Biloxi, Mississippi during the Hurricane Katrina recovery. From 1997 to 2007 he served as a forensic anthropologist with DMORT, and he is also a forensic anthropologist for several national and international disaster teams. From 1973 to 1980 he served as a patrolman with the Dekalb County Police Department in Decatur, Georgia. He received his Master's degree and Ph.D. in anthropology from the University of Tennessee.

Kris Sperry

Kris Sperry graduated from Kansas State College of Pittsburgh in Pittsburgh, Kansas in 1975 and completed medical school at the University of Kansas School of Medicine in Kansas City, Kansas in 1978. Following an internship in Allentown, Pennsylvania, Dr. Sperry served as a commissioned officer for 2 years in the United

States Public Health Service, specifically in the Indian Health Service on the reservation of the Red Lake Band of Chippewa Indians in Red Lake, Minnesota. He completed a pathology residency at the University of New Mexico School of Medicine in 1985, followed by a fellowship in the forensic pathology with the office of the Medical Investigator for the State of New Mexico. Dr. Sperry was Associated Medical Investigator and later became Medical Investigator for the Office of the Medical Investigator for the State of New Mexico from 1986 to 1989. He assumed the position of Associate Medical Examiner and later the position of Deputy Chief Medical Examiner for the Fulton County Medical Examiner's Office in Atlanta, Georgia from 1989 to 1997. He was appointed Chief Medical Examiner for the State of Georgia, Georgia Bureau of Investigation Division of Forensic Science in 1997 and currently serves in the position/capacity. Dr. Sperry is a nationally recognized expert in the fields of forensic pathology and childhood injury, and has lectured extensively concerning the evaluation of childhood injury and abuse.

Dawnie Wolfe Steadman

Dawnie Wolfe Steadman is an Associate Professor at Binghamton University whose teaching and research interests include bioarchaeology, paleopathology, and forensic anthropology. She is a Board Certified forensic anthropologist and serves as a consultant for a number of agencies in the United States. She is a member of the Disaster Mortuary Operational Response Team (DMORT) and has assisted with the identification of victims from the World Trade Center disaster on September 11, 2001, and the Tri-State Crematorium incident in 2002. Dr. Steadman is also involved in human rights investigations and has worked in Argentina, Cyprus, and Spain.

Hugh Tuller

Hugh Tuller is a Forensic Anthropologist in the Joint POW/MIA Accounting Command's Central Identification Laboratory on Hickam Air Force Base, Hawaii. He received his BA in Criminal Justice from Michigan State University and his MA in Anthropology from Louisiana State University. In the past he has assisted in and/or directed the excavations of individual, multiple, and mass graves with the International Criminal Tribunal for the former Yugoslavia (ICTY), the International Commission on Missing Persons (ICMP), and, under the sponsorship of the Argentine Forensic Anthropology Team (EAAF), the Committee on Missing Persons (CMP). He has published and presented several works on mass grave/fatality processing strategies.

Silvana Turner

Silvana Turner has an advanced degree in Anthropology from Universidad de Buenos Aires. Since she joined the staff of EAAF (Equipo Argentino de Antropología Forense) 18 years ago, she has acted as expert witness for the judiciary, special commissions of inquiry, and international tribunals. She has worked for EAAF in Argentina and other Latin American countries, the Balkans, Ethiopia, South Africa, Zimbabwe, and the Philippines on the application of forensic anthropology and archaeology to the investigation of human rights cases. She has conducted training seminars, presentations, and lectures on the application of Forensic Sciences at both academic and legal venues all over the world.

Douglas H. Ubelaker

Douglas H. Ubelaker is a physical anthropologist who conducts research on methodology as well as applications of human skeletal biology to remains recovered from both archeological and forensic contexts. He received his Ph.D. from the University of Kansas in 1973 and currently holds the position of Curator in the Smithsonian Institution's National Museum of Natural History. Since 1977, he also has served as consultant in forensic anthropology for the Federal Bureau of Investigation in Washington, D.C. and Quantico, Virginia.

Mark Viner

Mark Viner is Senior Clinical Advisor at St Bartholomew's and The Royal London Hospitals, London, UK. He is a Fellow of the Cranfield University Institute of Forensic Science at the Defence Academy of the United Kindom, where he is Director of Operations and Programmes for the International Forensic Centre of Excellence (INFORCE). He has over 23 years experience as a radiographer and radiology manager in the United Kingdom and his interests are in forensic imaging and the management of major incidents. He has acted as radiography consultant for a number of high-profile cases in the United Kingdom and overseas. He has extensive experience of organizing forensic radiography response to mass fatality incidents including the London Suicide Bombings, the Tsunami Disaster, and United Nations war crimes investigations in the Former Yugoslavia and Sierra Leone. He is a forensic radiography advisor to the United Nations International Criminal Court, the UK Home Office, the Government Office for London and is a consultant radiographer for LGC forensics and team member of Kenyon International Emergency Services. In 1998, he formed the forensic subcommittee of the Trauma Imaging Group and is a founder member and first Chairman of its successor, the Association of Forensic Radiographers (AFR), currently holding the position of Honorary Secretary.

In 2005 he was awarded a Winston Churchill Travelling Fellowship to study the role of radiography in forensic medicine in South Africa, Argentina, and the United States. He is a College of Radiographers Assessor and Validator and was awarded an Honorary Fellowship of the College of Radiographers in 2005.

Michael Warren

Michael Warren is an Associate Professor of Anthropology at the University of Florida, with research interests in forensic identification, human variation, and trauma analysis. He is a Fellow of the American Academy of Forensic Sciences and a Diplomate of the American Board of Forensic Anthropology. Dr. Warren serves as a consultant for several Medical Examiners in the state of Florida.

Laura Yazedjian

Laura Yazedjian completed a BSc in Biology at the University of Victoria (Victoria, BC) in 1998, a BA in Anthropology at the University of Manitoba (Winnipeg, MB) in 2001, and an MSc in Forensic Science at King's College London (London, UK) in 2002. She has been working for the International Commission on Missing Persons since 2002, primarily at the Podrinje Identification Project in Tuzla, Bosnia–Herzegovina.